PHARMACOKINETICS OF ANAESTHESIA

Pharmacokinetics of Anaesthesia

EDITED BY

C. PRYS-ROBERTS

PhD, MA, DM, MB BS, FFARCS, DA
Professor of Anaesthesia
The Royal Infirmary
Bristol BS2 8HW

AND

C. C. HUG JR

MD, PhD
Professor of Anesthesiology and Pharmacology
Emory University Medical School
Atlanta, Georgia 30322, USA

BLACKWELL SCIENTIFIC PUBLICATIONS
OXFORD LONDON EDINBURGH
BOSTON MELBOURNE

© 1984 by
Blackwell Scientific Publications
Editorial offices:
Osney Mead, Oxford, 0X2 0EL
8 John Street, London, WC1N 2ES
9 Forrest Road, Edinburgh, EH1 2QH
52 Beacon Street, Boston
    Massachusetts 02108, USA
99 Barry Street, Carlton
    Victoria 3053, Australia

First published 1984

Set by Macmillan India Ltd, Bangalore
Printed and bound in Great Britain by
Butler & Tanner Ltd, Frome, Somerset

DISTRIBUTORS

USA
  Blackwell Mosby Book Distributors
  11830 Westline Industrial Drive
  St Louis, Missouri63141

Canada
  Blackwell Mosby Book Distributors
  120 Melford Drive, Scarborough
  Ontario, M1B 2X4

Australia
  Blackwell Scientific Book Distributors
  31 Advantage Road, Highett
  Victoria 3190

British Library
Cataloguing in Publication Data

Pharmacokinetics of anaesthesia.
  1. Pharmacokinetics   2. Anesthesia
  I. Prys-Roberts, C.   II. Hug, C. C.
  615′.7′024617   RM301.5

ISBN   0–632–00905–5

Contents

List of Contributors

John A. Clements BSc, PhD, Lecturer in Pharmacy, Herriot Watt University, Chambers Street, Edinburgh EH1 1HX

Benjamin J. Covino PhD, MD, Chairman, Department of Anesthesia, Brigham and Women's Hospital, and Professor of Anesthesia, Harvard Medical School, Boston, MA 02115, USA

Carl C. Hug MD, PhD, Professor of Anesthesiology and Pharmacology, Emory University Hospital, Atlanta, Georgia 30322, USA

C. J. Hull MB, BS, MRCS, LRCP, FFA, RCS, Lecturer in Anaesthesia, Newcastle University Medical School, Newcastle-upon-Tyne

H. L. J. Makin MA, PhD, CChem, FRCS, Senior Lecturer in Chemical Pathology, The London Hospital Medical School, Turner Street, London E1 2AD

W. W. Mapleson DSc, FInstP, Professor of the Physics of Anaesthesia, Welsh National School of Medicine, Cardiff CF4 4XN

Ronald D. Miller MD, Professor of Anesthesia and Pharmacology, University of California Medical Center, San Francisco, CA 94143, USA

Walter S. Nimmo BSc, MB, ChB, MRCP, Senior Lecturer in Anaesthetics, University of Glasgow, Western Infirmary, Glasgow G11 6NT

John Norman PhD, MB, ChB, FFA, RCS, Professor of Anaesthesia, Southampton University Medical School, Southampton

C. Prys-Roberts PhD, MA, DM, MB, BS, FFA, RCS, DA, Professor of Anaesthesia, The Royal Infirmary, Bristol BS2 8HW

J. G. Reves MD, Professor of Anesthesiology and Director of Anaesthesia Research, School of Medicine, University of Alabama, 619 19th Street South, Birmingham, Alabama 35294, USA

J. W. Sear BSc, MB, BS, FFA, RCS, DObst, RCOG, Clinical Reader in Anaethetics, The Nuffield Department of Anaesthesia, The John Radcliffe Hospital, Oxford

P. J. Simpson MD, MB, BS, MRCS, LRCP, FFA, RCS, Consultant Anaesthetist, Frenchay Hospital, and Senior Clinical Lecturer, University of Bristol, Bristol

Donald R. Stanski MD, Assistant Professor of Anesthesia and Medicine, Stanford University School of Medicine, and Staff Anesthesiologist, Department of Anesthesia, Veterans Administration Hospital, Palo Alto, California 94304, USA

D. J. H. Trafford MIBiol, PhD, CChem, MRCS, Lecturer in Chemical Pathology, The London Hospital Medical School, Turner Street, London E1 2AD

E. M. Walsh MB, BS, BSc, FFA, RCS, Consultant Anaesthetist, Southmead Hospital, Bristol BS10 5NB

Preface

As a prelude to the 7th World Congress of Anaesthesiology in Hamburg in 1980, the Association of Anaesthetists of Great Britain and Ireland held their Annual Meeting at the Royal Festival Hall in London. The meeting took the form of an Anglo-American gathering to which American visitors to the Hamburg Congress were invited to contribute to the scientific proceedings. One whole day was devoted to a symposium on 'Pharmacokinetics of Anaesthesia' organised by one of us (C. P-R). Kind comments from many clinical practitioners and teachers of anaesthesiology, prompted us to produce a book in which the science of pharmacokinetics could be applied to anaesthesia for the benefit of trainees and practicing anaesthesiologists alike. This book is *not* a collection of lectures representing the proceedings of the symposium, indeed not all the contributors to this book took part in the symposium.

Pharmacokinetics is a science, not a form of 'pop art' as suggested by Feldman. It may well have reached a state of popularity among anaesthetists, largely because an understanding of the disposition of drugs in the body is essential for the full appreciation of how anaesthetics act. The term *pharmacokinetics* implies the application of *kinetics*, the rate of change in a system, to *pharmakon*, the Greek word for drugs and poisons. Specifically, it refers to the rate of change in drug concentration within a biological system: the body and its component organs, tissues and fluids. The practice of pharmacokinetics describes the relationships between drug dose and drug concentration in blood, plasma, or other body components. The kinetics of drug disposition cannot be viewed in isolation from the allied science of *pharmacodynamics*, which describes the relationships between drug concentration and drug response. These terms can be related as follows:

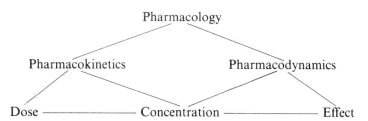

The anaesthesiologist is interested primarily in the effect produced by the dose administered. However the relationship between dose and effect varies from patient to patient, and even within the same patient under different conditions. We can categorise this variability, either according to pharmacokinetic factors affecting the relationship between dose and concentration, or pharmacodynamic factors affecting the responsiveness of the tissue or organ system to a particular drug concentration. As pharmacokinetic processes determine the rate of change of drug concentration over time during or following drug administration, they are consequently the determinants of the onset, intensity and duration of drug effect.

Pharmacokinetic processes include all those that affect the drug during its sojourn through the body: *absorption* into blood (plasma) from sites of administration; *distribution* throughout the body to tissues and organs; and *elimination* of the drug from the body by biotransformation and excretion. Anaesthesiologists need an understanding of the pharmacokinetics of the drugs they administer if they are to meet the challenges of rapid and safe anaesthesia of patients, maintenance of satisfactory levels of anaesthesia for as long as necessary, and prompt recovery of the patient after the operation. Pharmacokinetics can help the anaesthesiologist to:

1 Understand dose–effect relationships especially in terms of onset, intensity and duration of drug action;

2 Recognize dispositional factors as a cause of variability in the responses to a given dose;

3 Predict the consequences of different dosage regimens and to design more efficient ones that are optimally effective with minimal side-effects and toxicity;

4 Design comparative investigations of the potency and efficacy of drugs. This is most readily accomplished by maintaining stable drug concentrations in plasma and at sites of action during the periods of measurements of drug effects.

Perhaps the science of pharmacokinetics has been sullied in the minds of many anaesthesiologists by the over-zealous concentration by some authors on models of drug action. It is certainly true that some investigators in this field have concentrated on trying to fit data from man or experimental animals to a preconceived model rather than finding a model which closely approximates and explains the data. Models play a role in so many areas of scientific activity that their value in the field of kinetics cannot be ignored. Firstly it must be established that a model, whether mathematical, electrical or mechanical, fits the behaviour of physiological or pharmacological data derived under clinical conditions in man. Thereafter the model has enormous value as its behaviour can be perturbed and its performance assessed *as if* one was testing the behaviour of a human patient in response to the same perturbation. The predictive value of such a model is clearly of great value to the clinician who wishes to use a drug in a new mode. The use of such models in the prediction of drug disposition and action during continuous infusion of the drug has tremendous value and this aspect is covered by a number of contributors in this book.

Acknowledgements are due to Miss Lynne Breeze and Dr Hug's secretary for their assistance, and to Curig Prys-Roberts for help with the index.

Cedric Prys-Roberts
Carl C. Hug Jr.

1 General Principles of Pharmacokinetics

C. J. HULL

DRUG UPTAKE AND ELIMINATION
Drug uptake
Drug disposition in blood
Kinetics of drug transfer
The influence of ionisation, protein binding and lipid solubility upon
 redistribution
Volume of distribution
Drug elimination

PHARMACOKINETIC MODELS
The two-compartment model
The three-compartment model
Curve fitting

APPENDIX
The two-compartment 'open' model

Unlike the discipline of respiratory physiology, which has accepted a logical set of symbols[10] for all publications, pharmacokinetics enjoys no such uniformity. While offering eloquent testimony to authors' imagination, the numerous and frequently conflicting systems of symbols in the literature would almost appear to be a form of collective obscurantism. The symbols used in this work conform with those standardised by the *British Journal of Anaesthesia*[5]. Each symbol is defined when first used in each chapter, and also appears in a glossary of terms (Appendix).

Early pharmacological texts stated that if a drug were given in a certain dose, then a corresponding effect would follow. A later refinement stated that since a large subject often needs more drug than a small one, doses should be scaled to body weight. It was also accepted that some subjects would be 'sensitive', and others 'resistant' to the drug. Naturally, 'strong' drugs should be given in smaller doses than 'weak' ones. This static concept of the dose-effect relationship has retreated before the understanding that for most reversible drugs, a fundamental pharmacodynamic relationship exists between drug concentration at the site of action, or biophase, and the intensity of effect. The relationship between *dose* and *biophase concentration* is complex, multifactorial, and often tenuous. This is particularly true in the case of oral administration, where the viscissitudes of gastrointestinal uptake are added to those applying to the intravascular route. Once present in plasma, the drug will be distributed to a wide variety of tissues and will be excreted and/or metabolised (Fig. 1.1). These processes are dependent upon the chemical nature of the drug and upon its partition between different elements of the blood.

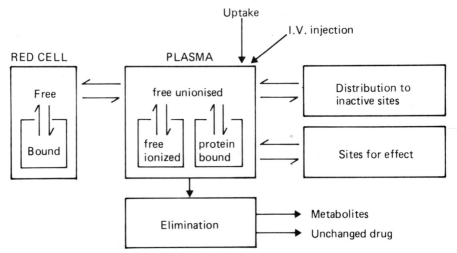

Fig. 1.1   The overall relationships between uptake, distribution and elimination of drugs.

DRUG UPTAKE AND ELIMINATION

Drug uptake

The proportion of administered drug which appears in plasma, and the route by which it does so, depends upon the route of administration. If given by *intravenous* or *intra-arterial* injection, the entire dose is immediately 'available'.

Following *intramuscular* or *subcutaneous* injection, uptake may be expected to be complete, but delayed. The primary determinant of uptake is the rate at which the injection site is perfused with blood. Vascular tissues may absorb drug very rapidly, while tissues with poor blood supply can sequester large quantities of drug for long periods. Drug solubility is also an important factor. If the agent is insoluble in water at the tissue pH, then uptake will be very slow. A drug which is prepared at an unphysiological pH in order to promote solubility may result in an initially rapid uptake, which declines as the depot pH moves towards that of the tissue.

Orally administered drugs are subject to numerous influences en route to the plasma. Only drugs in solution can be absorbed, so that many preparations are subject to delay at this stage. Solid formulations (tablets, granules, etc.) may dissolve rapidly, or may resist disintegration and dissolution and enter solution more gradually, releasing the drug solution over a prolonged period. Once in solution, absorption depends largely upon the gastrointestinal zone concerned. In the stomach, pH is generally very low (pH 1–3.5). Some drugs may be destroyed, but those which are acidic or basic will be subject to partition into ionised and non-ionised forms, according to the Henderson–Hasselbalch equations:

$$\text{(for a base)} \quad \log \frac{[\text{non-ionised}]}{[\text{ionised}]} + \text{pKa} = \text{pH}$$

$$\text{(for an acid)} \quad \log \frac{[\text{ionised}]}{[\text{non-ionised}]} + \text{pKa} = \text{pH}$$

Thus for a base, the non-ionised fraction (fn) is expressed by:

$$\text{fn} = \text{antilog (pH} - \text{pKa), so} \quad \%\text{n} = \left(\frac{\text{fn}}{\text{fn} + 1}\right) \times 100 \tag{1.1}$$

and for an acid, the ionised fraction (fi) is expressed by:

$$\text{fi} = \text{antilog (pH} - \text{pKa), so} \quad \%\text{i} = \left(\frac{\text{fi}}{\text{fi} + 1}\right) \times 100 \tag{1.2}$$

Thus salicylic acid (pKa = 3) is 9% ionised at pH 2, but 99.99% at pH 7.4, whereas diazepam (pKa = 3.5) is 97% ionised at pH 2, and 0.01% at pH 7.4.

Most drugs (except those of very low molecular weight) are absorbed by passive diffusion through the lipoidal outer layer of cells lining the gastrointestinal tract. Since the non-ionised form of a drug has very much higher lipid solubility than the ionised form, it should be regarded as the *absorbable fraction*[16]. Thus salicylic acid is well absorbed from the stomach, whereas diazepam (of which only 3% is diffusible at pH 2) is poorly absorbed. Further down the tract, as the pH rises progressively, the non-ionised fraction of a basic drug rises also. Clearly, absorption of non-ionised drug leads to re-association of ionised drug within the lumen in order to maintain the ratio of ionised to non-ionised molecules. This in turn provides further non-ionised drug for absorption, so that ultimately a high proportion of the administered dose may be absorbed. However, since the passive absorption rate at a given site is likely to be proportional to the non-ionised concentration in that particular absorption zone of the gut, the degree of ionisation may be expected to have a major effect upon the absorption *rate*.

If, by virtue of slow dissolution or high ionisation, the rate of absorption is slow, then factors such as gastric emptying rate, bowel motility or inflammatory disease may influence the overall absorbed dose. The absorbed fraction of an oral dose is defined as the *bio-availability*, and is usually given the symbol F. The effective absorbed dose may be even lower, since a further fraction will be removed by the liver before reaching the systemic circulation. Such *first-pass* elimination may be of great signficance in the case of drugs with rapid hepatic excretion (see Chapters 12 and 13).

Drug disposition in blood

After intravenous injection, it may be assumed that the drug will be well mixed with plasma water within a few circulation times. Most acidic and basic drugs will be present in both ionised and non-ionised forms, according to equations 1.1 and 1.2. Thus at pH 7.4, thiopentone (pKa 7.6) is 30% ionised, whereas diazepam (pKa 3.5) is only 0.01% ionised. Strong acids and bases (e.g. quaternary ammonium compounds such as pancuronium) are fully ionised at pH 7.4. Only the non-ionised form will penetrate lipid membranes or dissolve in lipid substances, so that as in the gut, this may be regarded as the active, diffusible fraction. Since there is very rapid equilibration between ionised and non-ionised forms, ionisation will not influence the partition of drug between tissues of equal pH; merely the rate of transfer. Partition (e.g. into erythrocytes) is influenced by lipid solubility: thus fentanyl, being highly lipid soluble[21], passes freely into erythrocytes, whereas pancuronium, being very poorly lipid soluble, does not.

Many drugs are reversibly bound to plasma proteins—usually to albumen, but also to other fractions. Each albumen molecule may provide more than one binding site; these may not necessarily possess the same affinity for the drug.

Thus the detailed relationship for a single drug may be extremely complex. The equilibrium between free and bound forms of drug is governed by the mass-action equation:

$$K_A = \frac{[\text{bound}]}{[\text{free}] \cdot \left[\begin{array}{c} \text{vacant} \\ \text{sites} \end{array}\right]} \tag{1.3}$$

where K_A is the equilibrium association constant. As the drug concentration rises, the proportion of bound drug falls, since the shift to the right of the equilibrium:

$$[\text{free}] + \left[\begin{array}{c} \text{vacant} \\ \text{sites} \end{array}\right] \rightleftharpoons [\text{bound}] \tag{1.4}$$

is limited by the diminishing number of vacant binding sites. However, the free drug concentration is often very small in relation to [vacant sites], so that drug binding may not, in fact, diminish [vacant sites] significantly. Thus the binding ratio may, as in the case of fentanyl[1], remain virtually constant over a very wide range of molar concentrations. Only when very high concentrations are reached (such as in an intravenous bolus before mixing is complete), or when two or more drugs compete for the same binding site, will the binding ratio diminish with increasing drug concentration. However, care must be taken that this simplification is not assumed without verification, since the binding ratios for some drugs (e.g. phenylbutazone) *do* diminish within the clinically attainable concentration range.

Protein-bound drug cannot be regarded as freely diffusible to other sites, since it must first dissociate into the free form. The binding ratio may have a profound effect upon the *rate* at which redistribution occurs, since the transfer rate of drug across a permeable membrane is almost always proportional to the free drug concentration. Thus lignocaine (30% free) is greatly favoured in comparison with diazepam (3% free)[13].

Kinetics of drug transfer

The processes concerned can frequently be characterised by the simple rate equation:

$$dC/dt = -k.C^n$$

(1.5)

where dC/dt represents the rate (with respect to time t) at which the concentration difference C across a membrane declines, k is a constant, and n an exponent of value 0 or 1. When $n = 0$, $C^n = 0$, so that the rate of concentration change is constant at $-k$. When $n = 1$, the rate of decline is $-k.C$, so that at any time t, the rate is directly proportional to the concentration. The exponent n determines the *order* of the equation, so that when $n = 0$ the process is zero-order, and when $n = 1$, first order. Passive drug transfer is almost always first order, but zero-order kinetics may apply when an active process (such as an enzyme reaction) is saturable, so that increasing drug concentration above a threshold level cannot increase the rate further. (The hepatic uptake of alcohol is a good example.) The first-order rate constant k simply states by what proportion C will decline in time t. Thus if the units of time are hours, $k = 0.5$ states that C will decline by a factor of 0.5 (i.e. 50%) per hour, *at the present level of C*. As C declines, it follows that the rate also will decline.

Having the dimension of a *rate*, k has the units 1/time, which will be hours^{-1} in the above case. The declining value of C can be characterised by integrating equation (1.5), thus:

$$C = C^0.e^{-kt}$$

(1.6)

where C^0 is the value of C at $t = 0$, and $t = 2.718$ (simplified), the base of the natural logarithm. The equation is that of a simple exponential decline.

Equation (1.6) can be simplified by taking natural logarithms of both sides:

$$\ln C = \ln C^0 - kt$$

(1.7)

This is a linear equation, so that a graph of $\ln C$ vs. t will be a straight line, of intercept $\ln C^0$ (Fig. 1.2).

The characteristics of an exponential decline are often defined by alternative parameters in the time domain. The *half-time* $(T_{\frac{1}{2}})$ describes the time taken for C to decline by a half, and is constant at any part of the curve. Since equation (1.7) can be rearranged to:

$$t = \frac{\ln (C/C^0)}{-k}$$

solution for $C/C^0 = 0.5$ yields

$$T_{\frac{1}{2}} = \frac{0.693}{k} \tag{1.8}$$

The *time constant* (τ) is more directly related to the exponential process, and describes the time taken for C to decline by a factor of e (i.e. 2.718). Since $\ln 2.718 = 1$,

$\tau = 1/k$.

It is now clear that $T_{\frac{1}{2}} = 0.693\,\tau$, so that both terms express the same relationship.

Far from being mathematically exotic, exponential change represents the natural order of things, and must be regarded as the foundation upon which the whole discipline of pharmacokinetics is built. When two or more first-order processes combine, the mathematics become arduous, but this does not make the process any less valid; we are, after all, struggling to use linear mathematics to describe an exponential world!

The influence of ionisation, protein binding and lipid solubility upon redistribution

We have seeen that drug transfer across a membrane is essentially a first order process, with regard to the non-ionised, free fraction of drug dissolved in plasma water. If the conditions on both 'plasma' and 'tissue' sides of the membrane are identical, then at equilibrium the drug concentrations also will be equal. However, when conditions are not equal, major deviations will occur.

Lipid solubility

It must be remembered that drug molecules constantly bombard both sides of a semi-permeable membrane, and cross in numbers proportional to their respective chemical potentials. Thus in identical solvents equilibrium occurs at equal molar concentrations, but if drug is more soluble in 'tissue' than in 'plasma' then the concentration on the 'tissue' side will have equal chemical potential at $\lambda.C$, where λ is the partition coefficient between 'tissue' and 'plasma'. Thiopentone is a good example, since the fat:plasma partition coefficient $\lambda = 11$. Thus at equilibrium, lipoid tissues contain 11 times as much thiopentone as plasma[14].

Protein binding

If $\lambda = 1$, and there is no protein binding on the 'tissue' side, then *free* drug may reach equal concentrations on both sides, but there will be 'bound' drug only on the 'plasma' side. If total drug concentrations are considered, then the 'tissue' conccentration may appear to reach equilibrium at a very low level. In practice, tissue proteins are often avid binders of drug molecules, so that drug distribution may be relatively unaffected. However, since only 'free' drug is diffusing across the membrane, the *rate of equilibration* may be very slow for highly bound drugs.

Drug ionisation

If there is a large pH gradient across the membrane, then the proportions of relatively diffusible non-ionised drug will differ greatly, i.e. if fentanyl (pKa 7.8) is diffusing from plasma to a zone of very low pH (say pH 2 in the gastric lumen) then the unionised fractions will be 28.5 % and 0.00016 % respectively. Thus 1 mg of drug in plasma at pH 7.4 equilibrates across a membrane with 178 g at pH 2! This provides an explanation for the observed accumulation of both fentanyl and pethidine in gastric secretions[19, 20].

Volume of distribution

At equilibrium, drug will be dispersed into a wide variety of tissues, each with a unique combination of ionisation, solubility, and binding. Clearly, a vast amount of detailed information (much of which is unknown) would be required to characterise the distribution pattern. As a gross simplification, the degree to which a mass of drug *appears* to be diluted (as indicated by the plasma concentration at equilibrium) may be used to derive an *apparent volume of distribution*. Thus

$$V_D = \frac{Xd}{C} \tag{1.9}$$

where Xd is the mass of drug given. C is the 'fully distributed' plasma concentration at time zero, and can be estimated by extrapolating the concentration-time curve (ignoring the distributive phase) back to $t = 0$. The apparent volume of distribution is assumed to be homogeneous, so that it does not attempt to indicate a real, anatomical volume, but represents a single *hypothetical* compartment consisting entirely of 'plasma'. The volume is determined principally by the nature of the drug rather than the size of the subject, and may vary over a very wide range. For example, drugs which are very highly bound to plasma protein (e.g. warfarin) do not leave the plasma in significant quantities, and therefore have small (approx. 10 l) distribution volumes[9]. By contrast, basic drugs such as pethidine are lipid-soluble and bound to tissue proteins, conferring large (> 200 l) distribution volumes[8]. During the elimination of drugs of this type, concentration gradients inevitably develop between peripheral tissues and plasma, so that the parameter V_D is an over-estimate. If distribution volume is calculated at an infusional equilibrium, then no such gradients exist, and a lower value is obtained. This is given the symbol V^{ss}, indicating that it applies to steady-state conditions. As elimination rate rises, so the discrepancy between V_D and V^{ss} also will rise. In the unusual case where the assumption of homogeneity does in fact apply, no concentration gradients will develop, so $V_D = V^{ss}$. However, the assumption does not readily apply to the majority of drugs, so that the single-compartment hypothesis (and so, also, V_D) is of very limited value. More sophisticated concepts of distribution will be introduced later.

Drug elimination

Elimination processes are frequently multiple, and additive in nature. They can be considered to *clear* the body of drug. The concept of clearance is very simple, and is considered here in relation to plasma.

Plasma clearance is the rate at which drug is eliminated *per unit of plasma concentration*, and is therefore a measure of elimination *efficiency*.

Since in dimensional terms, rate of removal = mass/time, and concentration = mass/volume, clearance = mass/time ÷ mass/volume, which simplifies to volume/time, i.e. litres per hour. Plasma clearance can be estimated by measuring plasma concentrations repeatedly after a single dose of drug, until it is entirely eliminated. Clearance can be stated as: mean rate of removal/mean plasma concentration. The mean rate of removal = dose/total time, and the mean concentration = area under curve/time, so that the clearance equation simplifies to:

$$Cl = \frac{\text{dose}}{\text{area under curve}} \tag{1.10}$$

In dimensional terms, dose = mass, and the area under the concentration-tissue plot = mass × time/volume, so that clearance = volume/time, as before. Clearance estimation by this method depends upon frequent, accurate estimations of concentration over an extended period, and requires computation of area, but makes no pharmacokinetic assumptions.

For the moment, let us assume that drug is dispersed into a single homogeneous compartment of apparent volume V_D, from which drug is eliminated in a first-order manner. Drug concentration will decline exponentially after a single i.v. dose according to equation (1.6). The mass of drug (X) remaining in the body at any time (t) will decline similarly: $dX/dt = k.X$. Since $X = V.C$, this may be rewritten as: $dX/dt = k.V.C$. Clearance, being the ratio of elimination rate to concentration, can now be expressed as

$$Cl = \frac{k.V.C}{C} = k.V \tag{1.11}$$

Also since $\quad k = \dfrac{0.693}{T_{\frac{1}{2}}}$ (equation 1.8) $\quad Cl = \dfrac{0.693}{T_{\frac{1}{2}}}$ and $T_{\frac{1}{2}} = \dfrac{0.693\,V}{Cl}$

Thus while half-life and clearance both describe the elimination process, they are by no means identical. While clearance indicates the efficiency of removal, half-life defines the rate at which *concentration* falls. For a given rate of drug elimination, this clearly depends upon the distribution volume. Thus a drug with high clearance and a large volume of distribution (i.e. fentanyl) may have an extended half-life[17]. Clearance can also be considered in terms of renal and hepatic function, which together account for most elimination processes.

Renal clearance can be determined conveniently by considering the rate of appearance of drug in the urine to represent drug output. Thus

$$Cl_R = \frac{C_U \cdot \dot{U}}{C_P} \qquad (1.12)$$

where C_U is the concentration of drug in urine, $\dot{U}$ the rate of urine flow, and C_P the drug concentration in plasma.

During renal excretion of drug, three distinct processes may be involved, viz. glomerular filtration, passive tubular reabsorption, and active tubular secretion. Glomerular filtrate contains all the components of plasma except protein, and the process of filtration does not 'strip' drug from protein-binding sites. Thus the concentration of drug in the filtrate is identical with the *free* (i.e. unbound) fraction in plasma. If no drug is reabsorbed (or secreted) in the tubule, free drug clearance will equal the glomerular filtration rate (i.e. 130 ml.min^{-1}).

Many drugs, especially those which are lipophilic and, being weak acids or bases, have significant unionised fractions at the intratubular pH, will be extensively reabsorbed by the distal tubule. Clearly, the pH partition principle applies here, so that acid urine will facilitate reabsorption of weak acids, thereby extending their half-lives; alkaline urine will have the same effect on weak bases. Renal clearance of drugs which are reabsorbed (but not actively secreted) will always be less than the glomerular filtration rate.

However, some drugs (e.g. penicillins) *are* actively transported across the tubular wall by specific carrier systems. As drug diffuses from plasma into the tubular cell, the free plasma concentration falls, and very rapidly reaches a new equilibrium with the protein-bound fraction (i.e. some drug dissociates and becomes free). Thus, if uptake is rapid, both free and bound drug are cleared from plasma. If, by this means, tubular capillary blood is entirely stripped of drug, clearance will equate with renal plasma flow, regardless of glomerular filtration.

Consideration of the renal clearance for a particular drug may give some indication of the mechanisms involved, but great care must be taken since it may represent the resultant of several processes. However, renal elimination will usually be a first-order process with respect to the amount of drug remaining in the plasma, so that renal elimination can be assigned a first-order rate constant. (This will not be the case if an active tubular secretion mechanism is presented with a drug concentration in excess of its Michaelis constant*.)

Hepatic clearance of drug can be considered in the same terms as before, but is also frequently defined as an extraction ratio ER_H. This is simply the fraction of drug contained in hepatic afferent blood which is removed as it passes through the liver. Thus if $ER_H = 1$, all drug is removed at each pass, and if $ER_H = 0.5$, only 50% is removed. The extraction ratio can also be conceived as that fraction of hepatic blood flow which is totally cleared of drug during each pass. Therefore, clearance must equal that fraction of hepatic blood flow: $Cl_H = ER_H \times Q_H$, where Q_H = hepatic blood flow. Many drugs are able to diffuse into hepatic cells, where they may be metabolised or actively excreted (unchanged) into bile. Such processes may be expected to follow Michaelis–Menten kinetics, so that as stated above, first-order elimination at low drug concentrations may become zero-order at higher levels.

The drug concentration which is presented to the active pathway may be assumed to be in equilibrium with the *free, non-ionised fraction in plasma*. If uptake of free drug is very small then very little re-equilibration with ionised or bound drug will take place, and the elimination rate will be proportional to the concentration of free drug in plasma. Consequently, the extraction ratio will be very low. At higher levels of free drug uptake, significant 'stripping' of bound drug may take place, so that the degree and tenacity of protein binding influences the overall elimination rate. The extraction ratio will be intermediate.

At very rapid uptake rates, hepatic blood will be nearly or completely stripped of drug (unless protein binding is very tenacious), so that the extraction ratio will approach 1 and clearance will approximate to hepatic blood flow. Here, elimination is strictly first-order, since the elimination rate will be proportional only to plasma

---

* The velocity V at which an enzyme reaction proceeds is given by the Michaelis–Menten equation

$$V = \frac{V_{max} \cdot C}{Km + C} \qquad (1.13)$$

where V_{max} is the maximum attainable velocity governed by enzyme availability, C is the molar concentration of substrate, and Km is the Michaelis constant. This is numerically equal to the substrate concentration at which the reaction velocity $= 0.5\ V_{max}$. Although the relationship between C and V is hyperbolic, velocity is proportional to substrate concentration when, as is usual, $Km \gg C$, $Km + C \simeq Km$, and equation (1.13) reduces to:

$$V = \frac{V_{max} \cdot C}{Km} \qquad (1.14)$$

Here, the transport reaction approaches a maximum attainable velocity, regardless of further increases in plasma concentration, so that excretion kinetics will be first order at low concentrations, becoming zero order as Km is reached).

concentration and hepatic blood flow. Drugs of this type may be expected to show high 'first pass' clearance after oral administration, so that it is difficult to attain effective concentrations in the systemic circulation by this route.

Although hepatic clearance is a useful concept in terms of overall performance, it tells us little in terms of actual metabolic efficiency. This is due to the effect of protein binding, since the rate of drug uptake and metabolism is proportional to the *free* drug concentration, but clearance is computed in terms of total (free + bound) concentration.

If Clearance = rate of metabolism/free drug concentration, and equation (1.14) defines rate of metabolism as $V_{max}.Cf/Km$, then dividing equation (1.14) by concentration yields:

$$Clf_H = \frac{V_{max}.Cf}{Km.Cf} = \frac{V_{max}}{Km} \tag{1.15}$$

Clf_H is the *intrinsic hepatic clearance*, and is a true measure of removal per unit of concentration. Like overall hepatic clearance, it has the units 'litres per hour', but refers to *free* drug only. Clearly, changes in plasma protein concentration, or in the number of available binding sites will have a direct effect upon hepatic clearance, but *intrinsic clearance* will remain unchanged. It should be remembered that equation (1.15) applies only at low free drug concentrations, where $Km \gg Cf$. At higher concentrations equation (1.13) applies; when $Cf \gg Km$ it reduces to $V = V_{max}$, and the kinetics become zero order.

PHARMACOKINETIC MODELS

So far we have considered distribution and elimination as separate processes. In practice, they occur simultaneously, so that the time-course of plasma drug concentration becomes complex, even after a single i.v. bolus. If the processes of uptake from depot sites at the gut are also to be considered, then the difficulties become immense. However, systems which seem to defy analysis can often be represented by conceptually simple *models*. These are simply analogues (mathematical, mechanical, or even electrical) which appear to be governed by similar rules.

As an example, we can consider some models for a drug whose deposition can be represented by a single homogeneous compartment (a few drugs, i.e. warfarin[9], which is very highly protein bound, do in fact behave in this way). The log-concentration of drug in plasma declines linearly (Fig. 1.2) and therefore can be satisfied by a first-order rate constant k. In pharmacokinetic terms this behaviour is characteristic of a one-compartment 'open' mathematical model (Fig. 1.3a) (open because drug can leave the model), with a first order elimination pathway. The apparent volume of distribution is clearly Xd/C° litres, the clearance $V.k$ litre.s^{-1}, and the half-life $0.693/k$ seconds.

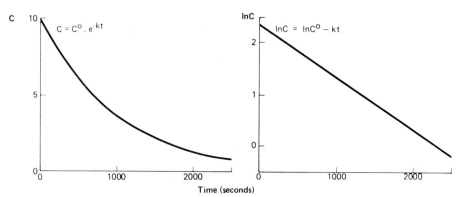

Time (seconds)

Fig. 1.2 Linear and semi-logarithmic plots for an exponential decay function where $C^0 = 10$, and $k = 10^{-3}\,s^{-1}$. Since $\tau = \dfrac{1}{k}$, the time constant is 1000 s. This function applies to the models shown in Fig. 1.3.

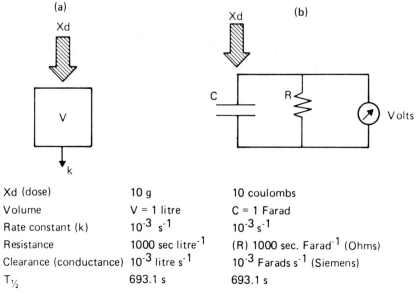

Xd (dose)	10 g	10 coulombs
Volume	V = 1 litre	C = 1 Farad
Rate constant (k)	$10^{-3}\,s^{-1}$	$10^{-3}\,s^{-1}$
Resistance	1000 sec litre^{-1}	(R) 1000 sec. Farad^{-1} (Ohms)
Clearance (conductance)	10^{-3} litre s^{-1}	10^{-3} Farads s^{-1} (Siemens)
$T_{1/2}$	693.1 s	693.1 s

Fig. 1.3 A one-compartment kinetic model (a), and its electrical equivalent (b). Time units are seconds, to avoid the use of multipliers. The time courses of both models are identical and are plotted in Fig. 1.2.

Similarly, a capacitor and resistor, connected as shown in Fig. 1.3b, will behave in a mathematically identical manner, and therefore form a valid electrical model[7]. C Farads $\equiv$ V litres, and Q Coulombs $\equiv$ X grams, so Drug concentration $\equiv$ Coulombs per Farad (i.e. Volts). Since resistance = flow (i.e. Coulombs/time = amps) per unit of concentration (i.e. Coulombs/Farads = Volts), the units will be seconds.litre^{-1} in the kinetic model, and seconds.Farad^{-1} in the electrical model. However, since Coulombs/time ÷ Coulombs/Farad also simplifies to Amps/Volts = Ohms, the resistance in the electrical model can be assigned familiar units.

Clearance can be considered in similar terms. Since Cl = mass/sec per mass/volume, i.e. volume per second in the kinetic model:

$$\frac{\text{Coulombs}}{\text{secs}} \text{ per } \frac{\text{Coulombs}}{\text{Farads}} = \text{Farads per second} = \text{Siemens}$$

Since this is clearly the reciprocal of resistance (defined above as seconds per Farad), clearance is equivalent to the *conductance* of the elimination pathway. Since conductance of the resistor is dependent only upon the physical characteristics of the resistor itself, so it is with clearance, which describes only the elimination pathway. In electrical terms, conductance is expressed in Siemens (i.e. 1/Ohms). The kinetic model has no such convenient unit, and expresses conductance in dimensional terms (e.g. litre.h^{-1}).

When applicable, the one-compartment model can be used to predict the time-course of concentration following different dosage regimes. Since a bolus dose yields $C^0 = Xd/V$, solution of equation (1.6) yields the plasma concentration at any time t. Similarly, the results of an infusion can be predicted. The zero order rate constant k′ represents the rate at which drug enters the model:

$$C = \frac{k'}{V.k}(1 - e^{-kt}) \qquad (1.16)$$

It will be noted that this is a wash-in exponential function, in which concentration gradually approaches the asymptotic value:

$$C^{ss} = \frac{k'}{k.V} \qquad (1.17)$$

Since k.V = Cl, the final concentration is simply the ratio of infusion rate to clearance. The system requires 4 half-times to reach 90% of C^{ss}, and seven half-times to reach 99%. If at any time the infusion is stopped, concentration simply declines according to the corresponding washout function:

$$C = \frac{k'}{V.k}(1 - e^{-kt^1})(e^{-kt^2}) \qquad (1.18)$$

where t^1 = time at which infusion stopped, and t^2 is the time since it stopped[3]. At infusional equilibrium, the steady state volume of distribution can be calculated:

$$V^{ss} = \frac{k'}{k.C^{ss}} \qquad (1.19)$$

From equation (1.18) it is evident that very simple systems may be characterised by quite complex mathematics. This complexity discourages some, and leads others to declare the equation false. Not so; it is simply the way things are. When the principles of the one-compartment model are applied to multi-compartment systems, it is to be expected that the mathematics will be more arduous. The reader will find that this is indeed the case.

The two-compartment model

The simple model so far considered takes no account of drug distribution; indeed it assumes that drug is instantaneously and perfectly mixed with the distribution volume on administration. Clearly this is a gross over-simplification for most drugs. In many cases, the plasma concentration curve following a single i.v. dose (Fig. 1.4) shows evidence of distribution in the form of a rapid initial decay, which then gives way to a slower terminal phase during which elimination is the dominant process. On

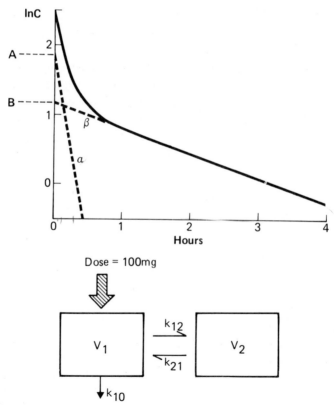

Fig. 1.4   A two-exponential decay plotted in semi-logarithmic form and its corresponding two-compartment open model.

examination it can be seen that this curve consists of the algebraic sum of two simple exponential decay curves, usually designated the α and β components. For this reason, the curve is often described (non-mathematically) as bi-exponential, and is characterised by the equation:

$$C = A.e^{-\alpha t} + B.e^{-\beta t} \tag{1.20}$$

where A, B are the zero-time intercepts and α, β the rate constants for the two exponential terms (see Fig. 1.4). From each rate constant a corresponding half-time can be calculated so that:

$$T_{\frac{1}{2}}^{\alpha} = \frac{0.693}{\alpha} \quad \text{and} \quad T_{\frac{1}{2}}^{\beta} = \frac{0.693}{\beta}$$

In particular, $T_{\frac{1}{2}}^{\beta}$ is widely quoted, being a useful indicator of the plasma concentration decay rate during the post-distributive phase. Equation (1.20) is also characteristic of a two-compartment open model[18], which has 'central' (1) and 'deep' (2) compartments, the latter representing distribution. Elimination is assumed to take place only from the central compartment.

Following a bolus dose, drug is both eliminated and distributed, according to rate constants k_{10} and k_{12}. The *efficiency* of the two pathways can be compared by calculating the two clearances $V_1.k_{10}$ and $V_1.K_{12}$. (Remember that clearance is a *conductance*, and can perfectly well be applied to an intercompartmental route.) As drug concentration in compartment 2 rises (Fig. 1.5), distribution slows down until concentrations in both compartments are equal, and drug movement stops. Continuing elimination then lowers the concentration in the central compartment still further, so that the distributive process reverses, and drug begins to return from compartment 2. From this point, concentrations in both compartments decline together, with the

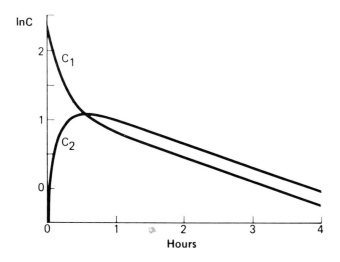

Fig. 1.5 Log-concentrations in both compartments of a two-compartment open model following a bolus dose.

difference in concentration declining as the rate of drug movement approaches zero (on a semi-logarithmic plot the concentrations decline in parallel). The rate constant for drug leaving compartment 2 is k_{21}. Since the intercompartmental clearance defines the pathway conductance (i.e. $Cl_{12} = V_1.k_{12}$) and must be the same in both directions, (i.e. $Cl_{12} = Cl_{21}$), it follows that:

$$V_1.k_{12} = V_2.k_{21},$$

and so
$$V_2 = \frac{V_1.k_{12}}{k_{21}}$$

Thus k_{21} will equate with k_{12} *only* when $V_1 = V_2$. It is emphasised that inequality of k_{12} and k_{21} *does not* imply that drug transfer occurs more readily in one direction than the other, or that the compartments differ in any respect other than their apparent volumes. Since A, B, α and β are not direct parameters of the model, some simple calculations must be made in sequence (see Appendix) in order to determine the volumes and rate constants.

Very frequently, drugs are given as short, rapid, intravenous infusions in order to facilitate mixing within the central compartment. As before, the plasma concentration curve declines in a two-exponential manner, with α, β unchanged. However, since drug is differently distributed at the end of infusion to that at time zero following a bolus, the intercept values A, B will be different. Therefore, post-infusional decay equations require correction before derivation of the two-compartment model[3]. The observed intercepts are designated A', B'. Then if t = infusion period, Xd = total dose, and k'_{01} = infusion rate,

$$A = \frac{A'.Xd.\alpha}{k'_{01}(1-e^{-\alpha t})} \qquad B = \frac{B'.Xd.\beta}{k'_{01}(1-e^{-\beta t})} \qquad (1.21)$$

Now the model can be calculated from A, B, α, β as before.

Given a model and a specified dose Xd, the concentration time course in both central and deep compartments can be calculated easily.

First, the constants A and B are calculated:

Given
$$C_1^0 = \frac{Xd}{V_1},$$

then
$$A = \frac{C_1^0(k_{21}-\alpha)}{\beta-\alpha} \qquad (1.22)$$

$$B = \frac{C_1^0(\beta-k_{21})}{\beta-\alpha} \qquad (1.23)$$

Then the corresponding constants L and M are calculated for the deep compartment.

$$L = \frac{C_1^0.k_{21}}{\beta-\alpha} \qquad (1.24)$$

$$M = -L \qquad (1.25)$$

Now the equations for drug concentrations in central (C_1) and deep (C_2) compartments can be written:

$$C_1 = A.e^{-\alpha t} + B.e^{-\beta t} \quad \text{and} \quad C_2 = L.e^{-\alpha t} + M.e^{-\beta t}$$

Clearly, the same time constants apply to both equations; it is only the constants A, B and L, M which differ. If it is remembered that at time-zero $(t = 0)$, the concentration in the deep compartment is zero, and $e^{-\alpha t} = e^{-\beta t} = 1$, constants L and M must be equal, but of opposite sign (equation 1.25).

These simple equations apply only to an 'empty' model given a single bolus dose. For applications where the model is not empty, and where a combination of bolus and infusional doses are required, or where the inverse solution is required (i.e. to find the dose required to yield a specified result) the more complex equations in the appendix are applicable.

The apparent volume of distribution in a two-compartment model can be considered in several ways. Since the decay curve after a bolus dose is essentially mono-exponential during the β phase, this slope $(B.e^{-\beta t})$ can be extrapolated back to $t = 0$ and the apparent volume expressed as

$$V \text{ (extrap)} = \frac{Xd}{B} \tag{1.26}$$

Alternatively, the distribution volume can be expressed as the quantity of drug remaining in the body in relation to the plasma concentration during the β phase. This proportionality factor is usually referred to as V^β.

$$V^\beta = \frac{V_1 . k_{10}}{\beta} \tag{1.27}$$

V^β can also be estimated by an infusion method, but relies upon reaching equilibrium:

$$V^\beta = \frac{k'_{01}}{C^{ss}.\beta} \tag{1.28}$$

Both V (extrap) and V^β over-estimate the distribution volume at all but very low clearances, so that changes in k_{10} also may result in spurious changes in distribution volume[12].

Of much greater value is the *apparent distribution volume at steady state* (V^{ss}). If an infusional equilibrium is achieved, V^{ss} can be calculated from the concentration at steady state (C^{ss}), the area under the curve to the end of infusion (AUC^t), and the area under the curve to complete elimination (AUC^∞):

$$V^{ss} = \frac{Xd}{C^{ss}} \left(1 - \frac{AUC^t}{AUC^\infty} \right) \tag{1.29}$$

However, this may be a very protracted procedure, so that it is more convenient to derive a two-compartment model (from a decay curve) and then make use of the simple relationship:

$$V^{ss} = V_1 + V_2 \qquad (1.30)$$

V^{ss} does not depend upon other model parameters, and therefore is preferable to V^β and V (extrap). While referred to in many texts as a 'model independent' parameter, this is only the case when estimated by the AUC method. The relationships between V^β, V (extrap) and V^{ss} are illustrated by Fig. 1.6, in which the effects of changing clearance upon these functions are plotted. It is clear that at high clearances, only V^{ss} is of practical use.

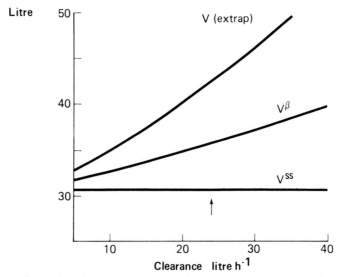

Fig. 1.6 The effects of variation in clearance on the apparent volume of distribution. A volunteer was given alfentanil $170\,\mu\text{g}$ i.v., and a two-compartment model derived from the plasma concentration data (0–6 h): $V_1 = 8.96$ l, $V_2 = 21.50$ l, $k_{10} = 2.66\,\text{h}^{-1}$, $k_{12} = 7.99\,\text{h}^{-1}$, $k_{21} = 3.33\,\text{h}^{-1}$. Model clearance was varied over the range 5–$401\,\text{h}^{-1}$ by substituting new values of k_{10}, and the apparent volume of distribution re-calculated by three methods described in the text: V(extrap), equation 1.26; V^β, equation 1.27; V^{ss}, equation 1.30. Clearly, distribution volume is overestimated by V^β, and grossly so by V(extrap) at high clearances. The arrow indicates the observed clearance $(V_1.k_{10})$.

Clearance from the two-compartment model is readily understood by application of the 'conductance' principle. Model clearance is quite independent of the second compartment, since it describes only the elimination pathway,

Thus: $$Cl = V_1.k_{10} \qquad (1.31)$$

Clearance can also be estimated by a model-free method, in which the area under the whole concentration-time curve is measured. Then

$$Cl = \frac{Xd}{AUC} \qquad (1.32)$$

Finally, an intermediate method uses the area under a fitted curve. Since

$$AUC = \frac{A}{\alpha} + \frac{B}{\beta}$$

(1.33)

the clearance can be calculated using equation (1.32). As in the one-compartment system, the time-course of a constant rate infusion can be predicted. Equation (1.34)[3] characterises the wash-in curve for drug concentration in the central compartment during an infusion of rate k'_{01}.

$$C_1 = \frac{k'_{01}}{V_1 . k_{10}} \left(1 + \frac{(\beta - k_{10})}{(\alpha - \beta)} . e^{-\alpha t} + \frac{(k_{10} - \alpha)}{(\alpha - \beta)} . e^{-\beta t} \right)$$

(1.34)

At equilibrium, this simplifies to:

$$C_1^{ss} = \frac{k'_{01}}{V_1 . k_{10}}$$

(1.35)

which is, of course, identical to equation (1.17) for the one-compartment model. Thus the final concentration is simply the ratio of infusion rate to clearance in all cases. If, at any time, the infusion is discontinued, the plasma concentration falls according to a complex wash-out equation. For practical purposes, it is advisable to use the segmented general solution in the appendix, by which it is possible to model any desired administration pattern (however irregular), and subsequent decay curves.

The three-compartment model

Some drugs result in plasma curves which are best satisfied by three-compartment models (see Fig. 1.7). These curves are characterised by equations with 3 exponential terms, i.e.

$$C = P.e^{-\pi t} + A.c^{-\alpha t} + B.e^{-\beta t}$$

(1.36)

Since it is conventional to use β as the slowest rate constant in equations of this kind, π is introduced as a new 'fast' constant, and α characterises the intermediate term. Concentrations in the deep compartments are characterised by similar, but more complex equations to those of the two-compartment model. These equations can be derived from a given compartmental model, but involve the solution of a cubic equation and some very tedious computation. The reader is referred to a detailed account[6].

Curve fitting

Up to this point we have ignored the task of fitting an n-exponential function to a set of concentration-time data following a bolus dose or infusion. This is a major topic in its own right, and full of statistical pitfalls[2, 4, 12, 15]. In essence, a whole series of exponential functions may be fitted to a set of data (i.e. for n = 1 to 3), and the most

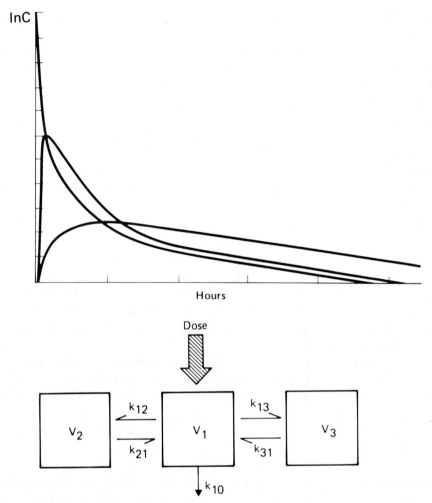

Fig. 1.7 Log-concentrations in all compartments of a three-compartment open model, and the corresponding model diagram.

probable chosen. Curve fitting can be performed very simply by means of the 'feathering' or 'stripping' method, but this should be regarded as a rough estimate, and more reliance placed on iterative, weighted, non-linear regression computer programmes which are now in widespread use.

Saunders[15] pointed out that since the derivation (see appendix) of a compartmental model from an equation (i.e. 1.20) is a *sequential* process (k_{21} is calculated first, then k_{10} from α, β and k_{21}, and finally k_{12} from α, β, k_{21} and k_{12}), the confidence limits for k_{12} are much wider than for k_{21}. Clearly the '*line of best fit*' is not identical with the '*model of best fit*'. This problem can be overcome[11] by a numerical technique which fits a *model* directly to the data, so that the rate constants have similar confidence intervals.

Given a set of fitted curves, each corresponding to a model of n-compartments, choice of the most probable can be a major task. As the number of terms increases, the actual 'sum of the differences' will decrease, but the number of degrees of freedom will diminish by two for every added term. Thus the 'fit' improves but the *probability* diminishes! The simplest possible model should always be chosen, never adding additional compartments unless statistically justified. In the case of a possible two-compartment model, an intuitive approach may suffice if $\alpha > 5\beta$, but for smaller differences than this, and in cases where data points are few, and/or experimental error is high, it is necessary to use complex statistical criteria which are outside the scope of this work[2].

When the data shows some degree of scatter, it frequently occurs that a number of equally probable curves may be derived, each of which corresponds to a different model. This is the problem of *non-uniqueness*, which has challenged mathematicians for many years (and still does). Thus when a compartmental model is chosen, the user must be aware that it is only an estimate, and that other models may be equally likely. He must also be confident that the model is linear, i.e. that giving a different dose of drug would not yield a quite different model. In the event of such *dose-dependent kinetics*, a more complex approach is required.

A model, once derived, can be used to predict the behaviour of the system following any conceivable dosage regime (see Appendix). However, it must be appreciated that if derived on the basis of a six-hour observation period, the model can state how it would behave during the same period, given any input. It will not *predict* accurately how the *subject* will behave in the future, and will be even less able to predict behaviour over a longer period.

Inspection of the equations in the Appendix shows that computation of model behaviour is fairly complex. However, errors will not be compounded by these manipulations, since they simply state, *without error*, how the model responds to a given input. The only error involved lies in the kineticist's choice of model in the first place!

APPENDIX

The two-compartment 'open' model

Although it is widely used in pharmacokinetic studies, many workers find the model difficult to handle in practice, since working equations are rarely quoted. Here, a method is presented which requires only substitution of values and a good deal of simple arithmetic, permitting computation of concentrations in both compartments for any dosage regime, and calculation of the infusion rate required to yield any specified concentration-time result.

To derive the parameters of a two-compartment open model from an equation of the form $C = A.e^{-\alpha t} + B.e^{-\beta t}$

$$V_1 = Xd/(A+B)$$
$$k_{21} = (A.\beta + B.\alpha)/(A+B)$$
$$k_{10} = \alpha.\beta/k_{21}$$
$$k_{12} = \alpha + \beta - k_{21} - k_{10}$$
$$V_2 = V_1.k_{12}/k_{21}$$

To calculate drug concentrations in a two-compartment open model, given any initial conditions, and to which any combination of bolus or infusion is given at any time

1   Find exponents α, β (if not already known for this model). α and β are the real roots of a quadratic equation, so that:

$$\alpha = \frac{b + \sqrt{b^2 - 4c}}{2} \quad \text{and} \quad \beta = \frac{b - \sqrt{b^2 - 4c}}{2}$$

where $\qquad b = k_{12} + k_{21} + k_{10}, \quad \text{and} \quad c = k_{21}.k_{10}$

2   Let ψ_1 and ψ_2 be the initial concentrations in compartments 1 and 2. For an 'empty' model, $\psi_1 = \psi_2 = 0$. If following a previous segment, they equate with terminal concentrations C_1 and C_2.

3   Compute the effect of any bolus dose

$$\psi_1 = \frac{Xd}{V_1} + \psi_1 \text{ (if none, then } \psi_1 = \psi_1)$$

4   For any constant rate infusion of rate k'_{01}, let $Z = \dfrac{k'_{01}}{V_1}$

If no infusion, $Z = 0$.

5   Let
$$Y_1 = \psi_1.k_{21} + \psi_2.k_{12} + Z$$
$$Y_2 = \psi_2(k_{12} + k_{10}) + \psi_1.k_{21}$$

6   Then:
$$A = \frac{\psi_1.\alpha^2 - Y_1.\alpha + Z.k_{21}}{\alpha(\alpha - \beta)}$$

$$B = \frac{\psi_1.\beta^2 - Y_1.\beta + Z.k_{21}}{\beta(\beta - \alpha)}$$

$$C = Z/k_{10} \text{ (zero if no infusion)}$$

$$L = \frac{\psi_2.\alpha^2 - Y_2.\alpha + Z.k_{21}}{\alpha(\alpha - \beta)}$$

$$M = \frac{\psi_2.\beta^2 - Y_2.\beta + Z.k_{21}}{\beta(\beta - \alpha)}$$

7 Now at any time t

$$C_1 = A.e^{-\alpha t} + B.e^{-\beta t} + C$$
$$C_2 = L.e^{-\alpha t} + M.e^{-\beta t} + C$$

8 For any change of conditions, return to (2), ensuring that after calculating terminal concentrations, and then $\psi_1 = C_1$ and $\psi_2 = C_2$, t restarts at zero for next segment. For a simple decay following any regime, simply specify $k'_{01} = 0$ and $Xd = 0$. Note that any change in the model itself necessitates recomputation of α, β.

To calculate the infusion rate required to yield a specified concentration in the central compartment at a specified time, for any initial conditions

1 Calculate α, β if not known (i.e. step b(1)).
2 specify ψ_1 and ψ_2. (zero for empty model, or C_1 and C_2 if following a previous segment)
3 Add a bolus dose if required:

$$\psi_1 = \psi_1 + Xd/V_1$$

4 Let C'_1 be the desired concentration at time t
5 Let $W = e^{-\alpha t}/\alpha(\alpha - \beta)$ and $Z = e^{-\beta t}/\beta(\beta - \alpha)$

6 $k'_{01} = V_1 \left(\dfrac{C'_1 + \psi_1.W.\alpha(k_{21} - \alpha) + \psi_1.Z.\beta(k_{21} - \beta) + \psi_2.k_{12}(W.\alpha + Z.\beta)}{k_{21}(W + Z) - W.\alpha - Z.\beta + 1/k_{10}} \right)$

NB. If the result is negative, this states the rate at which drug must be withdrawn to yield the desired result, i.e. the 'target' cannot be attained.
7 If the time course of this segment is required, or final concentrations C_1 and C_2 are needed for a subsequent segment, then return to step 4 of previous section, and insert this value of k'_{01} as before.

These calculations, although too tedious for manual calculation, are readily handled by any programmable calculator or small computer, and can run the model for any conceivable requirement. A similar method can be applied to the three-compartment model, but the equations, being very cumbersome, are not shown here[6].

However, programmes are available in BASIC for both two- and three-compartment models, by application to the author.

REFERENCES

1. BOWER S. (1981) Plasma protein binding of fentanyl. *J. Pharm. Pharmacol.* **33**, 507.

2. BOXENBAUM H. G., RIEGELMAN S. &

ELASHOFF R. M. (1974) Statistical estimations in pharmacokinetics. *J. Pharmacokinet. Biopharm.* **2**(2), 123.

3. GIBALDI M. & PERRIER D. (1975) *Pharm-*

acokinetics. Marcel Dekker, New York.

4. GLASS H. I. & DE GARRETA A. C. (1971) The quantitative limitations of exponential curve fitting. *Phys. Med. Biol.* **16**, 119.

5. HULL C. J. (1979) Symbols for compartmental models (Editorial). *Br. J. Anaesth.* **51**, 815.

6. HULL C. J., ENGLISH M. J. M. & SIBBALD A. (1980) Fazadinium and pancuronium, a pharmacodynamic study. *Br. J. Anaesth.* **52**, 1209.

7. HULL C. J. & MCLEOD K. (1976) Pharmacokinetic analysis using an electrical analogue. *Br. J. Anaesth.* **48**, 677.

8. KLOTZ U., MCHORSE T. S., WILKINSON G. R. & SCHENKER S. (1974) The effect of cirrhosis on the disposition and elimination of meperidine in man. *Clin. Pharmacol. Therap.* **16**, 667.

9. NAGASHIMA R., LEVY G. & O'REILLY R. A. (1968) Comparative pharmacokinetics of coumarin anticoagulants, IV. *J. Pharm. Sci.* **5**, 1888.

10. PAPPENHEIMER J. R. & COMMITTEE (1950) Standardisation of definitions and symbols in respiratory physiology. *Fed. Proc.* **9**, 602.

11. PFEFFER M. (1973) COMPT. a time-sharing program for non-linear regression analysis of compartmental models of drug distribution. *J. Pharmacokinet. Biopharm.* **1**, 137.

12. RIGGS D. S. (1963) *The mathematical approach to physiological problems.* Williams and Wilkins, Baltimore.

13. ROUTLEDGE P. A., BARCHOWSKY A., BJORNSSON T. D., KITCHELL B. B. & SHAND D. G. (1980) Lidocaine plasma protein binding. *Clin. Pharmacol. Ther.* **27**, 347.

14. SAIDMAN L. J. & EGER E. I. (1966) The effect of thiopental metabolism on duration of anaesthesia. *Anesthesiology* **27**, 118.

15. SAUNDERS L. & NATUNEN T. (1972) A statistical approach to pharmacokinetic calculations. *J. Pharm. Pharmacol.* **24**, Suppl. 94P.

16. SCHANKER L. S. (1959) Absorption of drugs from the rat colon. *J. Pharmacol. Exp. Ther.* **126**, 283.

17. BOWER S., HOLLAND D. E. & HULL C. J. (1976) The pharmacokinetics of fentanyl in man. *Br. J. Anaesth.* **48**, 1121.

18. SHEPPARD C. W. (1948) The theory of the study of transfers within a multicompartment system. *J. Appl. Physics.* **19**, 70.

19. STOECKEL H., HENGSTMANN J. H. & SCHUTTLER J. (1979) Pharmacokinetics of fentanyl as a possible explanation for recurrence of respiratory depression. *Br. J. Anaesth.* **51**, 741.

20. TRUDNOWSKI R. J. & GESSNER T. (1975) Gastric sequestration of meperidine following intravenous administration. *Abstracts, A. S. A. Meeting,* Chicago, p. 327.

21. VON CUBE B., TESCHEMACHER H. J., HERZ A. & HESS R. (1970) Permeation of morphine-like acting substances to their sites of antinociceptive action in the brain after intravenous and intraventricular application and dependence upon lipid solubility. *Naunyn-Schmiedebergs Arch. Pharmak.* **265**, 473.

GENERAL REFERENCES

GIBALDI M. (1977) *Biopharmaceutics and clinical pharmacokinetics,* 2nd Edition. Lea and Febiger, Philadelphia.

NOTARI R. E. (1980) *Biopharmaceutics and clinical pharmacokinetics: an introduction,* 3rd Edition. Marcel Dekker, New York.

2 Drug Receptor Reaction

JOHN NORMAN

Pharmacokinetics deals largely with the ways with which the body absorbs, distributes, metabolises and eliminates drugs. The quantitation of the relationship between drug dosage and the pharmacological effects produced is termed pharmacodynamics. Whilst much of the original work assessing the relationships between dose and effect was based on work done using isolated organs and tissues *in vitro*, with the recent development of pharmacokinetics it is now becoming possible to quantitate the relationships between dose and response in man. This chapter describes what sort of relationships might be expected in such dose-response studies.

With the possible exception of general anaesthesia most actions of drugs are due to chemical interactions between the drug and some specific component of the body. These components (*receptors*) were originally only a convenient concept, but now are being isolated from cell components. The original ideas of such specific receptors came from the knowledge that the chemical structure of a drug needed to be highly specific for an action to occur: with some drugs stereospecificity also occurs. Further, compounds of similar structure often produce similar effects. Finally, some drugs of similar structure interact to produce additive or competitive effects. All these lines of evidence point to the nature of the drug action being describable by chemical reactions. A drug in molar concentration [D] reacts with a receptor in a concentration [R] to produce a complex [DR] which then leads to an effect.

$$[D] + [R] \rightarrow [DR] \rightarrow \text{Effect} \tag{2.1}$$

The effects produced by drugs are of many varieties. At a biomolecular level a drug may combine with a receptor in the cell membrane, leading to a change in its shape perhaps letting it open or close an ion channel in the membrane (Fig. 2.1). Such changes in ionic permeability will have marked effects on excitable cells.

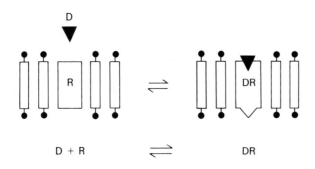

D + R $\rightleftharpoons$ DR

Fig. 2.1 Diagram showing the binding of a drug molecule to a receptor in a cell membrane with a consequent change in shape.

A second possibility is that the change in shape of the receptor in the membrane will act on other membrane structures, such as enzymes. When activated, beta-adrenergic receptors change the conformation of the enzyme adenylate cyclase, which then catalyzes the conversion of ATP (see Chapter 13). Drugs which are lipid soluble (e.g. steroids) will cross cell membranes easily and produce their actions on receptors in the cell, which lead eventually to alterations in protein synthesis. This variety of possibilities adds difficulties to the interpretation of the time-course of drug actions in the whole body: whilst the pharmacokinetic data may reasonably allow a prediction of the time of arrival and departure of drug from a receptor site, the time course of the action may be short (with actions on ionic permeability they may be fractions of a second) or very much longer (i.e. changes in protein synthesis). Some of the complexities at the fastest systems are described for acetylcholine receptors by Dreyer[2].

Most drugs used by anaesthetists produce actions which are reversible: once the drug concentration is lowered sufficiently the effect disappears. The first equation should therefore be rearranged.

$$[D] + [R] \rightleftharpoons [DR] \rightleftharpoons Effect \tag{2.2}$$

DEFINITIONS

Drugs which combine with receptors are said to possess *affinity* for the receptor: if the resulting combination leads to an effect then the drug also has *efficacy*. Such a drug is called an *agonist*. Some agonists even in very high concentrations do not produce the maximal effect seen with other drugs: they have lower efficacies and are called *partial agonists*. Some drugs combine with the receptor but do not produce any effect and, further, they block the effect of an agonist. These drugs are *antagonists*. They can be classified as *competitive* if their actions are surmountable by increasing the concentration of agonist and *non-competitive* if they are not.

REACTION MODELS

Langley–Clark Model

This model, described initially by Langley in 1907 and refined by Clark in 1933, deals with the simplest reaction[1, 7]. It assumes that the effect produced will be directly proportional to the amount of receptor which has drug bound to it. This can be related to the drug concentration at the receptor site as follows. At equilibrium the Law of Mass Action can be applied to relate the concentrations of drug [D], free receptor [R] and the combination [DR] such that

$$\frac{[D][R]}{[DR]} = K_d \tag{2.3}$$

where square brackets denote molar concentrations and K_d is the dissociation constant. High values of K_d indicate a low affinity of the drug and low values high affinity. To calculate the fraction of all receptors (R_t) that have drug bound the following development is needed:

$$R_t = [R] + [DR]$$

or

$$[R] = R_t - [DR]$$

By substitution and rearrangement from (2.3)

$$[D](R_t - [DR]) = K_d[DR] \tag{2.4}$$

and

$$[D]R_t - [D][DR] = K_d[DR]$$

and

$$[D]R_t = [DR]([D] + K_d)$$

and, finally

$$\frac{[DR]}{R_t} = \frac{[D]}{[D] + K_d} \tag{2.5}$$

Provided the efficacy of the drug is maximal and the maximum effect is produced only when all the receptors have drug bound, then the effect seen (E) is given by $[DR]/R_t$, i.e.

$$E = \frac{[DR]}{R_t} = \frac{[D]}{[D] + K_d} \tag{2.6}$$

The relationship between effect and drug concentration is shown in Fig. 2.2a. The curve is a rectangular hyperbola. The drug concentration at half maximum effect has the same value as the dissociation constant. There are problems in using Fig. 2.2 in practice in that only a small range of drug concentrations can be examined. Alternative

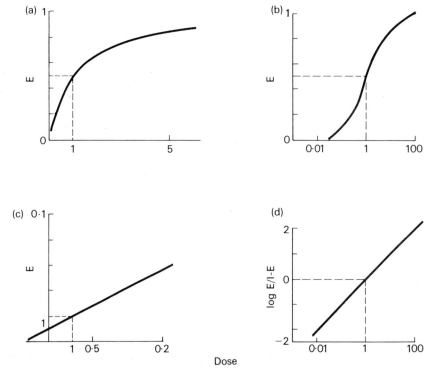

Fig. 2.2 *Dose–response curves* (a) Relationship between drug concentration and effect (equation (2.6) in text). (b) Relationship between drug concentration expressed on a logarithmic scale and the effect. (c) Lineweaver–Burke relationship between the reciprocals of the drug concentration and the effect (equation (2.6)). (d) The Hill plot relating the logit of the effect and the logarithm of the drug concentration (equation (2.18)).

plots are shown in Fig. 2.2b, c and d. The logarithm-dose response plot (Fig. 2.2b) is perhaps the commonest. It produces a symmetrical S-shaped curve and the portion covering effects at 20–80 % of maximal is almost linear. Thus it leads itself to fairly simple satistical analysis.

Lineweaver–Burke plot

One transformation which leads to a straight line is commonly used by biochemists who measure rates of reaction which are proportional to the amount of enzyme taking up a substrate—a situation analogous to receptor binding drugs. The graph (Fig. 2.2c) plots the reciprocal of the velocity of reactions (effect) as a function the reciprocal of the substrate (drug) concentration. The relationship can be developed from equation (2.6).

Invert
$$\frac{1}{E} = \frac{[D] + K_d}{[D]}$$

and
$$\frac{1}{E} = 1 + K_d \frac{1}{[D]} \qquad (2.7)$$

The dissociation constant K_d is the slope of line. In using this relationship to calculate K_d there are problems in that the results can be heavily weighted by results obtained at lower concentrations of drug. Riggs (1963) describes these[14] and gives alternative approaches.

A more useful transformation was derived by Hill[4] in 1909 in his studies of the oxyhaemoglobin dissociation curve. Equation (2.7) is further changed:

$$\frac{1}{E} - 1 = \frac{K_d}{[D]}$$

and by rearranging and inverting

$$\frac{E}{1-E} = \frac{[D]}{K_d}$$

Finally logarithms are taken

$$\log \frac{E}{1-E} = \log[D] - \log K_d \qquad (2.8)$$

This produces a straight line relationship (Fig. 2.2d) with a slope of unity. Should two molecules of drug be needed for each receptor, i.e.

$$2D + R \rightleftharpoons D_2 R$$

then the equation becomes

$$\log \frac{E}{1-E} = 2\log[D] - \log K_d \qquad (2.9)$$

With four molecules of drug per receptor the slope would go to four. The dissociation curve for haemoglobin plotted this way has a slope of about 2.7; the simple model does not seem to work for haemoglobin[3].

Probit scales

The term $\log(E/1 - E)$ is referred to as the logit transformation. There is an alternative approach which looks at the response as being due to statistical summation of probabilities that any individual receptor-drug combination will produce the effect. One concentration of drug produces a 50% effect (the ED_{50}). Assuming the probabilities of effect are distributed normally about this point of the log dose scale, $\pm 1\,SD$ will give 84% and 16% response respectively. $\pm 1.96\,SD$ correspond to the 95% and 5% points.

The effect ordinate is transformed from percentage of maximal on a linear scale (e.g. Fig. 2.2a, b) to this probability scale. The scale runs from minus infinity to plus infinity but gives a linear relationship between probability and log dose. In practice the difference between expressing results using probit scales and using logit transformations is minimal.

Effects of antagonists

The effects of antagonists can also be quantitated. Non-competitive drugs act in such a way that their effects cannot be overcome by increasing the concentration of agonist. In effect they reduce the concentration of receptor free to combine with agonist. If 50 % of receptors become blocked then the maximal effect is reduced by half (Fig. 2.3a).

With competitive drugs the antagonist actions can be overcome by increasing the concentration of agonist. Presumably all the reactions with the receptors are reversible and the effect produced will still be proportional to the fraction of receptors which have agonist drug bound ($[DR]/R_t$). The factors involved are the concentration of agonist $[D]$ and antagonist $[A]$ and the two dissociation constant K_d and K_a.

For the agonist equation (2.6) applies, and for the antagonist A:

$$A + R \rightleftharpoons AR$$

$$\frac{[A][R]}{[AR]} = K_a$$

At equilibrium with both drugs the concentration of free receptors $[R]$ is given by

$$[R] = K_d \frac{[DR]}{[D]} = K_a \frac{[AR]}{[A]} \tag{2.10}$$

The concentration of antagonist-receptor $[AR]$ can be calculated:

$$[AR] = [DR] \frac{K_d}{K_a} \frac{[A]}{[D]} \tag{2.11}$$

The total receptor concentration R_t is given by

$$R_t = [R] + [DR] + [AR]$$

$$= [R] + [DR] + [DR] \frac{K_d}{K_a} \frac{[A]}{[D]} \tag{2.12}$$

This can be arranged to calculate $[R]$ and in turn this can be substituted in equation (2.3)

$$K_d[DR] = [D] \left(R_t - [DR] - [DR] \frac{K_d}{K_a} \frac{[A]}{[D]} \right)$$

$$= [D]R_t - [D][DR] - [DR] \frac{K_d}{K_a} [A] \tag{2.13}$$

Collecting all the [DR] terms:

$$[DR]\left(K_d + [D] + [A]\frac{K_d}{K_a}\right) = [D]R_t \qquad (2.14)$$

The fraction of receptor occupied by drug becomes:

$$\frac{[DR]}{R_t} = \frac{[D]}{[D] + K_d\left(1 + \frac{[A]}{K_a}\right)} \qquad (2.15)$$

Increasing the concentration of antagonist or using a more potent one (with a lower K_a) will increase the denominator and lower the effect of the agonist. Fig. 2.3b shows the effect on a logarithm-dose response curve. Competitive antagonists produced a curve shifted to the right but parallel to the original. Such a parallel shift implies that in order to get a given effect (say a 50% contraction of a muscle) the concentration of agonist must be raised by a constant proportion. Schild[12] introduced a term pAx which allows a comparison of the potencies of series of antagonists. With the parallel shift there will be concentrations of each antagonist which necessitate the dose of agonist be increased by the x-factor to produce the original effect. Using a notation similar to that of the pH scale (pA $= -\log [A]$) Schild defined pA_{10} as the negative logarithm of the concentration of antagonist necessitating a 10-fold increase in agonist and pA_2 as that needing a two-fold increase. pA_2 is also numerically equal to the negative logarithm of the dissociation constant of the antagonist ($pA_2 = -\log K_a$). High pA_2 values are associated with potent antagonists.

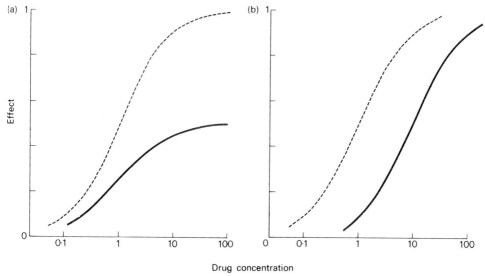

Fig. 2.3 Log-dose response curves for non-competitive (a) and competitive (b) antagonists.

SUBUNIT MODELS

The classic theory developed by Clark[1] does not account for all the responses seen with agonists and antagonists. There is now interest in alternative models which consider the receptor as being composed of a number of subunits which may each bind drugs. When one subunit has a drug bound to it there can be a resulting change in the relationships of the whole array of units. Such a total change in shape could lead to opening or closing of pores in membranes or to exposing other reacting groups, leading to changes in enzyme activity.

A similar situation exists with haemoglobin which can carry one oxygen molecule per subunit. 2,3-diphosphoglyceric acid binds to a site different to the oxygen-carrying site and yet by changing the whole shape of the haemoglobin alters the affinity for oxygen. Such effects are called *allosteric*.

There are a number of models which show how subunits can interact and how changing drug concentrations can alter the state of the whole molecule[6, 9, 10]. In 1969 Monod *et al*[8] described a somewhat simpler system which starts by assuming each subunit to exist in one of two forms or shapes (Fig. 2.4). One is defined as the tense structure (T), and one the relaxed (R).

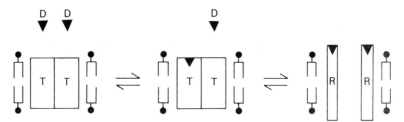

Fig. 2.4 Diagram showing the binding of drug molecules to a receptor composed of two subunits.

The simplest model starts by assuming there are two subunits and that the whole molecule exists either as TT or RR. If we also assume that drugs bind only to the R form of the subunit we can work out the relationship between drug concentration and the fraction of the total molecules in the RR form. It may be that the RR form is the active one, allowing an ion channel to open or an enzyme to be active.

To begin: there will be an equilibrium in the absence of drug between the tense and relaxed forms

$$TT \rightleftharpoons RR$$

At equilibrium, applying the Law of Mass Action

$$L = [TT]/[RR] \qquad (2.16)$$

(L is the conventional term for this ratio. High values indicate a low concentration in the relaxed form).

Assume the drug (D) binds only to the R form, how does changing [D] influence the ratio?

Binding the first molecule:

$$RR + D \rightleftharpoons RD.R$$

To apply the Law of Mass Action remember that each molecule of RR has two binding sites for D. Thus

$$\frac{2[RR][D]}{[RD.R]} = K$$

where K is the dissociation constant. By rearrangement

$$[RD.R] = 2[RR][D]/K$$

Binding a second drug molecule is represented by

$$RD.R + D \rightleftharpoons RD.RD \tag{2.17}$$

and

$$\frac{[RD.R][D]}{2[RD.RD]} = K \tag{2.18}$$

Again each RD.RD molecule has two molecules of drug bound to it. Therefore

$$[RD.RD] = [RD.R][D]/2K$$

and by substitution

$$[RD.RD] = 2[RR]\frac{[D]}{K} \cdot \frac{[D]}{2K}$$

$$= [RR]\frac{[D]^2}{K^2} \tag{2.19}$$

To derive the fraction of all the receptor molecules in the RR form start with the total sum R_t

$$R_t = [TT] + [RR] + [RD.R] + [RD.RD]$$

Substituting from equations (2.16), (2.17), (2.19).

$$R_t = L[RR] + [RR] + 2[RR]\frac{[D]}{K} + [RR]\frac{[D]^2}{[K]^2}$$

which simplifies to

$$R_t = [RR]\left[L + \left(1 + \frac{[D]}{K}\right)^2\right] \tag{2.20}$$

The number of receptors in the relaxed form is given by the sum of $[RR]$ and $[RD.R]$ and $[RD.RD]$ and is given by:

$$[RR]+[RD.R]+[RD.RD] = [RR]+\frac{2[RR][D]}{K}+[RR]\frac{[D]^2}{[K]^2}$$

$$= [RR]\left(1+\frac{[D]}{K}\right)^2 \qquad (2.21)$$

The fraction of all the receptor in the relaxed from (Y) is then given by the ratio of equations (2.20) and (2.21).

$$Y = \frac{[RR]\left(1+\dfrac{[D]}{K}\right)^2}{[RR]\left[L+\left(1+\dfrac{[D]}{K}\right)^2\right]}$$

$$= \frac{\left(1+\dfrac{[D]}{K}\right)^2}{L+\left(1+\dfrac{[D]}{K}\right)^2} \qquad (2.22)$$

The fraction in the relaxed form, and as with the Clark model, the effect, is thus a function of the drug concentration, its dissociation constant and the ratio L. Provided L does not equal zero the curve relating drug concentration to effect will be sigmoid (Fig. 2.5). Antagonists can still act competitively with effect of modifying K as will the Clark model or may act at other sites to alter the balance between tense and relaxed forms, thereby changing L.

If more than two subunits are involved the effect is to increase the power term: with 4 subunits interacting the power becomes 4 and so on[9].

If the effect is proportional to the fraction of receptor in the relaxed form it is possible to use the logit transformation to estimate n—the number of subunits involved. From equation 2.22 using the same route as described earlier for the Hill equation:

$$\log\frac{Y}{1-Y} = n\log\left(1+\frac{[D]}{K}\right)-\log L \qquad (2.23)$$

At low drug concentrations ($[D] \ll K$) the curve is flat but at high concentrations ($[D] \gg K$) the slope of the curve is almost equal to n. Fig. 2.6 shows the types of picture that emerge. Over the readily measured response range (10–90%) the logit log dose plot is virtually a straight line of slope just under n in value.

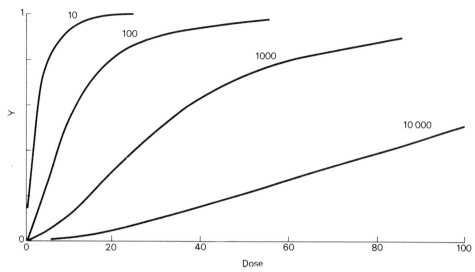

Fig. 2.5 The dose response curve for the subunit model showing the effect of changing L—the ratio of the numbers of receptors in the tense and relaxed forms.

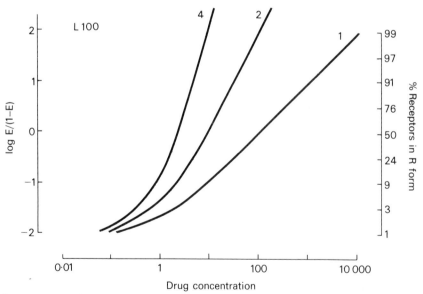

Fig. 2.6 Hill plot of the relationship between the logit of the effect and the logarithm of the drug concentration. At high drug concentrations the slope is almost the same as n. Four curves are shown for n values of 1, 2 and 4. L was set at 100. The right hand axis shows the percentage of receptors in the relaxed form (equation (2.22) in the text with the selected n values).

DANGERS OF DYNAMIC MODELLING

In applying models of agonist and antagonist action much success has been gained with *in vitro* studies. Organ bath drug concentrations will be close to the free drug concentrations and effects can be measured readily. Increasing sophistication of measurement of the effects such as is now possible at the neuromuscular junction with conductance measurements[2] allow precise estimates of many of the parameters to be made. It is now also possible to assay the minute concentrations of drug present in blood from patients and the kinetic models presented elsewhere in this book let us derive what may be happening in various tissues of the body. However, the relative crudeness of our techniques of measuring effects in man can lead to many problems in marrying the kinetic and dynamic data. Attempts have been made with clinical neuromuscular block[5, 13, 14].

From relationships between theoretical receptor site drug concentration and the paralysis produced it is possible to use the logit transformation and estimate values for the slope. These cannot be equated with the 'n' values of the subunit model. The problems first arise from the measurement of effect. With neuromuscular block the effect is the antagonism of the evoked muscle contraction produced by acetylcholine released at the nerve terminal. Equating block with effect is suspect. In addition if it is remembered that there are more receptors for acetylcholine at any neuromuscular junction than are needed to produce a muscle contraction, the situation becomes even more complex. Whilst the models presented here give insight at a biomolecular level they must be used with great caution in clinical practice.

REFERENCES

1. CLARK A. J. (1933) *The Mode of Action of Drugs on Cells.* Edward Arnold, London.
2. DREYER F. (1982) Acetylcholine receptor. *Br. J. Anaesth.* **54**, 115.
3. GILLIES I. D. S. (1974) Anaesthesia and anaemia. *Br. J. Anaesth.* **46**, 589.
4. HILL A. V. (1910) The possible effect of the aggregation of the molecules of haemoglobin on its dissociation curve. *J. Physiol.* **40**, iv.
5. HULL C. J., ENGLISH M. J. M. & SIBBALD A. (1980) Fazadinium and pancuronium: a pharmacodynamic study. *Br. J. Anaesth.* **52**, 1209.
6. KOSHLAND D. E. (1973) Protein shape and biological control. *Sci. Am.* **229** (4), 52.
7. LANGLEY J. N. (1907) On the contraction of muscle, chiefly in relation to the pre-sence of 'receptive' substances. *J. Physiol.* **36**, 347.
8. MONOD J., WYMAN J. & CHANGEAUX J. P. (1965) On the nature of allosteric transitions. *J. Mol. Biol.* **12**, 86.
9. NEWSHOLME E. A. & START C. (1973) *Regulation in Metabolism.* John Wiley, London.
10. NORMAN J. (1979) Drug-receptor reactions. *Br. J. Anaesth.* **51**, 595.
11. RIGGS D. S. (1963) *The Mathematical Approach to Physiological Problems.* Williams & Wilkins, Baltimore.
12. SCHILD H. O. (1974) pA, a new scale for the measurement of drug antagonism. *Br. J. Pharmacol. Ther.* **2**, 189.
13. SHANKS C. A., SOMOGYI A. A., RAMZAN M. I. & TRIGGS E. J. (1980) Tubucurarine

and pancuronium: a pharmacokinetic view. *Anaesth. Intensive Care* **8**, 4.

14. SHEINER L. B., STANSKI D. R., VOZEH S., MILLER R. D. & HAM J. (1979) Simultaneous modelling of pharmacokinetics and pharmacodynamics: applications to d-tubocurarine. *Clin. Pharmacol. Ther.* **3**, 358.

3 General Methods of Measuring Drug Concentrations in Plasma, Urine and other Tissues

J. W. SEAR, D. J. H. TRAFFORD and H. L. J. MAKIN

METHODS OF DETECTION AND QUANTITATION
Spectrophotometry and colorimetry
Spectrofluorimetry
Saturation analysis

PURIFICATION PRIOR TO QUANTITATION

COMBINED SEPARATION AND QUANTITATION OF CHEMICALS AND
  DRUGS
High pressure liquid chromatography
Gas chromatography
Capillary column chromatography
Mass spectrometry
Isotope derivative assays
Determination of total drug concentration and free or unbound concen-
  tration in plasma

In order to measure the concentration of a drug or its metabolite(s) in plasma, urine or a tissue, it is necessary to isolate the drug from other substances which may interfere in the quantification method chosen. When choosing the method of quantification for use in any given circumstances two factors, sensitivity and specificity, have to be considered. It is clear that a quantitative method of high specificity is inadequate if it does not have the required sensitivity, although it may be useful in giving a rough estimate of the level of the drug in question.

If a method has sufficient sensitivity, even though it may lack specificity, it can be used, provided that the required degree of purification is achieved prior to quantification. This is not always easy to demonstrate and even the best methods occasionally give spurious results due to unforeseen interference. Radioimmunoassays using antisera of high specificity (e.g. for aldosterone) can be carried out directly on plasma without any prior extraction. In renal disease, aldosterone glucuronide, which has a metabolic clearance rate (MCR) equal to the renal blood flow, is not cleared as rapidly

38

as usual. Thus, it accumulates in the plasma and cross-reacts with the antiserum used causing spuriously high results[35]. Specificity is therefore never absolute and each patient may have something present in the plasma, urine or tissue of interest which can interfere in the final assay.

Some methods of quantification are more suspect in terms of specificity than others. Simple UV absorption at a fixed wavelength is clearly less specific than the use of a high resolution mass spectrometer. The methods of purification prior to quantification are therefore just as important as the method of quantification itself. Since the latter determines the degree of purification required, these methods will be considered first of all.

The correct choice of internal standard, which allows a correction for losses incurred during purification in individual samples rather than relying on average recoveries for a number of samples, is also an important consideration when setting up an assay. The more complex the purification required prior to quantification, the more necessary a good internal standard becomes. Internal standards can be the compound itself, radiolabelled usually with ^{3}H, or a chemically related compound which is not usually found in the sample to be analysed. Provided the radiolabelled compound is available, and has sufficiently high specific activity to enable radioactivity (counts/minute) to be added without significantly increasing the mass of compound present in the sample, radiolabelled internal standards are probably to be preferred. The use of chemically related compounds as internal standards can cause problems since they may not always behave in the same way as the compound being analysed and may separate during purification.

As a result of improvements in technology, and the development of specific radioimmunoassay systems, the volume of the biological sample needed for the analysis may be reduced. Early assays for ACTH used a bioassay method[17, 53] which required 500–1000 ml of blood. By contrast, the modern radioimmunoassay for fentanyl, alfentanil, +-tubocurarine and morphine may use as little as 20 μl of plasma.

METHODS OF DETECTION AND QUANTITATION

Spectrophotometry and colorimetry

These methods rely on the principle of light absorption and have been in use for many years. The absorption of incident light is related to the concentration of solute and to the length of the light path by the Beer–Lambert Law. This states that if the light path is fixed, the concentration of the solute is proportional to $\log_{10}$ incident light/transmitted light. The ratio is termed the absorbance (extinction or optical density) of the solution. Unfortunately, not all solutes obey this law and it is necessary to establish whether or not the absorbance is proportional to concentration over the solute concentration range likely to be encountered. Creatinine is one such compound which does not show such proportionality when measured by the Jaffe reaction involving the formation of a red complex with picric acid.

A spectrophotometer is a device in which a prism or a diffraction grating is used to select a specific wavelength of incident light within the range 200–800 nm, whereas a simple colorimeter uses filters to select the incident light and covers only the visible range 400–800 nm. Sensitivity depends almost exclusively on the compound being measured since the absorbance of different compounds varies widely. Many assays depend on measurement in the ultraviolet (UV) range, at wavelengths less than 400 nm. Using very small volume cells, nanogram amounts of some compounds can be measured with satisfactory precision. As with all methods of quantification the specificity depends upon the relative concentration of the compound of interest and the degree of purification carried out prior to assay. A compound present in plasma in high concentration, such as cholesterol (2 mg ml^{-1}), can be measured directly after formation of a coloured complex. In urine, 17-oxosteroids have been measured by colorimetry after formation of coloured complexes using the Zimmermann reaction[24]. While these simple colorimetric procedures may give useful information, they lack specificity and many other compounds may interfere if present in elevated amounts.

On the other hand, compounds present in low concentration must be purified before quantification and provided adequate purification is achieved, specific answers can be obtained using spectrophotometry. The use of linked enzyme systems for the generation of coloured compounds, or for the oxidoreduction of nicotinamide adenine dinucleotide (NAD) or reduced nicotinamide adenine dinucleotide (NADH) can confer an extra degree of specificity depending upon the specificity of the enzyme used. Glucose oxidase, a highly specific enzyme, can be used for the measurement of blood glucose, by measuring the oxygen uptake or by linking the hydrogen peroxide formed to the oxidation of a colourless compound (such as o-toluidine) to a coloured compound, catalysed by the enzyme peroxidase. The absorbance can be measured and the glucose quantified by comparison to a standard. Glucose can also be measured using the enzyme hexokinase plus ATP to form glucose-6-phosphate, followed by the second enzyme, glucose-6-phosphate dehydrogenase, measuring the reduction of NADP at 340 nm. There are many similar procedures which have been applied to a wide variety of compounds without prior purification, as described for glucose, or after purification. Examples of anaesthetic drugs which have been measured using spectrophotometry include thiopentone[11], methohexitone[10], and di-isopropylphenol measured after high pressure liquid chromatography (HPLC)[1].

Apart from its use as a method of quantification, UV and visible spectra can provide a valuable insight into the nature of unknown compounds. In the steroid field, for example, UV spectra are commonly used for the detection of double bond systems (the Δ4-ene-3-one system absorbs strongly at 240 nm, whereas the Δ4, 6-diene-3-ones absorb at 280 nm). Lists of the absorption spectra of a wide variety of steroids have been published[22] and similar data has been published for other compounds.

Spectrofluorimetry

Some compounds absorb light and emit it at a different wavelength. This is called fluorescence, i.e. the amount of light emitted is small, and very sensitive detectors incorporating photomultipliers are required. Theoretically, fluorescence measurements can be 60–100 times more sensitive than simple UV measurements, although the full increase in sensitivity is not always achieved. Sensitivity depends on the nature of the compound, and the amount of fluorescence emitted can vary widely. Not all compounds have a native fluorescence but it can sometimes be induced by reaction with other compounds. Plasma 11-hydroxy-corticosteroids exhibit a fluorescence when treated with concentrated sulphuric acid and this fact has been used for the development of a useful but relatively non-specific method for plasma cortisol[44]. Compounds containing $1°$ and $2°$ amines, imidazole or phenolic groupings can be linked to dansyl chloride, producing fluorescent conjugates[74]. Peptides or proteins can be measured at very low levels using this procedure. There are other fluorescent probes (such as fluorescein) which can be used in a similar fashion.

NAD and NADH can be measured by their fluorescence and this fact has been put to good use in the development of very sensitive assays. For example, the enzyme-catalysed oxidation or reduction of a compound is linked to the oxido-reduction of NAD, which is measured by the change in fluorescence. The degree of specificity of these reactions depends on the specificity and purity of the enzyme which is used. A typical example is the measurement of 3α- and 3β-hydroxysteroids (e.g. bile acids—3α-hydroxysteroids) using the enzymes 3α- and 3β-hydroxysteroid dehydro-genase. These reactions are extremely valuable in that they can be coupled with further oxidoreduction cycles of NAD/NADH and the sensitivity can be amplified 5000–20 000 times. The use of hydroxysteroid dehydrogenase, with amplification by NAD(H) cycling, to measure steroids has recently been described by Payne, Shikita and Talalay[56] and is illustrated in Fig. 3.1. A similar system has been described to estimate vitamin D metabolites with sensitivities down to 0.2–0.5 pmol[27]. One problem with this type of assay is that most of the dehydrogenases used in these systems are relatively non-specific, and hence some prior purification is still required[56].

Spectrophotometry or spectrofluorimetry as the detection system for the effluent of HPLC systems have been described for a number of compounds. Using small volume cells (ca. 6 μl) very small changes in UV absorbance at fixed wavelength can be detected. The amount will obviously depend on the molar extinction coefficient of the compound of interest at the wavelength chosen. The use of sequential detectors monitoring the HPLC effluent at different wawelengths can also be useful, as can a stopped flow tech-nique which allows the UV scan of an isolated peak as it emerges from the HPLC column.

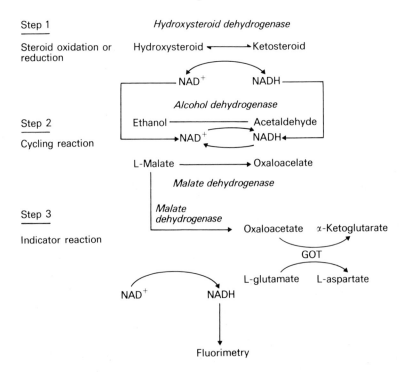

Fig. 3.1 Schematic presentation of the estimation of hydroxy- and keto-steroids using hydroxysteroid dehydrogenases in conjunction with NAD(H) cycling. (From Payne D. W., Shikita, M. and Talalay, P. (1982) *Biol. Chem.* **257**, 633.) Reproduced by permission of the authors and the publisher.

Anaesthetic drugs which have been assayed using HPLC assay linked to UV absorbance include thiopentone[67] using a UV detector at 254 nm. However, the sensitivity of the method, compared with other methods using UV spectrophotometry or colorimetry, was not reported. More recently, an HPLC assay for di-isopropyl-phenol has been reported. This method uses UV detection at 276 nm of an intensely absorbing indophenol derivative produced by the reaction of the drug with Gibbs reagent (2,6-dichloroquinone-4-chloroimide) giving a minimum detection limit of around 25 ng ml^{-1}[1].

Fluorescent techniques have also been described for the determination of the neuromuscular blocking drugs, +-tubocurarine[16], pancuronium bromide[37, 73, 76], and more recently fazadinium[55]. All these drugs contain one or more bisquaternary ammonium radicals with which a fluorescent conjugate can be prepared by the technique of ion-pair extraction into chloroform using Rose Bengal.

Saturation Analysis

This is a general term which covers a wide variety of assays, all of which are based on the interaction between the molecule in question, and some kind of binding protein. Three types of analysis may be used:

1   *Receptor binding assays* are those which use cytoplasmic or nuclear receptor proteins (e.g. for steroid or thyroid hormones), or receptor proteins from cell membranes (for peptide or protein hormones).

2   *Competitive protein binding assays* are those which use binding proteins which occur naturally (e.g. in plasma).

3   Also included in this group are *immunoassays* in which the binding protein involved in the assay is an antibody, usually used in an unpurified state as a heterogenous antiserum raised in an experimental animal in response to the injection of an immunogen. Protein molecules may be immunogenic themselves but many of the small molecules which might be of interest are not natural immunogens. They can however be joined by covalent bonds to protein such as bovine serum albumin (BSA), and when this complex is injected into an experimental animal, antibodies may be produced which will bind with the small molecule even when it is not linked to BSA. The small molecule (described as a hapten) therefore acts as an antigen in the antigen–antibody reaction, although it is not itself immunogenic.

There is a bewildering variety of different immunoassay systems and the interested reader is best referred to a review on the available methods of immunoassay[33, 64]. Although there is some controversy about the mathematics of these saturation analysis methods, a simple approach is to regard the system as a competition between the compound in question and a labelled compound (which may be the same compound or another compound) for the binding site on the binding protein. For a fixed amount of binding protein and labelled compound, increasing amounts of unlabelled compound indicate that an increasing proportion of unlabelled compound will be bound to the protein. A simple graph which illustrates this is given in Fig. 3.2.

In heterogenous radioimmunoassays an essential stage is the separation of the bound and unbound label (Fig. 3.2). This separation is necessary to determine the proportion of label bound to the protein. A wide variety of methods have been described to effect this separation [58] varying from a second antibody for insulin[25], to ammonium sulphate precipitation of the bound label[14], absorption of the bound label onto hydroxyapatite[69], and absorption of the free unbound protein onto Florisil[50]. A very commonly used procedure is the absorption of the free unbound protein onto dextran-coated charcoal[6]. Once separated, the label can then be apportioned between the free and the protein bound.

Fig. 3.3 illustrates the point that these binding proteins will also bind other compounds although this interference (cross-reactivity) may occur only at higher concentrations of other compounds. Various mathematical manipulations can be made, allowing different representations of the change in binding with increasing

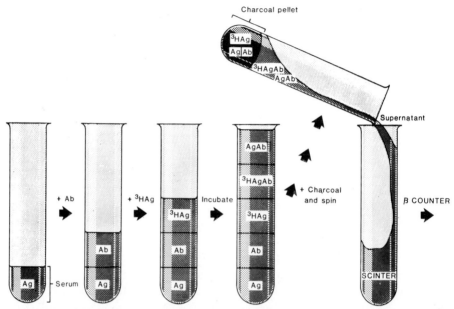

Fig. 3.2　Principle of radioimmunoassay. The drug to be assayed is regarded as an antigen (Ag) to which is added an antibody (Ab) produced by repeated dosing of an animal with the appropriate drug bound to bovine serum albumin. Tritiated drug (^{3}HAg) is added to the mixture and after incubation, the mixture partitions further with the formation of a drug–antibody complex (AgAb) and tritiated drug–antibody complex (^{3}HAgAb). The two latter complexes are separated by absorption of free drug (Ag), unbound antibody (Ab) and unbound tritiated drug (^{3}HAg) on to charcoal. The supernatant liquid containing the bound complexes are then added to scinter fluid and the radioactivity measured in a β counter.

ligand concentration. A ligand can best be defined as the small molecule which binds to the protein, and in a radioimmunoassay method it would be identical to the antigen in the antigen–antibody reaction. In this circumstance the ligand may or may not be the same as the hapten.

Radioimmunoassay uses a radioactive label, usually ^{3}H or some emitting isotope such as ^{125}I and the label is quantitated by liquid or solid scintillation counting. There are, however, a variety of labels other than radioactivity which can be used. For example, an immunoassay for morphine using spin labelling, quantitated by measuring electron spin resonance (ESR) has been described[39] and there are increasing numbers of fluorescence-labelled and enzyme-labelled immunoassays being described[54, 63]. The use of some of the alternative labels has led to the development of simpler homogenous immunoassays which do not require the bound and free to be separated. For example the antibody can be labelled and the label itself is found to be altered in some way when the hapten is bound to the antibody. Binding of the hapten might therefore change the fluorescence of a fluorescent-labelled antibody, and the decrease or increase of the

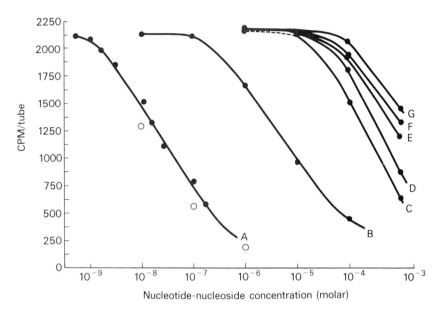

Fig. 3.3 Graph showing the reduction in binding of radiolabelled antigen (succinyl-cAMP-tyrosine methyl ester-^{125}I) to the cAMP antibody by various nucleotides. (From Steiner A. L. *et al.* (1969) *Proc. Nat. Acad. Sci.* (*USA*) **64**, 367.) Reproduced by permission of the authors and the publisher.

fluorescence is thus an indication of the amount of binding to the antibody which has occurred. Strictly this is not perhaps a competitive binding assay. Competitive binding assays and immunoassays are of varying specificity and generally require some purification steps before quantification. Immunoassays are however usually more specific than competitive binding assays and some highly specific antisera, such as the one described for aldosterone, have been described which allow assay of the plasma without extraction. Of drugs used in anaesthesia, fentanyl and its congeners, alfentanil and sufentanil may be assayed by RIA using ^{3}H-fentanyl of the congener as the labelled ligand[45, 46]. The high specificity of these assays has recently allowed Hull and his colleagues to measure fentanyl and alfentanil in the same samples after the simultaneous administration of the two drugs[9]. This depends on the cross-reactivity of each drug for the other in the assays being negligible; in the case of fentanyl and alfentanil, the cross-reaction is less than 10^{-4} molar. The absolute sensitivity of the two assays allows the measurement of as little as 2 pg ml^{-1} of plasma[8]. This approach to comparative pharmacokinetics within a single subject should help to overcome the immense biovariability that exists between individuals.

Other opioid drugs for which radioimmunoassays have been developed include the mixed agonist–antagonist buprenorphine[2] and the archetypal opioid morphine. Early assays for morphine[5] have been questioned as to their cross-reactivity with the main metabolite, morphine-3-glucuronide. An improved assay has been described by Catlin[13] with the ability to detect as little as 1 ng ml^{-1} serum. The availability of these techniques overcomes the problems of variable extraction ratios, column losses and extensive sample preparation required for both spectral and chromatographic analyses. However, the preparation of a suitable antiserum does not ensure a satisfactory assay, as evidence must be obtained to show that the antiserum does not significantly cross-react with any of the known metabolites of the drug. The suitability of an antiserum will also depend on the molar ratio of metabolites to parent drug in the biological tissue under investigation.

Receptor binding assays

The pharmacological effect of any drug depends on the interaction of the free unbound fraction with specific cellular receptors. Assays have been developed to determine the density or concentration of these receptor binding sites, and the kinetics of drug-receptor interaction (Chapter 2). Simply, drug receptor interaction may be described by the equation

$$[L] + [R] \underset{K_2}{\overset{K_1}{\rightleftharpoons}} [LR]$$

where R = free receptor site concentration, L = drug or ligand concentration and K_1 and K_2 are the respective rate constants.

At equilibrium:
$$\frac{[L][R]}{[LR]} = K_D = \frac{1}{K_A}$$

where K_A = association constant, K_D = dissociation constant.

If free drug and bound drug concentrations are determined by techniques described earlier, there are two main methods of data analysis for studying drug-receptor binding at different free drug concentrations[32].

The Scatchard plot

The Scatchard plot allows the measurement of the density of binding sites without requiring the use of a saturating concentration of ligand or drug. The relationship between the free drug concentration and the drug-receptor bound concentration is described by a rectangular hyperbola.

By extrapolation,
$$\frac{[LR]}{[L]} = \frac{[LR]}{K_D} + \frac{RT}{K_D}$$

where RT = total number of binding sites available for drug interaction ([L] and [LR]). If [LR][L] is plotted against [LR], the slope will be equal to $-1/K_D$, and the abscissa intercept RT.

The Hill plot

This requires a pre-existing knowledge of the binding site concentration [RT]. From the Hill equation, it is possible to calculate the free drug concentration at which 50 % is bound, i.e. $K_{0.5}$. This is described as:

$$\log \frac{[LR]}{[RT - LR]} = n \log [L] - n \log K_{0.5}$$

where n = Hill constant.

If $\log [LR]/[RT - LR]$ is plotted against $\log [L]$, the slope will be equal to n, and the intercept $K_{0.5}$. Because of the non linearity of the Hill Plot, it is necessary to use the central linear portion of the bound drug-receptor concentration range (10–90 %).

The ratio of [LR]/RT is referred to as the *receptor site occupancy* (Y).

Thus: $$Y = \frac{[L]}{[L] + K_D}$$

If 50 % of the receptors are occupied, $K_D = [L]$. K_D has been determined experimentally for many drugs, including the neuromuscular relaxants pancuronium and + -tubocurarine, where values of 25.1 and 34.5 nmol respectively have been found (see Chapter 2).

In many cases, the interaction of a drug and its receptors are more complex than that described by the original equation; and may therefore reflect changes in binding affinity at different drug concentrations, or a heterogeneity of binding sites.

Use of the technique of receptor binding site assay has been described for the β-adrenoceptors by Levitzki[38]. However, the assay was unreliable due to high non-specific binding of the cathecholamines. Marker substances for these receptors are usually radiolabelled β-adrenoreceptor antagonists. Most commonly used examples are ^{125}I iodinated hydroxybenzylpindolol and ^{3}H-dihydroalprenolol[41]. These compounds show low non-specific binding, high β-receptor binding, and can be obtained with a high specific activity.

If the radiolabelled compound is added to the membrane fraction under study, total binding will comprise both specific and non-specific binding. When non-labelled drug is now added in concentrations in excess of the receptor concentration, the radiolabelled drug is specifically and competitively removed from the receptor sites. Thus, on recounting the sample, the remaining radioactivity must be due to the non-specific binding. From the difference of total minus non-specific, the specific β-adrenoreceptor binding activity can be determined. Using the Scatchard plot method of analysis, varying concentrations of added non-labelled drug can be plotted against the bound drug, and hence the receptor site, activity. From the plot [LR]/[L] against [LR], the intercept will give the number of binding sites RT. This method has also been used by Hedberg[28] to categorise the β receptors and their $\beta 1$ and $\beta 2$ subtypes in the cat and guinea pig left ventricle and right atrium. The non-linearity of both the Scatchard and Hill plots in this study confirmed the presence of the two different populations of binding sites.

Receptor binding assays may be adapted to study the interaction of both endogenous and other compounds within the central nervous system. Receptors have been demonstrated for diazepam[48], and for both morphine and endogenous opioids[31, 57, 66].

PURIFICATION PRIOR TO QUANTITATION

An organic extraction of plasma, urine or tissue of interest, largely removes a hydrophobic compound from protein. Sequential washing of the organic extract with acid and alkali provides a means of fractioning the extract into basic, acidic and neutral fractions. Differential solvent extraction systems[43] can also be employed to give a considerable degree of separation of different compounds (see Table 3.1). Simple chemical procedures can also be used, such as the precipitation of 3 β-hydroxysteroids by the formation of the digitonide, which does not occur with the 3α-hydroxysteroids. Compounds which are not extracted by organic solvents may be absorbed onto solid phases such as ion-exchange resins, silica, alumina or Sep-pak cartridges.

Table 3.1 Differential solvent extraction systems for steroids from plasma (adapted from ref. 43).

Solvent	Steroid extracted in organic phase (%)			
	Cortisol	*Corticosterone*	*Progesterone*	*17 hydroxy-progesterone*
Carbon tetrachloride	12	90	—	—
Hexane	1	1	85	7
	Aetiocholanolone		*11β-OH Aetiocholanolone*	
Isopentane	96		2.5	
	Oestradiol	*Oestrone*	*Oestriol*	
Benzene/L.P. (1:1)	96	97	4	

A wide variety of chromatographic techniques may be used to purify the sample further. These include thin layer chromatography (TLC), column and paper-chromatography, and perhaps electrophoresis, if the compounds of interest can be separated by virtue of their differential migration in an electric field. Although classical electrophoretic separations were carried out in solution, use of solid or semi-solid supporting media for the solution will reduce the separation of molecules by heat convection currents. The supporting phase may also obstruct the free migration of ions.

Electrophoresis may be coupled with immunological methods of protein identification, such as occurs in the immunoelectrophoretic detection of the complement proteins.

COMBINED SEPARATION AND QUANTITATION OF CHEMICALS AND DRUGS

The techniques of high performance (or high pressure) liquid chromatography (HPLC) and gas–liquid (GLC) or gas–solid (GSC) chromatography provide methods of separation, and, when coupled to suitable detectors, simultaneous quantitative measurement.

High pressure liquid chromatography (HPLC)

HPLC developed from an application of the principles of liquid chromatography and an attempt to maximise the separation achieved during conventional gravity-fed column chromatography. The conventional irregular-shaped celite or silica support materials were carefully graded into regular and very small sizes (5–10 μm) and indeed in some applications replaced by synthetic spherical support materials. Smaller regular-shaped particles allow greater distribution of the solute between the mobile and aqueous phases, but because they are packed tightly, the resistance to solvent flow is greatly increased. In order to achieve realistic flow rates, it becomes necessary to use pumps to produce the higher solvent pressures which have to be used to overcome the resistance of regular and tightly packed support materials. Support materials fall into two classes—straight phase and reverse phase.

1   *Straight phase* systems are usually based on silica, alumina or some synthetic material (Spherisorb). The polarity of these columns can be increased by bonding components to the silica packing (e.g. cyano-NO_2 or NH_2). Straight-phase columns are eluted with a variety of non-polar organic solvents.

2   *Reverse-phase columns* are produced by bonding octadecasilane (ODS) or similar organic, hydrophobic substance to the silica. Solutes can be eluted with more polar solvents such as water: methanol and methyl cyanide. These straight and reverse phase columns are usually of high efficiency.

The efficiency is dependent upon maximising the number of theoretical plates—which are considered to be those small and theoretical areas of the column where the solute is in equilibrium with the mobile and stationary phases—such that partition occurs. In the case of columns used for HPLC, the number of theoretical plates maybe as high as 10 000–25 000 per metre of column length.

Ion exchange HPLC systems can also be used, as can gel filtration (sometimes called exclusion chromatography), but they are not as efficient as the absorption (straight-phase) and reverse-phase columns. Ion-exchange columns usually give around 10 000 theoretical plates per metre.

Fig. 3.4 shows an example of the sort of separation which can be achieved for some closely related antidepressant and antiarrhythmic drugs using a reverse-phase system. This figure also shows the variation in the sensitivity of the procedures since Fig. 3.4a is detecting 50 ng and Fig. 3.4b is detecting 1.1 μg.

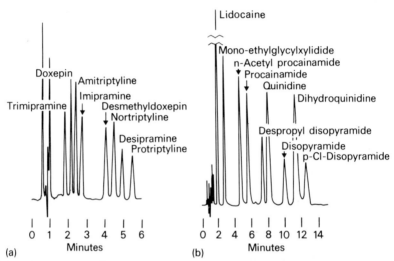

Fig. 3.4 High pressure liquid chromatography of some drugs. Figure 3.4a shows the separation of some of the tricyclic antidepressant drugs, and Fig. 3.4b separation of the antiarrhythmic agents. Reproduced by permission of Dr. W. Supina, Supelco Corporation, Bellefonte, Ca. USA.

HPLC has also found use in the estimation of vitamin D and its metabolites both directly and as a purification stage prior to RIA[7, 70].

One considerable advantage of HPLC is that it does not use high temperature, which destroys thermolabile compounds. Thus volatile derivatives do not always have to be made. Detection systems are attached to the end of the HPLC column and a variety of systems are available. UV detectors are normally employed, although fluorometric, refractive index and electrochemical detectors have been used. Electrochemical detection has been applied to the measurement of plasma and urinary catecholamines after HPLC[49]. Many systems for the separation of catecholamines have been used but reverse-phase ion pair systems have given the best results. At the carbon electrode of the detector a potential of around 0.6 V is applied and an oxidoreduction occurs (Fig. 3.5) giving a change in current which is then amplified and recorded. This principle is similar to the polarograph used for measuring partial pressures of oxygen. Any similar molecule which can be induced to undergo oxido-reduction can be detected in a similar fashion. The electrochemical detector can be extremely sensitive and 50 pg of catecholamine standards have been detected after HPLC (Fig. 3.6). Unfortunately, this

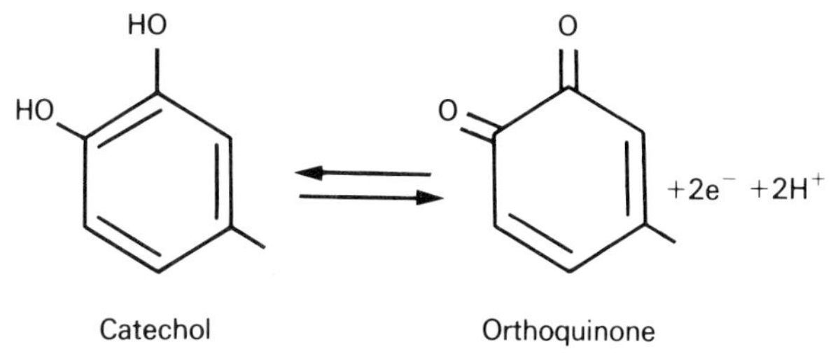

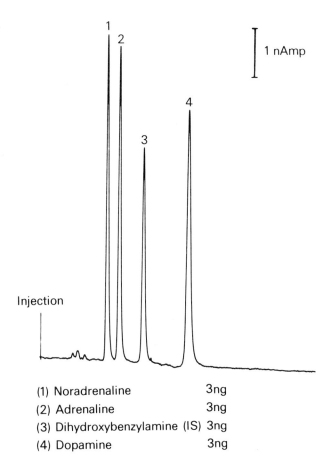

Fig. 3.5 Oxido-reduction of catechols.

Catechol

Orthoquinone

$+2e^- +2H^+$

1 nAmp

1

2

4

3

Injection

(1) Noradrenaline   3ng
(2) Adrenaline   3ng
(3) Dihydroxybenzylamine (IS) 3ng
(4) Dopamine   3ng

Fig. 3.6 High pressure liquid chromatogram (electrochemical detector) of a mixture of catecholamines. Reproduced by permission of Dr John Low.

detector can only be used with aqueous solvents and is thus not applicable to the analysis of lipophilic substances not soluble in aqueous media.

Many compounds which can be separated by HPLC do not absorb in the UV or are not susceptible to electrochemical detection. It is sometimes possible in these cases to form derivatives which may fluoresce or absorb UV. Bile acids, for example, have been analysed by HPLC by forming the p-bromophenacyl esters which absorb in the UV at 250 nm[47].

Gas chromatography

Gas chromatography depends upon the solute being in the vapour phase and thus being able to partition between the gaseous mobile phase and the solid (gas–solid chromatography, GSC) or liquid (gas–liquid chromatography, GLC) stationary phase. For molecules of molecular weight greater than around 200–300 daltons, this requires that the separation must be carried out at elevated temperatures. In general, therefore, substances for analysis by GLC require to be volatile and resistant to thermal changes during the chromatography. Substances of molecular weight in excess of around 700 daltons are not generally suitable for analysis by GC. Compounds with polar groups are very susceptible to absorption and loss during chromatography, and it is advisable to minimise this loss by forming derivatives before GLC. A common derivative for hydroxyl groups is the trimethylsilyl ether formed by a variety of reagents but trimethylsilylimidazole has, in our hands, given the best results with both sterically and non-sterically-hindered groups. Oxo groups can be reacted with methoxyamine hydrochloride forming o-methyloximes[60]. Many other derivatives, such as per-fluoroacyl esters, which have good electron capturing properties, have also been used.

Gas–solid chromatography uses molecular sieves or absorbants such as charcoal and silica gel, but, in general, the use of GSC has had very limited application apart from the analysis of some gases using thermal conductivity detectors. Anaesthetic gases have also been analysed by using GLC, and an example of the sort of separation which can be achieved is shown in Fig. 3.7 (see also references [20, 42, 68, 77]).

Gas–liquid chromatography is more versatile than GSC and has found more application in the analysis of many of the common drugs found in plasma and urine, and in human tissues. Two types of GLC are in common use, using conventional packed columns and capillary columns. Conventional columns are coiled glass or metal columns of internal diameter 0.2–0.4 cm, around 1.5–2.5 m long, packed with an inert support which is coated with the stationary phase. Capillary columns on the other hand are very long (around 50–100 metres) with internal diameter 0.2–0.4 mm. The stationary phase is coated onto the walls of the glass, fused silica, or metal (wall-coated open tubular column, WCOT). Support-coated (SCOT) capillary columns, where the stationary phase is coated onto support material which itself adheres to the wall, have also been used. In both open tubular and support-coated capillary columns, there is unrestricted carrier gas flow through the middle of the column. Capillary columns have much greater resolving power than the conventional packed columns and usually give around 3000 theoretical plates per metre. Capillary columns have, however, limited capacity and the amount of sample which can be applied is restricted. This may require special injection techniques to be used. A common stationary phase widely used for

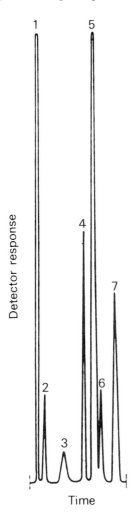

Fig. 3.7 Gas-liquid chromatographic separation of some of the anaesthetic gases. 1. oxygen, nitrous oxide, carbon dioxide, cyclopropane unresolved; 2. ether; 3. fluothane; 4. oxygen; 5. carbon dioxide; 6. cyclopropane. This is a composite trace of the same sample injected into two GLC columns connected in parallel. Peaks 1–3 are separated on a dinonyl phalate column, and peaks 4–6 are separated on a dimethyl sulfoxide column. Both stationary phases were coated onto suitable support media at around 15–20% (from Adlard E. R. and Hill. D. W. (1960) *Nature* **186**, 1045). Reproduced by permission of the authors and the publisher.

GLC analysis is SE30, or the more thermostable OV1, both of which are simple methylsiloxane polymers of different size. These stationary phases are described as being non-selective in that they separate mainly according to molecular size and shape. By substituting other chemical groups on to the methylsiloxane group, a variety of stationary phases with differing properties can be produced. QF1 (FS1265—a trifluoropropyl–methylsiloxane polymer) is a more polar (or selective) phase, showing increased retention of hydroxylated compounds, and behaving in a similar fashion to the more stable OV17 (phenylmethylsiloxane). Cyanomethylsiloxane phases (XE60) are also used. Highly polar stationary phases are available which can be mixed substituted polymers (e.g. OV225 which is a 50% substituted methylsiloxane: 25% phenylmethyl and 25% cyanopropylmethyl). Different stationary phases can be mixed together and coated onto the column support material, giving rise to differing retention characteristics derived from both components of the mixture.

Polyester stationary phases (DEGS: diethyleneglycol succinate; PEGA: polyethleneglycol adipate; neopentyl-glycerol succinate, etc.) are available and are used for the separation of compounds containing one or more polar functional groups.

Support phases are usually graded Celite (80–100 or 100–120 mesh) which has been treated in various ways (acid and alkali washed, silanised by treatment with dimethyldichlorosilane or hexamethyldisilazane) to render it inert. The proper treatment of these support materials is essential for good chromatography using conventional packed columns, otherwise the 'inert' support will absorb material, making quantification difficult, particularly at very low concentrations.

GLC detection

Various detection systems have been described for the quantification of peaks as they emerge from the GLC. In the drug analysis field, apart from the use of the mass spectrometer, which will be discussed separately, there are three main systems which have been used.

1 *The flame ionisation detector (FID)* which is sensitive down to levels around 0.1 µg of most compounds.

2 *The electron capture detector (ECD)* which normally requires the use of derivatives containing halogen atoms to enhance the electron-capturing ability of the compound of interest, although some compounds may be detectable without derivatisation. The ECD can detect pure standards at levels as low as 5 pg but is very susceptible to interference if reagents are not absolutely pure. The detection system can easily be poisoned, necessitating removal and cleaning.

3 *The alkali flame ionisation (AFI) detector* which gives a selective response to compounds containing nitrogen or phosphorus at levels around 1–5 ng. It thus falls into the range between the FID and the ECD.

For all these detection systems, the linear response range for the compound in question must be established before use. Plasma alphaxalone[60] has been measured by GLC using conventional packed columns with OV17 stationary phase and running O-methyloxime acetate derivatives using AFI detection, although GLC-FID systems have also been described[19, 61]. Similarly, fentanyl, and its analogues sufentanil and alfentanil, and some of their metabolites in plasma have been analysed by GLC using 3% OV17 coated onto an inert support in conventional packed columns[23, 72] using a selective nitrogen/phosphorous detection system.

Capillary column chromatography

This has been widely used for the development of 'profiling' (or separation of numbers of closely allied compounds all of which are present in a biological fluid), such as steroid metabolites in urine, bile acids, amino acids, organic acids in urine, sugars, etc. Good separation of enantiomers of some sympathomimetic drugs and free underivatised acids and bases (e.g. diazepam and nitrazepam) has been described[62].

Mass spectrometry

Another detection system which can be attached to the end of a gas chromatograph is the mass spectrometer (MS). This has similar sensitivity to the EC detector, but has increased specificity with none of the difficulties found when using the EC detector. Gas chromatography–mass spectrometry (GC–MS) provides a means of separating (GC) and quantifying (MS), by focussing onto specific ion fragments produced in the MS and monitoring simultaneously by rapidly focussing onto each fragment sequentially (multiple ion detection MID). Alternatively, a single ion can be monitored (single ion monitoring: SIM). The MS can also be used for the identification of peaks emerging from the GC, monitored by measuring the total ion current (TIC), and by scanning peaks to obtain a mass spectrum. The MS can, of course, be used independently of the GC and unknown compounds can be introduced directly into the ion source and mass spectra produced. Attempts have been made, without much success, to link the MS to the effluent from an HPLC, giving rise to HPLC–MS.

Conventional GCs are usually joined to the MS by some sort of molecular separator which disposes of the light carrier gas and allows the higher molecular weight compounds to pass through to the ion source. Capillary columns, because of their significantly lower carrier gas flow (1–2 ml min^{-1}), can be connected directly to the ion source; or connected by a molecular separator after adding extra carrier gas to bring the total flow to the optimum for the separator (around 20–30 ml min^{-1}).

Several types of mass spectrometer can be used in this context but all are based on the same basic principle: molecules entering the ion source of the MS are ionised, the ions are then removed and separated, giving a spectrum which indicates the intensity of each ion against its mass/charge ratio. There are a number of different methods of achieving the initial ionisation, but only two are so far widely used; chemical ionisation (CI) and ionisation by electron impact (EI). Electron impact ionisation, as its name implies, produces positively-charged ions by bombarding molecules with relatively high energy electrons (around 70 eV). The degree and type of fragment produced depends upon the structure of the molecule, which may sometimes be completely fragmented, giving rise to undetectable levels of the molecular ion (M^+). With chemical ionisation, the ionisation of the compound of interest occurs by interaction with ions of a reagent gas which have been produced by high energy electron (500 eV) bombardment. CI produces ions which are more stable than those produced during EI. In particular, protonated molecular ions (MH$^+$) are produced and these are of particular value since they indicate the molecular weight. The reagent gas used during CI has a considerable effect on the type of ions produced, and this introduces an extra degree of flexibility.

The ions produced from the compound of interest must be separated and, although quadrapole instruments which rely on a combination of radiofrequency and DC have been used, most research instruments use either a single magnet separation (low resolution) or a magnetic system in series with electrostatic separation (high resolution). The ions produced from the compound of interest in the ion source are accelerated into the separating system and finally focussed onto an electron multiplier, which gives a measure of the intensity of the ion. Focussing in a magnetic sector, MS can be effected by altering either the accelerating voltage or by changing the magnetic field. Because of the hysteresis effect, changes in the magnetic field are primarily used for producing a mass spectrum by scanning from low to high mass. Rapid back and forth changes during multiple ion detection can only be made by changing the accelerating voltage, thus allowing different ions to be sequentially focussed for a fraction of a second (60 msec) onto the electron multiplier.

Mass spectrometers can be controlled by computers and as an alternative to focussing on different ion fragments and continuously monitoring their ion intensity (mass fragmentography), the GC effluent can be constantly scanned at short time intervals (say 5–10 sec), storing the mass spectra obtained in the data store of the computer. At the end of the chromatographic separation, a record of the intensity of any given ion with time can be recalled from the computer and displayed. This process is called mass chromatography. Depending upon the ion chosen, it should be possible to detect a peak of 50 pg.

The interpretation of mass spectra is not difficult provided that the fragmentation of chemical analogues is known. Like all quantitative procedures, an internal standard is required to correct for losses which occur during the pre-purification. For most quantification methods, a radioactive internal standard or a chemical analogue of the compound of interest are used. The MS, because it can distinguish between compounds of different mass, allows the use of standards labelled with stable isotopes (^{13}C, ^{15}N, ^{2}H), which can be added at the beginning of the procedure and only separated during the final quantification in the MS. An example of the use of GC–MS for both quantification and for identification is given in the paper of Holly *et al.*[30] where metabolites of Althesin were quantitated and identified. Fig. 3.8 shows a mass fragmentogram obtained from a pooled plasma extract from patients who had been infused with Althesin. Although the peak identified as alphadolone has the same retention time as 11,20-direduced alphaxalone, the mass spectrum of this peak clearly indicates that it is in fact alphadolone. Pregnenolone was used as an internal standard and the amount of each metabolite was quantitated by comparison with a standard

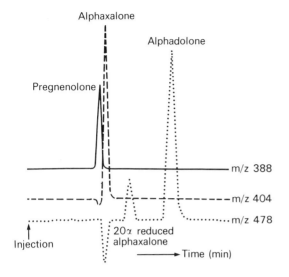

Fig. 3.8 Mass fragmentogram obtained after the extraction of pooled plasma from patients receiving Althesin by infusion. Trimethylsilyl ethers were prepared and run on OV1 at 250° (from Holly J. M. P., Trafford D. J. H., Sear, J. W. and Makin H. L. J. (1981) *J. Pharm. Pharmacol.* **33**, 427). Reproduced by permission of the authors and the publishers.

curve. This paper also describes the use of ΔRm analysis for the identification of unknown peaks during gas chromatography[21]. This kind of analysis can be used for any kind of chromatography and was originally described for paper chromatography[3]. Other examples of anaesthetic drugs that have been measured by gas chromatography–mass spectrometry include etomidate[71] and ketamine[18].

Other methods of quantification of drug or chemical compound

Isotope derivative assays

A group of assays which were popular some years ago in the steroid field, but have now largely been superseded by radioimmunoassay, were the isotope derivative assays. These assays used ^{14}C-labelled steroid as the internal standard, added at the start of the assay, and reacted an extract with ^{3}H- or ^{35}S-labelled reagent to produce a labelled product. Typical reagents used were tritiated acetic anhydride or ^{35}S-labelled thiosemicarbazide. The products were then submitted to extensive purification until the ^{14}C:^{3}H ration remained constant—an indication of purity. The number of ^{14}C and ^{3}H (or ^{35}S) counts were then measured separately. The ^{14}C counts were used to correct for losses during purification and the ^{3}H or ^{35}S counts enabled a calculation to be made of the amount of steroid in the original sample which had reacted with the labelled reagent. These procedures were cumbersome and time-consuming but gave values for many steroids in plasma which were later confirmed by more modern procedures. These procedures have been adapted to use enzymes instead of the relatively non-specific reagents, thus giving a higher degree of specificity and requiring less purification after reaction. These radioenzymatic assays are, for example, used for the measurement of catecholamines in human plasma using ^{3}H- adenosylmethionine as a methyl donor in the reactions catalysed by the enzymes phenylethanolamine-N-methyl transferase (PNMT), which uses adrenaline as a substrate, or catechol-o-methyl transferase (COMT) which uses adrenaline, noradrenaline and dopamine as substrates[34]. There are many other examples of the use of this type of assay.

Determination of drug kinetics and metabolism using isotopically labelled compounds

The absence of a suitable assay for a drug may necessitate early kinetic studies being carried out using radiolabelled drug. Examples in the literature include those of Welles *et al.*[75] studying the metabolism and excretion of methohexitone in the rat and the dog; Child *et al.*[15], and Strunin *et al.*[65] for the kinetics of Althesin (as $^{14}C_{21}$ labelled alphaxalone) in the rat and in man; and those of Hess *et al.*[29] and McClain and Hug[40] for fentanyl. Labelled compounds also allow whole body studies to be undertaken in animals to define the distribution of the drugs[12, 59]. The advantage of these methods are the lack of extensive sample preparation before analysis, and the rapidity of obtaining results. However, there are significant disadvantages including the administration of radiolabelled drug to volunteers or patients; a need for high radiochemical purity ($> 98 \%$), otherwise spurious results may occur possibly through counting of activity due to impurities; and a lack of absolute specificity about the results obtained. Total activity counting may include both parent drug and inactive metabolites such that further separatory techniques are needed[51].

Use of isotopic labelling in structural groups outside the main nucleus of a molecule (such as the $^{14}C_{21}$ labelling of alphaxalone) allows the possibility of radiolysis of the molecule, with release of the label as a small fragment. This may be one explanation for the apparent difference in the disposition of alphaxalone in man, as studied by Strunin *et al.* and Holly *et al.*[65, 30].

Another use of isotopically-labelled compounds is in the study of the organ extraction of an anaesthetic agent. Nicholas and his colleagues investigated the clearance and metabolism of ^{14}C alphaxalone by the isolated perfused rat lung. Identification of metabolites was carried out by a combination of thin layer chromatography, localisation of radioactivity by scanning the plate, and then scraping off these areas into vials for counting. Absolute characterisation of the metabolites was achieved by gas chromatography–mass spectrometry, using ether extracts of the areas of the thin layer chromatography plates[52]. In other experiments, the authors found a marked delay between infusing alphaxalone and its subsequent appearance in the venous effluent. By comparing the efflux of ^{14}C- alphaxalone with ^{3}H-dextran (which cannot leave the pulmonary circulation), the results suggest clearance occurs by a stochastic model of a physical process resembling the sequence of events that occur in a chromatography column. Thus, within the lung tissue, the alphaxalone concentration is not assumed to be spatially uniform[36].

Until now, it has always been assumed that drugs given intravenously together (such as atropine and neostigmine, fentanyl and droperidol, thiopentone and relaxant) will reach the systemic arterial circulation together. The experiments of Nicholas have shown that after passage through the lungs, this may not be true.

Determination of total drug concentration and free or unbound concentration in plasma

Knowledge of the extent of plasma protein binding of drugs is of importance in the interpretation of drug responses and drug kinetics. Most methods for the determination of plasma drug concentrations measure total drug (that is, free and bound). From a pharmacological point of view, only free drug has any pharmacodynamic effect. However, *in vitro* methods must be used if determination of free drug activity is required. Two main techniques of separation of free and bound drug have been employed:

1 Centrifugal ultrafiltration.
2 Equilibrium dialysis.

The two techniques have been compared for the binding of thiopentone to plasma proteins[4]. For added drug concentrations over the range 1–80 μg/ml, similar results were obtained (free drug concentration 18.3–21.2%). However, the technique of equilibrium dialysis against Sorensen's phosphate buffer is considerably more time-consuming compared to ultrafiltration through Amicon PM 50 cones (Amicon Corporation, Lexington, Mass 02173). More recently, both Hargrave[26] and Bower[8] have studied using equilibrium dialysis, the effects of pH, temperature, and competition by other drugs or endogenous ligands on the plasma protein binding of fentanyl. For this highly lipophilic weak base, they have found increased binding with increases in pH and increases in temperature. A significant decrease in plasma protein binding of fentanyl was found in the presence of four drugs, namely aspirin, sodium salicylate, phenylbutazone and quinidine. This competition for binding sites resulted in decreased binding to albumin in the case of the first three drugs, and to three lipoprotein fractions (very light density, light density, high density) in the case of quinidine.

REFERENCES

1. ADAM H. K., GLEN J. B. & HOYLE P. A. (1980) Pharmacokinetics in laboratory animals of ICI 35868; a new I. V. anaesthetic agent. *Br. J. Anaesth.* **52**, 743.
2. BARTLETT A. J., LLOYD-JONES J. G.,

RANCE M. J., FLOCKHART I. R., DOCKRAY G., BENNETT M. R. D. & MOORE R. A. (1980) The radioimmunoassay of buprenorphine. *Europ. J. Clin. Pharmacol.* **18**, 339.

3. BATE-SMITH E. C. & WESTALL R. G. (1950) Chromatographic behaviour and chemical structure. Some naturally occurring phenolic substances. *Biochem. Biophys. Acta* **4**, 427.

4. BECKER K. E. (1976) Gas chromatographic assay for free and total plasma levels of thiopental. *Anesthesiology* **45**, 656.

5. BERKOWITZ B. A., NGAI S. H., YANG J. C., HEMPSTEAD J. & SPECTOR S. (1975) The disposition of morphine in surgical patients. *Clin. Pharmacol. Ther.* **17**, 629.

6. BINOUX M. A. & ODELL W. D. (1974) Use of dextran coated charcoal to separate antibody bound from free hormone: A critique. *J. Clin. Endocr. Metab.* **36**, 303.

7. BOUILLON R., DEMOOR P., BAGGIOLINI E. G. & USKOKOVIC M. R. (1980) A radioimmunoassay for 1,25-dihydroxyl-cholecalciferol. *Clin. Chem.* **26**, 562.

8. BOWER S. (1981) Plasma protein binding of fentanyl. *J. Pharm. Pharmacol.* **33**, 507.

9. BOWER S. & HULL C. J. (1982) Comparative pharmacokinetics of fentanyl and alfentanil. *Br. J. Anaesth.* **54**, 871.

10. BRAND L., MARK L. C., SNELL M. M., VRINDTEN P. & DAYTON P. G. (1963) Physiologic disposition of methohexital in man. *Anaesthesiology* **24**, 331.

11. BRODIE B. B., MARK L. C., PAPPER E. M., LIEF P. A., BERNSTEIN E. & ROVENSTINE E. A. (1950) The fate of thiopental in man; and a method for its estimation in biological material. *J. Pharmacol. Exp. Ther.* **98**, 85.

12. CARD B., MCCULLOCH R. J. & PRATT D. A. H. (1972) Tissue distribution of CT1341 in the rat: an autoradiographic study. *Postgrad. Med. J.* **48** (suppl. 2), 34.

13. CATLIN D. H. (1977) Pharmacokinetics of morphine by radio-immunoassay: the influence of immunochemical factors. *J. Pharmacol. Exp. Ther.* **200**, 224.

14. CHARD T., MARTIN M. & LANDON J. (1971) In Kirkham K. E. & Hunter W. M. (eds.), *Radioimmunoassay Methods*, pp. 257–66. Churchill Livingstone, Edinburgh.

15. CHILD K. J., GIBSON W., HARNBY G. & HART J. W. (1972) Metabolism and excretion of Althesin (CT 1341) in the rat. *Postgrad. Med. J.* **48** (suppl. 2), 37.

16. COHEN E. N. (1963) Fluorescent analysis of d-tubocurarine hydrochloride. *J. Lab. Clin. Med.* **61**, 338.

17. DAVIES B. M. A. (1964) Blood corticotrophin in normal adults and patients with Cushing's syndrome. *Acta. Endocr.* **45**, 55.

18. DOMINO E. F., ZSIGMOND E. K., DOMINO L. E., DOMINO K. E., KOTHARY S. P. & DOMINO S. E. (1982). Plasma levels of ketamine and two of its metabolites in surgical patients using a gas chromatographic-mass fragmentographic assay. *Anesth. Analg.* **61**, 87.

19. DUBOIS M., ALLISON J. & GEDDES I. (1975) The determination of alphaxalone in human blood by gas-liquid chromatography. *Br. J. Anaesth.* **47**, 902.

20. DUECK R., RATHBUN M. & WAGNER P. D. (1978) Chromatographic analysis of multiple tracer gases in the presence of anaesthetic gas. *Anesthesiology* **49**, 31.

21. EDWARDS R. W. H. (1969) R_m and ΔR_m: making full use of R_m values. In Smith I. (ed.), *Chromatographic and Electrophoretic Techniques*, 3rd Edition, Vol. 1, p. 621.

22. ENGEL L. L. (ed.) (1963) *Physical Properties of the Steroid Hormones.* MacMillan, New York.

23. GILLESPIE T. J., GANDOLFI A. J., MAIORINO R. M. & VAUGHAN R. W. (1981) Gas chromatographic determination of fentanyl and its analogues in human plasma. *J. Anal. Toxicol.* **5**, 133.

24. GRAY C. H., BARON D. N., BROOKS R. V. & JAMES V. H. T. (1969) A critical appraisal of a method of estimating urinary 17-oxosteroids and total 17-oxogenic steroids. *Lancet i*, 124.

25. HALES C. N. & RANDLE P. J. (1963) Immunoassay of insulin with insulin-antibody precipitate. *Biochem. J.* **88**, 137.

26. HARGRAVE S. A. (1979) Estimation of binding of ³H-fentanyl to plasma proteins. *Br. J. Anaesth.* **51**, 569P.

27. HARKONEN M., ADLERCREUTZ H., DABEK J. T. & O'RIORDAN J. L. H. (1979) *In vitro* oxidation of vitamin D metabolites by steroid dehydrogenases. *J. Steroid Biochem.* **11**, 1205.

28. HEDBERG A., MINNEMAN K. P. & MOLINOFF P. B. (1980) Differential distribution of beta and beta$_2$-adrenoreceptors in cat and guinea pig heart. *J. Pharmacol. Exp. Ther.* **212**, 503.

29. HESS R., STIEBLER G. & HERTZ A. (1972). Pharmacokinetics of fentanyl in man and the rabbit. *Europ. J. Clin. Pharmacol.* **4**, 137.

30. HOLLY J. M. P., TRAFFORD D. J. H., SEAR J. M. & MAKIN H. L. J. (1981) The *in vivo* metabolism of Althesin (alphaxalone and alphadolone acetate) in man. *J. Pharm. Pharmacol.* **33**, 427.

31. HUGHES J., SMITH T. W., KOSTERLITZ H. W., FOTHERGILL L. A., MORGAN B. A. & MORRIS H. R. (1975) Identification of two related pentapeptides from the brain with potent opiate agonist activity. *Nature (Lond.)* **258**, 577.

32. HULL C. J. (1979) Pharmacokinetics and pharmacodynamics. *Br. J. Anaesth.* **51**, 579.

33. JAFFE B. M. & BEHMAN H. R. (eds.) (1979) *Methods of Hormone Immunoassay*, 2nd Edition. Academic Press, New York.

34. JOHNSON G. A., KUPIECKI R. M. & BAKER C. A. (1980) Single isotope derivative (radioenzymatic) methods in the measurement of catecholamines. *Metabolism* **29** (suppl. 1), 1106.

35. JONES J. C., CARTER G. D. & MACGREGOR G. A. (1981) Interference by polar metabolites in a direct radio-

immunoassay for plasma aldosterone. *Ann. Clin. Biochem.* **18**, 54.

36. JONES M. E. & NICHOLAS T. E. (1981) The pharmacokinetics of the intravenous steroid anaesthetic alphaxalone in the isolated perfused rat lung. *J. Pharmacokin. Biopharm.* **9**, 343.

37. KERSTEN U. K., MEIJER D. K. F. & AGOSTON S. (1973) Fluorimetric and chromatographic determination of pancuronium bromide and its metabolites in biological materials. *Clin. Chem. Acta* **44**, 59.

38. LEVITZKI A. (1978) Catecholamine receptors. *Rev. Physiol. Biochem. Pharmacol.* **82**, 1.

39. LEUTE R., ULLMAN E. F. & GOLDSTEIN A. (1972) Spin immunoassay of opiates and narcotics in urine and saliva. *J. Am. Med. Assoc.* **221**, 1231.

40. McCLAIN D. A. & HUG C. C. (1980) Intravenous fentanyl kinetics. *Clin. Pharmacol. Ther.* **28**, 106.

41. MAGUIRE M. E., ROSS E. M. & GILMAN A. G. (1977). Beta-adrenergic receptor: Ligand binding properties and the interaction with adenylate cyclase. *Adv. Cyclic Nucleotide. Res.* **8**, 1.

42. MAIORINO R. M., SIPES I. G., GANDOLFI A. J. & BROWN B. R. (1979) Quantitative analysis of volatile halothane metabolites in biological tissues by gas chromatography. *J. Chromatogr. (Biomed. Applications)* **164**, 63.

43. MAKIN H. L. J. (1975) Methods of steroid analysis I. Group estimations and separation techniques. In Makin H. L. J. (ed.), *Biochemistry of Steroid Hormones*. Blackwell Scientific Publications, Oxford.

44. MATTINGLY D. (1962) A simple fluorimetric method for the estimation of free 11-hydroxycorticoids in human plasma. *J. Clin. Path.* **15**, 374.

45. MICHIELS M., HENDRIKS R. & HEYKANTS J. (1977) A sensitive radioimmunoassay for fentanyl. *Eur. J. Clin. Pharmacol.* **12**, 153.

46. MICHELS M., HENDRICKS R. & HEYKANTS J. (1983) Radioimmunoassay of the new opiate analgesics, alfentanil and sufentanil. Preliminary pharmaco-kinetic profile in man. *J. Pharm. Pharmacol.* **35**, 86.

47. MINGROVE G., GRECO A. V. & PASSI S. (1980) Reversed-phase high-performance liquid chromatographic separation and quantification of individual human bile acids. *J. Chromatogr.* **183**, 277.

48. MOHLER H. & OKADA R. (1977) Benzo-diazepine receptor: demonstration in the c.n.s. *Science* (Wash.) **198**, 849.

49. MOYER T. P., JIANG N. S., TYCE G. M. & SHEDS S. G. (1979) Analysis for urinary catecholamines by liquid chromato-graphy with amperometric detection: methodology and clinical interpretation of results. *Clin. Chem.* **25**, 256.

50. MURPHY B. E. P. (1967) Some studies of the protein-binding of steroids and their application to the routine micro and ultramicro measurement of various steroids in body fluids by competitive protein-binding radioassay. *J. Clin. Endocr. Metab.* **27**, 973.

51. MURPHY M. R., OLSON W. A. & HUG C. C. (1979) Pharmacokinetics of ^{3}H-fentanyl in the dog anesthetised with enflurane. *Anesthesiology* **50**, 13.

52. NICHOLAS T. E., JONES M. E., JOHNSON D. W. & PHILLIPOU G. (1981) Metab-olism of the steroid anaesthetic alpha-xalone by the isolated perfused rat lung. *J. Steroid Biochem.* **14**, 45.

53. ORTH D. N. (1979) Adrenocorticotrophic hormone (ACTH). In Jaffe B. M. & Behrmann H. R. (eds.), *Methods of Hormone Radioimmunoassays*, 2nd edition, pp. 245–84. Academic Press, New York.

54. O'SULLIVAN M. J., BRIDGES J. W. & MARKS V. (1979) Enzyme immuno-assay: a review. *Am. Clin. Biochem.* **16**, 221.

55. PASTORINO A. M. (1978) Fluorimetric determination and pharmacokinetic studies of fazadinium bromide in dogs. *Arzneim Forsch.* **28**, 1728.

56. PAYNE D. W., SHIKITA M. & TALALAY P. (1982) Enzymatic estimation of steroids in subpicomole quantities by hydroxy-steroid dehydrogenases and nicotinamide nucleotide cycling. *J. Biol. Chem.* **257**, 633.

57. PERT C. B. & SYNDER S. H. (1973) Opiate receptor: demonstration in nervous tissue. *Science* (Wash.) **179**, 1011.

58. RATCLIFFE J. G. (1974) Separation tech-niques in immunoassay. *Br. Med. Bull.* **30**, 32.

59. RHODES C. & LONGSHAW S. (1977) Antoradiographic distribution study of a short acting anaesthetic, ICI 35868. *Acta Pharmacol. Toxicol.* **41**, 132.

60. SEAR J. W., HOLLY J. M. P., TRAFFORD D. J. H. & MAKIN H. L. J. (1980) Plasma concentrations of alphaxalone by gas chromatography: comparison with other gas chromatographic methods and gas chromatography-mass spectrometry. *J. Pharm. Pharmacol.* **32**, 349.

61. SEAR J. W. & PRYS-ROBERTS C. (1979) Plasma concentrations of alphaxalone during continuous infusion of Althesin. *Br. J. Anaesth.* **51**, 861.

62. SHACKLETON C. H. L. (1980) Chapter 16: Multicomponent analysis by capillary gas chromatography. In Lawson A. M., Lim C. K. & Richmond W. (eds.), *Current Developments in the Clinical Application of HPLC, GC and MS.* Academic Press, New York.

63. SMITH D. S., AL-HAKIEM M. H. H. & LANDON J. (1981) A review of fluo-roimmunoassay and immunofluori-metric assay. *Ann. Clin. Biochem.* **18**, 253.

64. SONKSEN P. H. (ed.) (1974) Radioim-munoassay and saturation analysis *Br. Med. Bull.* **30**, 30.

65. STRUNIN L., STRUNIN J. M., KNIGHTS K. M. & WARD M. E. (1977) Metabolism of 14C-labelled alphaxalone in man. *Br. J. Anaesth.* **49**, 609.

66. TERENIUS L. & WAHLSTROM A. (1975) Search for an endogenous ligand for the opiate receptor. *Acta Physiol. Scand.* **94**, 74.

67. TONER W., HOWARD P. J., DUNDEE J. W. & MCILROY P. D. A. (1979) Estimation of thiopentone. The use of high performance liquid chromatography and an ether extraction. *Anaesthesia* **34**, 657.

68. TONER W., HOWARD P. J., SCOTT M. G., BLACK G. W. & DUNDEE J. W. (1977). Estimation of blood enflurane concentrations by gas liquid chromatography. *Br. J. Anaesth.* **49**, 871.

69. TRAFFORD D. J. H. & MAKIN H. L. J. (1980) Use of hydroxyapatite in radioimmunoassay. *Methods Enzymol.* **70**, 291.

70. TURNBULL H., TRAFFORD D. J. H. & MAKIN H. L. J. (1982) A rapid and simple method for the measurement of plasma 25-hydroxyvitamin D_2 and 25-hydroxyvitamin D_3 using Sep-Pak C_{18} cartridges and a single high-performance liquid chromatographic step. *Clin. Chim. Acta* **120**, 65.

71. VAN HAMME M. H., AMBRE J. J. & GHONEIM M. M. (1977) Determination of etomidate plasma concentrations by mass-fragmentography. *J. Pharm. Sci.* **66**, 1344.

72. VAN ROOY H. H., VERMEULEN N. P. E. & BOVILL J. G. (1981) The assays of fentanyl and its metabolites in plasma of patients using gas chromatography with alkali flame ionisation detection and gas chromatography-mass spectrometry. *J. Chromatogr.* **223**, 85.

73. WATSON M. J. & MCLEOD K. (1977) A modified method for the fluorimetric determination of pancuronium bromide in plasma. *Clin. Chim. Acta* **79**, 511.

74. WEBER G. (1952) Polarization of the fluorescence of macromolecules 2: fluorescent conjugates of ovalbumin and bovine serum albumin. *Biochem. J.* **51**, 155.

75. WELLES J. S., MCMAHON R. E. & DORAN W. J. (1963) The metabolism and excretion of methohexital in the rat and dog. *J. Pharmacol. Exp. Ther.* **139**, 166.

76. WINGARD L. B., ABOULEISH E., WEST D. C. & GOEHL T. J. (1979) Modified fluorimetric quantitation of pancuronium bromide and metabolites in human maternal and umbilical serums. *J. Pharm. Sci.* **68**, 914.

77. YAMAMURA H., WAKASUGI B., SATO S. & TAKEBE Y. (1966) Gas Chromatographic analysis of inhalation anesthetics in whole blood by an equilibration method. *Anesthesiology* **27**, 311.

4 Effect of Renal and Hepatic Disease on Pharmacokinetics of Anaesthetic Agents

J. W. SEAR

MOLECULAR MECHANISMS OF DRUG METABOLISM

Drug and xenobiotic metabolism occurs primarily in the liver, and involves mainly oxidative reactions catalysed by the enzymes of the endoplasmic reticulum. In general, metabolism is aimed at inactivation of polar, lipophilic drugs by rendering the compound more hydrophilic, and thereby increasing urinary excretion. The general pathways of drug metabolism in the liver are shown in Table 4.1.

Most of these degradations may be considered as hydroxylation reactions. Brodie *et al.*[11] were the first researchers to suggest that reduced nicotinamide adenine dinucleotide phosphate (NADPH) and molecular oxygen were absolute requirements for metabolism to occur, as well as a microsomal hydroxylase, mono-oxygenase or mixed function oxidase enzyme. The oxygen combined with a specific microsomal component to form an 'active complex'. In turn, this complex hydroxylated drugs or other endogenous substrates. The involvement of cytochrome P450 as the terminal oxidase was based on the work of Klingenberg[47] and Garfinkel[30], while confirmation of the reduction of cytochrome P450 by NADPH was shown in experiments by Cooper and his colleagues[17]. These reductions were mediated by the enzyme

Table 4.1   General pathways of drug metabolism in the liver by non-specific enzymes.

Phase I reactions	Localisation of enzymes	Phase II reactions	Localisation of enzymes
Oxidations			
Hydroxylation	Microsomes	Glucuronidation	Microsomes
Dealkylation	Microsomes	Acylation	Mitochondria, soluble
Oxide formation	Microsomes	Methylation	Soluble
Desulphuration	Microsomes	Sulphate conjugation	Soluble
Dehalogenation	Microsomes	Mercapturic acid conjugation	Soluble
Alcohol oxidation	Soluble		
Aldehyde oxidation	Soluble		
Reductions			
Aldehyde reduction	Soluble		
Azoreduction	Microsomes		
Nitroreduction	Microsomes, soluble		
Hydrolyses			
De-esterification	Microsomes		
De-amidation	Microsomes		

NADPH–cytochrome c reductase. However, the relationship between cytochrome P450 and the reductase enzyme is not 1 : 1, but may be up to 2 : 1[27, 56].

The mixed function oxygenases may be divided into mono-oxygenases, which incorporate one atom of oxygen into the donor drug, and the di-oxygenases which incorporate both atoms of oxygen. The mixed functions oxidase enzymes are found in two main tissue areas of the body: the steroid synthesising tissue (ovary, testes and adrenal cortex), and the tissues involved in drug and xenobiotic metabolism (liver, and to a lesser extent, the kidneys, lungs, intestinal cells, skin, brain and placenta). In mammals, the enzymes are membrane-bound and therefore have proven difficult to characterise[17, 53, 62]. However, several separate components have been recognised.

Cytochrome P450

This is the terminal oxidase of the electron transport system, with a specific binding site for the substrate molecule. Numerous studies have shown there to be different forms of cytochrome P450 in liver microsomes. Changes in the catalytic activity towards various substrates, and in the spectral properties of cytochrome P450 after pretreatment with different inducing agents have been observed in microsomes isolated from hepatic tissue. Purified cytochromes P450 and P448 also show species differences with respect to their spectral properties, minimal molecular weights and substrate specificities in the presence of NADPH–cytochrome c reductase and phospholipid. Alterations in the proportions of these cytochromes within microsomal preparations may explain species, strain, age, tissue and sex differences seen in drug metabolism.

NADPH–cytochrome c reductase

This enzyme is a flavoprotein containing one molecule each of flavine adenine dinucleotide (FAD) and flavine mono nucleotide (FMN) per single polypeptide, and is responsible for the reduction by electron transfer of oxidised cytochrome P450. Like cytochrome P450, the enzyme is induced by agents such as phenobarbital.

Phosphatidyl choline

Although the membrane lipids are not necessary for the spectral properties of the cytochromes, phosphatidyl choline is essential for electron transfer from NADPH to cytochrome P450[85]. However it is clear that the lipid does not function as an electron carrier. Recent studies have suggested that the phospholipid enhances substrate binding[32].

Soluble factor, non-haem iron protein and selenium

Addition of a liver homogenate soluble fraction stimulates the metabolism of several substrates[52]. This is probably by a 'soluble factor', reversing the inhibitory effect of lipid peroxidation. The involvement of non-haem iron protein and selenium in cytochrome P450 mediated hydroxylations has also been proposed. However the adequate metabolism of a variety of substrates by purified reconstituted cytochrome systems has made the absolute need of these components seem unlikely.

Cytochrome b$_5$

This cytochrome also has a definite role in some, but not all of the NADPH-dependent reactions of drug metabolism. It is however, an essential component in reduced nicotinamide adenine dinucleotide-dependent hydroxylations, demethylations and hydroxylase reductions. Cytochrome b$_5$ has another function in the interaction between the NADPH-mediated electron transport pathways. The inter-relationship of these various co-factors and cytochromes as part of the microsomal drug metabolising enzyme is shown in Fig. 4.1. In general, the hydroxylation reactions in hepatic microsomes may be expressed in the following equation:

$$RH + O_2 + H^+ + NADPH \rightarrow ROH + H_2O + NADP$$

Accordingly, equivalent amounts of NADPH and oxygen should be utilised during the reaction. However, the reduction of cytochrome P450 receives only one electron

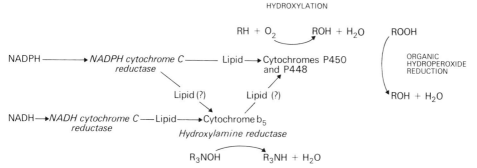

Fig. 4.1 Schematic arrangement of the liver microsomal electron transport systems[52].

from NADPH; so that the other electron must enter the electron transfer system at some point either during the reduction of the cytochrome P450 or during its reoxidation. Hildebrandt and Estabrook[33] have suggested that cytochrome b_5 may be involved as the mediator of the electron transfer after the formation of the cytochrome P450–substrate–oxygen complex. As indicated above, cytochrome b_5 may be reduced by either NADPH or NADH, with the necessary electron arising from either of these co-factors.

Effect of hepatic disease on microsomal mixed function oxidase activity

The literature contains many reports of the concentrations of the cytochromes in adult human liver microsomes. While Alvares *et al.*[2] and Darby *et al.*[19] have suggested that the concentration of cytochrome P450 was significantly lower in man than in the rat, more recent studies have failed to confirm this[1, 20, 64]. The results of Ahmed and Black[1] showed a human microsomal cytochrome P450 concentration of 0.6 ± 0.1 nmol mg^{-1} microsomal protein; which compares with their values for the laboratory rat of 0.75–0.9 nmol mg^{-1} protein. However, there was a wide variation in the results found in man. Similarly, the concentration of NADPH–cytochrome c reductase was slightly lower in man compared to the rat. The cytochrome b_5 concentration in man (0.49 ± 0.06 nmol mg^{-1} microsomal protein) is similar to that found in the rat. The differences in the concentrations of cytochromes and reductase between species may also be related to the marked variation in the drug metabolising capacity of the human liver[82, 93]. A synergistic effect of NADH with NADPH on the rate of morphine N-demethylation has provided evidence of the involvement of cytochrome b_5 in some of the cytochrome P450-mediated microsomal reactions in man[1]. Boobis *et al.*[9] have studied the microsomal mixed function oxidase activity of liver biopsy samples taken from patients with and without histological evidence of hepatic disease (e.g. fatty change, cirrhosis, hepatitis). There were no significant differences between the groups with respect to the protein yield or NADPH-cytochrome c reductase activity. However, there was a significant decrease of cytochrome P450 and aryl hydrocarbon hydroxylase activity in the liver disease group.

The effect of cholestasis on human liver drug metabolism has been studied by Ahmed and Black[1] who found no significant decreases of the concentrations of hepatic P450, b_5 and NADPH-cytochrome c reductase, nor of the rate of *in vitro* ethylmorphine-N-dimethylation. Thus, in contrast to earlier studies, it appears that prolonged cholestasis in man has little effect on either the cofactors of the microsomal mono-oxygenase system, or the associated *in vitro* rate of xenobiotic metabolism.

Studies by May *et al.*[57] and Schoene *et al.*[75] have failed to demonstrate any correlation between the cytochrome P450 content of human hepatic biopsy tissue, and the plasma half life of antipyrine. This would suggest that factors other than the concentrations of cytochrome P450 and NAPDH–cytochrome c reductase in the liver are the rate-limiting steps in hepatic drug metabolism in liver disease. Farrell, Cooksley and Powell[29] compared the hepatic microsomal cytochrome P450, aryl hydrocarbon hydroxylase and ethylmorphine N-demethylase activity in biopsy tissue with the *in vitro* half life of antipyrine. There was a good correlation (r = 0.79) between the cytochrome P450 content and the two enzyme activities *in vitro*. There was also a significant correlation between the antipyrine half life *in vitro* and hepatic drug metabolising activities *in vitro*. As in the studies of May and Schoene, there was a significant reduction in the microsomal cytochrome P450 content in patients with severe liver disease (chronic active hepatitis or active alcoholic cirrhosis). Many of these patients had jaundice and/or ascites. No reduction in the cytochrome content was found in patients with either inactive cirrhosis, or mild-to-moderate hepatocellular disease (less than 50% hepatocytes abnormal morphologically).

Influence of hepatic venous congestion on drug metabolism

Hepatic blood flow is influenced in experimental animals, and perhaps in man, by increases in the hepatic venous pressure. Under such conditions, the centrilobular hepatocytes are liable to pressure disruption. These are the liver cells with the highest cytochrome P450 concentration. However, experimental studies in the rat have shown no effect of venous congestion on cytochrome P450 content or NADPH-dependent cytochrome c reductase activity[51]. Increased hepatic venous pressure resulted in no effect on the *in vitro* hydroxylation of pentobarbital. However, there was a decrease in the rate of morphine glucuronidation and a reduction in the plasma protein binding of morphine from 12.0% to 7.9%, though no change in the elimination half life, volume of distribution, or clearance of morphine were found. As total hepatic blood flow decreased and there was no significant extra-hepatic metabolism, these results must indicate the ability for an increased hepatic extraction efficiency to compensate for the altered blood flow[51]. These findings of an unchanged rate of morphine glucuronidation, and hence no decrease in the clearance of morphine are in contrast to the clinical observations of Thomsen with respect to the clearance of lignocaine in patients with congestive cardiac failure[91].

Although these animal studies would suggest no effect of hepatic venous congestion on drug pharmacokinetics, Pessayre has shown that the clearance of propranolol in patients with cirrhosis was decreased to a greater extent than the decrease in the hepatic blood flow. This may be the result of a reduced ability of the liver to clear the drug from the blood[66]. In contrast, Patwardhan and his colleagues found no decrease in the clearance of morphine in patients with cirrhotic liver disease[63]. However, in viral hepatitis, there is a decreased clearance of high extraction ratio compounds (indo-cyanine green and lignocaine) in the presence of an unaltered hepatic blood flow[97]. Thus, factors other than changes in the blood flow to the liver, and the cytochrome P450 content, may significantly alter the clearance of drugs with a high extraction ratio in patients with liver disease.

Glucuronidation

Glucuronides are formed by the conjugation of glucuronic acid into several different functional groups, such as –OH, –COOH, –NH$_2$, and –SH. Of these, the ether type (–OH) and ester type (–COOH) are the most common. Before conjugation can be achieved in relatively non-polar compounds, groupings need to be introduced by the phase I reaction. Glucuronic acid is transferred to the drug from the donor, uridine diphosphoglucuronic acid. This reaction is catalysed by the microsomal enzyme, glucuronyl transferase. Glucuronidation normally leads to a reduction or absence of pharmacological activity as well as leading to strongly acidic compounds (pKa 3.5 to 4.0). These are fully ionised in the plasma and this aids their excretion in the urine. The glucuronides of some drugs are also excreted into the bile; the percentage depending on the chemical structure, molecular weight, the polarity of the glucuronide conjugate, and the species. Within the gastrointestinal tract, glucuronides may be broken down by microfloral β-glucuronidase. This allows the release and, therefore, reabsorption of the parent drug (enterohepatic recirculation). This enzymic hydrolysis can also be activated by lysosomal β-glucuronidase, which is present in most tissues of the body, including the kidney.

Examples of drugs that are excreted as glucuronides in the urine are chloram-phenicol, lorazepam and oxazepam, and propranolol. Of these, only oxazepam shows accumulation due to enterohepatic recirculation of parent compound that has been hydrolysed in the gut.

CLINICAL ASPECTS OF DRUG METABOLISM

The hepatic elimination of a drug usually proceeds via biotransformation into one or more metabolites; or in direct transport of the active compound into the bile without previous metabolism. Although hepatic metabolism may result in the conversion to a more active form of the drug (prednisone to prednisolone; azathioprine to 6-mercaptopurine), drugs are usually converted to less active, more polar (i.e. water soluble) products. Metabolism occurs in two phases. The initial phase (phase I reaction) consists of either oxidative, reductive, or hydrolytic alterations of the molecule. The second phase reaction involves the conjugation of the altered molecule to one or more organic acids (glucuronic acid, sulphonic acid). Other conjugates include acylation products and methyl compounds.

Effect of liver disease on drug disposition

The liver receives its blood supply from two sources—the hepatic artery (30%), and the hepatic portal vein (70%). Thus, drugs which are absorbed from the intestines following oral administration may be extensively metabolised before entering into the systemic circulation. This is termed hepatic first pass metabolism, and will alter the systemic bioavailability of the drug[8]. Altered patterns of drug availability can also occur through the enterohepatic recycling of drugs (e.g. diazepam, pethidine, fentanyl), where drugs that are eliminated in the bile without biotransformation may be reabsorbed further down the gastrointestinal tract. This may result in secondary peaks of plasma drug concentration during the elimination phase and possible pharmacodynamic effects. Despite many studies aimed at defining the effect of hepatic disease on drug pharmacokinetics and pharmacodynamics, it is often difficult to predict the exact response of a given individual with hepatic impairment; and whether there will be retardation, acceleration, or no change in the rate of drug elimination.

Effect of renal disease on drug disposition

Renal disease affects the rate of clearance of drugs mainly eliminated as unmetabolised, pharmacologically-active compounds[92]. In the absence of excretion, accumulation will occur with the resulting development of toxic effects. If biotransformation plays an important role in the elimination of the drug, the effect of renal disease on the disposition and metabolism of the compound is often unpredictable. The rate of hepatic metabolism of drug may be increased, decreased or unaltered in patients with renal failure[71]. In general, oxidations occur at the normal rate or slightly faster; reductive metabolism tends to be decreased; and hydrolytic reactions are also slowed from the normal rate. Conjugation with glucuronic acid or glycine is unaffected[92] while acetylation and sulphation are generally depressed. Other factors which may change drug disposition are alterations in tissue and plasma protein binding, with consequent changes of free drug concentration. Usually there is a reduction in plasma protein binding, with a resultant increase in the apparent volume of distribution and clearance rate of the drug. Thus either chronic administration of drugs, or administration by infusion can be associated with a lower total drug steady state concentration[31]. However, in the absence of concomitant liver disease, the steady-state free unbound drug concentration will be unaltered. Whereas anionic drugs (phenytoin) show such a decrease in plasma protein binding as do some of the basic drugs (morphine and diazepam)[61]; many other basic drugs (propranolol and +- tubocurarine) show no change in protein binding. Although most metabolites are pharmacologically inactive, certain drugs are biodegraded to active compounds. These include the metabolites of pethidine and α-methyl DOPA. Inactive metabolites may also affect drug pharmacokinetics by the displacement of parent compound from plasma and tissue protein binding sites, by competition for active transport mechanisms, and by inhibition of further drug metabolism[21].

Although the effects on drug biotransformation are of importance, other biochemical changes in renal disease may also affect drug pharmacokinetics.

Uraemia leads to changes in fluid compartment volumes, as well as alterations in tissue and plasma protein binding. This is presumably due to deconfiguration of the receptor site by the high circulating urea concentration.

Hypoalbumenaemia is found in patients with the nephrotic syndrome and other protein-losing diseases. This results in an increased free drug concentration for agents binding predominantly to albumen.

Changes in the molecular structure of proteins

Competition for binding sites with endogenous substrates that accumulate in renal failure.

The alterations in binding will increase the systemic clearance of highly bound drugs with a low hepatic extraction ratio.

Laboratory studies investigating microsomal metabolism in both acutely and chronically uraemic rats have shown there to be a decrease in oxidative, reductive and N-demethylase activities and in the cytochrome P450 activity[87]. Not all of these *in vitro* alterations in the metabolic rates are found *in vivo*, but there is some evidence in the literature to suggest that chronic uraemia in the rat results in alterations of *in vivo* hepatic xenobiotic excretion.

THE CLINICAL IMPORTANCE OF PHARMACOKINETICS

The profile of the graph of total blood concentration against time, associated with either an intravenous bolus or an infusion of a drug, is dependent on several factors including plasma protein and tissue binding, hepatic blood flow, intrinsic hepatic clearance and the route of drug administration. Increased intrinsic hepatic clearance secondary to enzyme induction will increase the systemic clearance of drugs with a low extraction ratio (E $\leqslant$ 0.10) to a greater extent than those with a high extraction ratio (E $\geqslant$ 0.90)[59, 96].

Protein binding

Hepatic extraction of drug can occur in two different ways: restrictive clearance of the free drug (unbound) alone, or non-restrictive clearance of both free and bound drug together. In the latter mechanism, the removal of free drug leads to a dissociation of bound drug and some fraction of this released drug is then extracted by the liver. When the free fraction of a given dose of drug is increased, the initial concentration of the drug is sufficiently raised that a pronounced pharmacodynamic effect may be observed. Subsequently, a more rapid decline occurs of the plasma free drug concentration, where the dissociation of bound drug occurs readily. Thus, although this increase in the free fraction may cause an increased intensity of the initial pharmacological effect, the duration of the effect may be increased or decreased depending on the minimum effective free drug concentration[7, 10].

Plasma drug concentration

This is governed by several independent factors. These include the rate and degree of absorption of orally administered drugs, the bioavailability of the drug, the distribution of the drug, and the rate of elimination by metabolism and/or excretion.

Distribution volume

The volume of distribution[48] may be defined in different ways (V_D^β, V_D area, V_D infusion), but only the volume of distribution under steady-state conditions (V_D^{ss}) is entirely independent of the elimination process. Distribution of a drug is governed by a number of individual variables:

1   The degree of protein binding of the drug: in general, the greater the binding, the smaller the volume of distribution.
2   Weight and body surface area of the patient.
3   Sex: for a given drug, the distribution volume tends to be greater in females.
4   Blood flow and cardiac output.
5   Patient age: there is good evidence that ageing results in a decrease in the clearance of drugs, and a decrease in the distribution volume.
6   Drug interactions: such as those involving drug displacement from binding sites.

Liver disease may influence the elimination half-life of a drug by altering either the volume of distribution, the intrinsic clearance of the drug, or both. Many drugs have been shown to exhibit decreased binding, and hence increases in the volume of distribution in the presence of liver disease. Examples include phenytoin, propranolol, sulphonamides, digitoxin, tolbutamide, diazepam and morphine[16, 36, 61]. The reduction in drug binding seems, in many instances, to be inversely correlated with the serum bilirubin concentration. Other factors contributing to this increased volume of distribution may include a decreased number of plasma binding sites due to hypoalbumenaemia, and an alteration in tissue binding capacity.

Hepatic clearance

Only free unbound drug is cleared from the blood by the liver. For flow-limited drugs, the rate of clearance is dependent on the hepatic blood flow. For capacity-limited drugs, it is dependent on the intrinsic ability of the liver to clear xenobiotics. Other factors include the extent of drug binding to plasma proteins and other cellular components.

Effects of changes in liver blood flow on drug pharmacokinetics

Hepatic blood flow, intrinsic clearance and the total drug concentration/time profile are interrelated. The intrinsic hepatic clearance of a drug is an index of the maximum possible clearance rate under conditions where the blood flow to the liver is not rate limiting. If the intrinsic clearance of a drug having an extraction ratio of 0.1 is doubled, as might occur during enzyme induction, then the major effect is an increase in the efficiency of hepatic extraction (from 0.1 to 0.18). However, for drugs with a high intrinsic clearance, and hence extraction ratios of 0.9 or greater, a doubling of the intrinsic clearance will only result in a small increase in the efficiency of hepatic extraction, from 0.9 to 0.95. Under these two contrasting conditions, and assuming a liver blood flow of $1.5 \, l \, min^{-1}$, the systemic clearance in the first instance will increase from 0.15 to $0.27/l \, min^{-1}$; while in the latter case, there will only be an increase from 1.35 to $1.42 \, l \, min^{-1}$. By contrast, the effects of altering hepatic blood flow will be greatest in the systemic clearance of drugs with a high extraction ratio[96].

These concepts have lead to the development of the physiological or 'perfusion limited' pharmacokinetic model. If there is minimal extrahepatic metabolism of a drug, the relationship between hepatic blood flow (expressed in terms of multiples of intrinsic clearance) and the systemic (hepatic) drug clearance may be described by the equation:

$$Cl_H = Q_H \frac{Cl_{int}}{Q_H + Cl_{int}}$$

where Cl_H = hepatic clearance of total drug, Cl_{int} = intrinsic clearance of total drug, and Q_H = hepatic blood flow.

When flow is high, the actual clearance rate approaches the intrinsic clearance; and then the change in flow has little effect on systemic clearance. When hepatic flow is small relative to the intrinsic ability of the liver to remove drug, then the actual clearance is solely dependent on hepatic blood flow. As hepatic blood flow does not vary greatly *in vivo*, only one part of the curve, relating actual clearance to intrinsic clearance, will be functional for any drug. When Cl_{int} is equal to the hepatic blood flow, the extraction ratio is 0.5. With lower intrinsic clearances, the extraction ratio will be less than 0.5, or higher if the Cl_{int} is greater than hepatic blood flow.

This theoretical approach has been studied *in vitro* using the isolated perfused rat liver. For propranolol, the clearance is dependent on the flow rate, exactly as predicted by the model.

Alterations in hepatic blood flow can occur through physiological, pathological or pharmacological factors (Table 4.2).

Table 4.2   Factors influencing hepatic blood flow.

	Increased blood flow	Decreased blood flow
Physiological	Supine posture Food intake, digestion	Upright posture Thermal stress Exercise Volume depletion
Pathological		Congestive cardiac failure Hepatic cirrhosis Circulatory collapse Renovascular hypertension
Pharmacological	Glucagon Isoprenaline Phenobarbitone	Propranolol Noradrenaline General anaesthesia

Adapted from[59] by permission of the authors and the publishers of *Clinical Pharmacokinetics*.

Physiological factors

Hypocapnia induced during controlled ventilation may also cause a decrease of hepatic arterial and hepatic portal venous flow[41]. The restoration of normal Pa_{CO_2} values whilst still maintaining hyperventilation results in a return of hepatic portal venous flow to normal but causes a further decrease in hepatic arterial flow. This indicates that the decrease in total hepatic blood flow found during hyperventilation is mainly attributable to the hypocapnia. The decrease of hepatic blood flow was accompanied by a small, although not significant, decrease in hepatic oxygen consumption and a reduction in hepatic aerobic metabolism. Whether this is also associated with a decrease in oxidative drug and xenobiotic metabolism does not appear to have been studied.

Hypercapnia causes splanchnic vasoconstriction during administration of most anaesthetic agents except halothane, which appears to suppress the constrictor reflex. Thus the clearance of flow-limited drugs should be unaltered during halothane anaesthesia in the spontaneously breathing individual.

However, recent studies suggest that in the greyhound total blood flow to the liver is increased at high values of Pa_{CO_2} during pentobarbitone/oxygen anaesthesia[40]. Thus, the peripheral smooth muscle relaxant effect of carbon dioxide appears to predominate over central sympathetic stimulation.

Under eucapnic conditions, increasing concentrations of nitrous oxide in oxygen result in decreases in hepatic artery, portal venous and total hepatic blood flow[90]. These occur despite a cardiac output-mediated increase of mean arterial pressure, and are due to increases in total peripheral resistance, as a result of the α-receptor stimulant effect of nitrous oxide. Whether the use of oxygen-enriched air in place of nitrous oxide in oxygen during total intravenous anaesthesia could be associated with an increased clearance of flow limited drugs is unknown.

Pathological factors

When the cardiac output is pathologically decreased, the splanchnic circulation becomes vasoconstricted. Under these conditions, the estimated fall in hepatic blood flow is proportional to or slightly greater than the fall in cardiac output. Thus, in congestive cardiac failure, there is a decreased clearance of substances with a high intrinsic clearance (lignocaine, aldosterone). In circulatory shock, Benowitz[40] found that the decrease in lignocaine clearance was greater than would be expected from analysis of the perfusion limited model. This suggests that hepatic ischaemia may also cause a simultaneous decrease in intrinsic clearing ability. Liver disease is usually associated with defects of hepatic blood flow and hepatocellular function, the former due to the existence of intra- and extra-hepatic shunting of blood. The decrease in metabolic activity of the liver results in a reduction in the efficiency of elimination of drugs with a low intrinsic clearance, such as antipyrine and phenylbutazone.

Pharmacological factors

There is no doubt that volatile anaesthetic agents causing myocardial depression will also cause a decrease in splanchnic blood flow[4, 5, 42, 43]. Studies in the greyhound have shown that, although both enflurane and halothane caused a dose-dependent decrease of mean arterial pressure and cardiac output, enflurane also induced a significant decrease of both total systemic and hepatic arterial vascular resistance[39]. Furthermore, anaesthetics may indirectly influence hepatic flow; for instance, the increase in sympathetic tone associated with cyclopropane and di-ethyl ether, which results in a decrease in hepatic blood flow. Methoxyflurane may decrease hepatic arterial and total hepatic blood flow as a result of myocardial depression of the cardiac output, combined with a direct active splanchnic vasoconstrictor mechanism.

Studies by Mather and his colleagues[56a] using a sheep model have allowed the direct determination of the effect of general and spinal anaesthesia on the clearance of flow-dependent drugs such as pethidine and chlormethiazole. General anaesthesia resulted in a decrease of hepatic blood flow of 80% and of renal blood flow of 50%; while there were only small changes following high spinal anaesthesia. Consequently, the clearance of pethidine was reduced by 50% under general anaesthesia. During the awake state 50% of the drug was cleared by the kidney, but this was decreased to zero under general anaesthesia. A similar decrease in the clearance of chlormethiazole was found during general anaesthesia.

Effects of hepatic and renal dysfunction on metabolism and clearance of drugs used in anaesthesia

Although hepatic and renal disease have been considered separately with respect to their effects on the pharmacokinetics of anaesthetic agents, many patients with systemic disease show both renal and hepatic dysfunction. In these circumstances, the disposition of an agent may be markedly altered, such that overdosage may occur on administration of normal doses, with the development of adverse side-effects. Similarly, the inappropriate administration of a drug to patients with liver or kidney disease may not only lead to altered pharmacokinetics, but also to organ toxic effects. Examples of the latter include methoxyflurane nephropathy when the agent is given to patients with impaired renal function; hepatic toxicity from halothane if administered to an hypoxic or ischaemic liver[13]; and the acceleration of hepatic encephalopathy by the administration of excess doses of sedatives or narcotics to patients in liver failure.

Barbiturates (see also Chapter 6)

The influence of renal and hepatic disease on the pharmacokinetics of the barbiturates is mainly related to changes in the plasma protein binding of the drugs. Although Saidman and Eger[73] suggested that metabolism may play a part in the decrease of the drug's pharmacodynamic action, the latter has since been shown to be primarily an effect of drug redistribution. In renal disease, the elimination half-life of thiopentone is unaltered; although the free drug fraction, systemic drug clearance, and the volume of distribution at steady state are increased[14]. Animal studies in the rat have failed to show any effect of administration of microsomal enzyme inhibitors or inducers on either the duration of action of a single dose of thiopentone, or the associated circulatory effects of the drug. Neither hepatic damage nor impaired intrinsic metabolising ability of the liver appear to alter the disposition of thiopentone (capacity limited clearance). This is in contrast to the marked effect on the duration of action of the steroid anaesthetic agent, Althesin (flow-limited clearance), when given under similar conditions[60]. Similarly, no significant decrease in the systemic clearance of methohexitone has been found in patients with cirrhotic liver disease in the absence of associated cardiovascular disturbances[72].

Etomidate

Few data have been available until recently on the pharmacokinetics and metabolism of etomidate in patients with hepatic and renal disease. However, Carlos *et al.*[15] have shown a significant decrease in the plasma protein binding of etomidate in patients with either uraemia or hepatic cirrhosis. In both conditions, the percentage binding correlated significantly with the serum albumen concentration. Bonnardot and his colleagues[8a] have given etomidate by infusion for surgery in patients with both normal and impaired hepatic function. Their results are shown in Table 4.3. The main changes in the patients with impaired hepatic function was a prolongation of the elimination half-life, and a decrease in the systemic clearance. Van Beem[91a] found similar results in patients given etomidate by infusion for the maintenance of anaesthesia for the endoscopic injection of oesophaegeal varices (Table 4.3). They too found a prolongation of the elimination half-life, but no decrease in the systemic clearance.

Table 4.3   Effect of liver disease on the pharmacokinetics of etomidate (mean ± SD).

Source	Normal patients			Patients with cirrhosis		
	Elim $T_{\frac{1}{2}}$	$V_D$area	Cl_P	Elim $T_{\frac{1}{2}}$	$V_D$area	Cl_P
Bonnardot	85 ± 55	3.6 ± 2.3	30.1 ± 10.2	152 ± 74	2.8 ± 1.4	13.1 ± 4.3
Van Beem	209 ± 65	3.7 ± 0.7	12.8 ± 2.3	540 ± 150	8.9 ± 1.3	12.7 ± 5.1

Elim $T_{\frac{1}{2}}$ = min; V_D area = 1 Kg^{-1}; Cl_P = ml kg^{-1} min^{-1}

The difference in the half-lives for both the normal patients, and those with hepatic cirrhosis, between the studies of Bonnardot and Van Beem, may be related to the longer period of post-infusion sampling in the latter studies. Van Beem and his colleagues also found an increase in the volume of distribution of etomidate in the patients with hepatic cirrhosis, probably due to a decrease in the plasma protein binding of etomidate[15].

Chlormethiazole

Chlormethiazole is frequently used in Intensive Care Units for the treatment of delirium tremens, also for the sedation of other patients requiring controlled ventilation[76]. To a lesser extent, the drug is used in the management of patients with pre-eclampsia. There has been some suggestion that accumulation of the drug could occur during prolonged infusion, but this has not been confirmed by the recent studies of Scott[76]. Both the clearance of chlormethiazole (8.7 ml kg^{-1} min^{-1}) and its volume of distribution (5.6 l kg^{-1}) in Scott's patients were considerably less than the values in healthy adults ($64.5\,ml\,kg^{-1}\,min^{-1}$ and $20.6\,l\,kg^{-1}$ respectively). The variations in hepatic blood flow which may occur in critically ill patients may account for the pharmacokinetic differences and influence the recovery of the patient.

In two other series of patients (one of elderly volunteers, the other of patients with proven cirrhosis of the liver), the clearance rates were similar to those determined by Scott. However, Pentikainen[65] found an 11-fold increase in the bioavailability of chlormethiazole after oral administration to patients with cirrhosis, coupled with a 33% reduction in the systemic clearance of the drug.

Steroid anaesthetics

Although Strunin et al.[86] have shown no significant effect of anuria or cholestasis on the clinical effects and plasma clearance of ^{14}C-labelled alphaxalone, du Cailar[22] reported a prolongation of recovery after administration of Althesin to patients with acute hepatic failure. The author and his colleagues have shown significant alterations in the pharmacokinetic disposition of Althesin when given to patients with compensated primary biliary cirrhosis undergoing surgery for the formation of a mesocaval H graft[78]. There was a significant increase in the volume of distribution of alphaxalone, and an increase in the systemic clearance of the total (free and bound) drug. This was probably due to a decrease in the plasma and tissue protein binding of the alphaxalone; but extra-hepatic sequestration and uptake cannot be excluded and may be of importance in the clearance of this lipophilic drug. In limited studies to date, similar kinetic profiles have been found for alphadolone as well as alphaxalone in both healthy patients and those suffering from cirrhosis (Table 4.4).

Further studies, where the plasma concentrations of alphaxalone has been measured 30–40 min after infusion at various rates, have compared the results in healthy and cirrhotic individuals[72, 77]. For given multiples of the minimum infusion rate (MIR) of Althesin up to $5 \times$ MIR, there was a consistently lower plasma concentration of alphaxalone in the patients with cirrhosis. Again, this can be explained by an alteration in the volume of distribution due to a decrease in plasma protein binding (Table 4.5).

Table 4.4 Effect of primary biliary cirrhosis on the disposition of alphaxalone[78, 80].

	$T_{\frac{1}{2}}^{\alpha}$ (min)	$T_{\frac{1}{2}}^{\beta}$ (min)	Cl_P (ml kg^{-1} min^{-1})	V_1 (l kg^{-1})	V_D^{ss} (l kg^{-1})
Healthy control group (n = 9)	2.84 ±0.86	90.9 ±7.5	16.9 ±1.7	1.49 ±0.30	2.18 ±0.37
Cirrhotic patients (n = 9)	3.93 ±0.86	127.0 ±35.3	17.9 ±1.7	2.41 ±0.51	6.61 ±2.95

Table 4.5 Plasma concentration of alphaxalone at different rates of infusion of Althesin in patients without clinical or biochemical evidence of hepatic disease (n = 22 patients), and a separate group of patients with histologically proven primary biliary cirrhosis (n = 15 patients). The infusion rates chosen were multiples of the minimum infusion rate (MIR) in healthy patients (13.5 μg alphaxalone kg^{-1} min^{-1}). Data points were obtained for each patient at each multiple of MIR (number in parenthesis indicates number of observations). The infusion rate was maintained as indicated for 30–40 minutes before sampling[77, 78, 79].

	Healthy patients		Patients with cirrhosis	
Multiple of MIR	Actual infusion rate	Plasma alphaxalone concentration	Actual infusion rate	Plasma alphaxalone concentration
1	13.5 ± 0.66	1.91 ± 0.09 (33)	15.1 ± 1.10	0.72 ± 0.13 (9)
2	26.7 ± 0.63	2.24 ± 0.15 (27)	23.2 ± 1.00	0.89 ± 0.17 (11)
3	38.7 ± 0.77	2.86 ± 0.17 (29)	35.9 ± 1.00	1.11 ± 0.16 (7)
4	52.4 ± 1.22	3.28 ± 0.09 (12)	50.2 ± 0.50	1.47 ± 0.22 (4)
5	67.8 ± 2.41	3.93 ± 0.28 (14)	70.0 ± 2.90	1.61 + 0.35 (3)

Infusion rate = μg Alphaxalone kg^{-1} min^{-1}; plasma concentration = μg alphaxalone ml^{-1}

Analysis of plasma and urine samples from patients with primary biliary cirrhosis showed no significant difference in the metabolites from those found in patients with normal hepatic function—with the parent steroids and their metabolites being excreted to about 90–95 % in the glucuronide fraction of the urine[34, 77]. Although Strunin was able to detect the presence of radioactivity in the bile of patients after injection of a single dose of Althesin, we have been unable to confirm the presence of alphaxalone, alphadolone acetate, alphadolone, or 20α-reduced alphaxalone in the bile using the technique of gas chromatography–mass spectrometry in the selective ion monitoring (SIM) mode. Thus, Strunin's results must be explained on the basis of radio-impurity, or the excretion of more polar compounds not detected by our extraction procedure. In a single patient with acute hepatic damage following ingestion of salicylates and paracetamol, there was a quantitative decrease in the excretion of the glucuronide conjugates of the component steroids, and an increase in the excretion of unconjugated alphaxalone and 20α-reduced alphaxalone. This is perhaps surprising as glucuronidation is often preserved until late in the natural history of hepatic damage[78].

In the cirrhotic patient and in the patient with chronic renal failure there is no significant prolongation of recovery after an anaesthetic dose of Althesin, given either as a bolus or by continuous infusion. However, the administration of thioacetamide or ethiomamide to produce liver damage in the rat results in a prolongation of sleep time to an intravenous dose. Similar increases in the duration of anaesthesia have been found by the author following the administration of intraperitoneal Althesin (33 mg kg^{-1}) to rats treated with carbon tetrachloride[77]. This agent and many other halogenated hydrocarbons cause degradation of the microsomal cytochrome P450, and a decrease in the rate of oxidative metabolism of the Althesin steroids. Previous studies showed a correlation between the rate of microsomal degradation of alphaxalone and hence the microsomal cytochrome P450 concentration, and the duration of sleep following Althesin[77]. This is in contrast to anaesthesia produced by the thiobarbiturates, where recovery is highly dependent on a redistribution of drug rather than on rapid metabolism to an inactive form within the liver and other drug metabolising tissues.

Narcotic analgesics (see Chapter 9)

Pethidine, pentazocine, fentanyl and morphine are all lipid-soluble drugs with high extraction ratios and a high intrinsic clearance. A decrease in drug clearance and an increased oral bioavailability has been observed during use of these drugs in patients with hepatic cirrhosis and acute viral hepatitis. There was, however, little change in the volume of distribution at steady state, and in the plasma protein binding of the drugs[50, 54, 59, 67]. Despite the presence of liver failure, the glucuronidation of morphine can still occur as a result of extrahepatic biotransformation[37]. The absence of this extrahepatic metabolism in the acutely anhepatic animal suggests that the alternate biotransformation pathway develops in parallel with the slow deterioration of hepatic function during end-stage cirrhosis[38]. Recent studies by Chan and his colleagues[44] have shown a similar prolongation of the elimination half-life, and decrease in the systemic clearance when phenoperidine is administered to patients with hepatic dysfunction.

β-adrenoceptor antagonists (see Chapter 13)

The elimination of both propranolol and metoprolol are unaffected by changes in renal function. However, in severe renal failure there is a decreased rate of clearance of propranolol and accumulation of inactive metabolites of metoprolol if the glomerular filtration rate falls below $20 \, ml \, min^{-1}$[89]. As the main metabolite of acetubolol is pharmacologically active, there is a significant increase in the pharmacodynamic effect of the drug in renal disease[58]. Similar increases in the efficacy of atenolol and sotalol are seen in renal failure; their clearance rate being directly related to the glomerular filtration rate.

Chronic liver disease influences the pharmacokinetics and disposition of several of the β-adrenoceptor antagonists by alterations in the extent of first-pass metabolism, the volumes of distribution, and the rates of systemic clearance of the drugs. Propranolol has been used by many workers as a model compound for studying the effects of liver disease on pharmacokinetics. It is extensively metabolised in the liver, as well as undergoing a significant first-pass metabolism in the liver after oral dosage.

Cirrhosis leads to an increased oral bioavailability, a decreased plasma protein binding, and hence increased free steady-state plasma drug concentrations[98]. Drug clearance decreases in parallel with the reduction in liver blood flow; a characteristic seen with all drugs having a high extraction ratio, and a clearance rate approximately equal to the hepatic blood flow. Similar changes have been found when metoprolol and labetolol were given to patients with hepatic cirrhosis[35, 45].

Benzodiazepines (see Chapter 8)

In cirrhosis, a decrease has been found in the plasma protein binding of diazepam, coupled with a small increase in the steady state volume of distribution[49, 88]. A decrease in the systemic clearance of diazepam was found in patients with either cirrhosis or chronic active hepatitis. In chronic renal disease, there was a similar decrease in the plasma protein binding from 98% to 92%[46]. However, no linear correlation has been found between the serum albumen concentration and the diazepam binding in patients with acute renal failure[3]. More recent pharmacokinetic studies of diazepam given to patients with chronic renal failure have shown an increased volume of distribution and a highly significant increase in the systemic clearance of the drug. This effect was entirely due to an increase in the free unbound fraction of the drug from 1.4% to 7.9%. All studies on the clearance of diazepam in hepatic cirrhosis have suggested that an impairment occurs in the formation of the primary metabolite, N-desmethyl diazepam. This will lead to a decrease in the systemic clearance of both diazepam and the metabolite.

Oxazepam shows unaltered disposition and elimination in viral hepatitis or cirrhosis[81]. As in the case of morphine disposition in acute liver disease, there is evidence of extra-hepatic biotransformation of oxazepam to the glucuronide, to such an extent as to compensate for the impaired hepatic metabolism. Alternatively, these disease processes may result in a greater decrease in mono-oxygenase activity than in the enzymes of glucuronidation. Support for the latter hypothesis has been obtained in that bilirubin conjugation is unaltered in patients with acute viral hepatitis or cirrhosis[6]. Altered disposition and excretion of oxazepam has been found in patients with renal failure.

Neuromuscular blocking drugs and their antagonists (see Chapter 11)

The effect of renal and hepatic dysfunction on the neuromuscular blocking drugs has been studied under a variety of conditions. In both cholestatic and cirrhotic liver disease in man, the elimination half-lives of fazadinium, pancuronium and gallamine were prolonged as a result of a decrease in the systemic clearance[23, 70, 84, 95]. Similar results were found following the administration of pancuronium to patients with acute hepatic failure[94]. Cirrhosis and cholestasis also increased the volume of distribution of pancuronium and fazadinium. However, although there was a 56% increase in the volume of distribution of fazadinium in liver disease, this appeared to have little effect on the duration of action of the neuromuscular blockade[26]. Cirrhosis does not appear to significantly alter the plasma protein binding of pancuronium, fazadinium, ORG NC 45, or +-tubocurarine. The biliary excretion of the muscular relaxants varies from about 10% for alcuronium, d-tubocurarine and pancuronium to 20–40% for fazadinium[25]. These percentages may not be of importance in the duration of action of the drugs. Duvaldestin has suggested that the role of the liver in the uptake and metabolism of fazadinium is probably less significant than would be expected by the high biliary excretion[26].

In chronic renal failure, the pharmacokinetics of fazadinium are less altered than those of pancuronium or +-tubocurarine, although the elimination of all three agents is decreased[24, 55, 83]. The cumulative urinary excretion of pancuronium or fazadinium constitutes only about 50% of the injected dose, as compared with approximately 80% for alcuronium or gallamine[69]. The pharmacodynamic effects of the neuromuscular blocking drugs may be prolonged in renal failure if drug accumulation occurs. This is especially important with the use of gallamine, which is wholly excreted unchanged, and with +-tubocurarine, which is excreted partially unchanged.

The two newer neuromuscular blocking drugs, NC ORG 45 and metocurine, have both been studied in healthy patients and in patients with renal failure. NC 45 does not appear to be dependent on either the kidney or the liver for recovery of muscle tone. It has a short elimination half-life compared to pancuronium; more as a result of a greater systemic clearance than its smaller volume of distribution. In patients with renal disease, there were no significant alterations of the volume of distribution, nor of the systemic clearance[28]. Metocurine, on the other hand, appears to be more dependent on the kidney for its excretion than does +-tubocurarine. In studies in patients with chronic renal failure, there was a prolongation of the elimination half-life, while the clearance was decreased by about 65–70%. There was no change in the central volume of distribution of the relaxant, but the total volume of distribution was smaller in the patients with chronic renal disease[12]. This is in contrast to the changes found with pancuronium, fazadinium and gallamine.

Recent studies with Atracurium has shown this relaxant to be non-cumulative and easily reversed both in the patient with normal renal function and in the patient undergoing renal transplantation (J. Hunter, pers. comm.). As the breakdown of this relaxant by Hoffman degradation is independent of either hepatic or renal mechanisms, Atracurium may become the agent of choice in the neuromuscular paralysis of patients with impaired liver or kidney function.

The effects of chronic renal disease have also been studied with reference to the neuromuscular blocking drug antagonists[18]. The volumes of distribution of neostigmine, pyridostigmine or edrophonium are not significantly altered in renal disease nor is systemic clearance decreased. However, hepatic metabolism occurs to a different extent for each of the three drugs; 25% for pyridostigmine, 30% for edrophonium, and 50% for neostigmine. Thus, in renal failure, the elimination half-lives are prolonged (pyridostigmine greater than neostigmine), and excretion is decreased. The mechanism of renal excretion is both by glomerular filtration and tubular secretion.

REFERENCES

1. AHMED N. & BLACK M. (1977) The hepatic microsomal mixed—function oxidase system in man: cofactor effects and the influence of cholestasis. *J. Pharmacol. Exp. Ther.* **203**, 397.
2. ALVARES A. P., SCHILLING G., LEWIN W. & KUNTZMAN R. (1969) Cytochromes P450 and b₅ in human liver microsomes. *Clin. Pharmacol. Ther.* **10**, 655.
3. ANDREASEN F. (1974) The effects of dialysis on the protein binding of drugs in patients with acute renal failure. *Acta Pharmacol. Toxicol.* **34**, 284.
4. ANDREEN M., IRESTEDT L. & ZETTERSTROM B. (1977) The different responses of the hepatic arterial bed to hypovolaemia and to halothane anaesthesia. *Acta Anaesthesiol. Scand.* **21**, 457.
4a. BENOWITZ N., FORSYTH R. P., MELMON K. L. & ROWLAND M. (1974) Lidocaine disposition kinetics in monkey and man. II. Effects of hemorrhage and sympathomimetic drug administration. *Clin. Pharmacol. Ther.* **16**, 99.
5. BENUMOF J. L., BOOKSTEIN J. J., SAIDMAN L. J. & HARRIS R. (1976) Diminished hepatic arterial flow during halothane administration. *Anesthesiology* **45**, 545.
6. BILLING B. & BLACK M. (1971) The action of drugs on bilirubin metabolism in man. *Ann. NY Acad. Sci.* **179**, 403.
7. BLATSCHE T. F. (1977) Protein binding and kinetics of drugs in liver disease. *Clin. Pharmacokin.* **2**, 32.
8. BLASCHKE T. F. & RUBIN P. C. (1979) Hepatic first-pass metabolism in liver disease. *Clin. Pharmacokin.* **4**, 423.
8a. BONNARDOT J. P., DESLAURIERS M., LEVRON J. C., BRULE M. L., FLAISLER B. & DELIGNE P. (1982) Pharmacokinetics of etomidate: Comparison in normal and

hepatic patients. *Anaesthesia*: Volume of summaries, Sixth European Congress of Anaesthesiology, London. Abstract **23** p. 15.
9. BOOBIS A. R., BRODIE M. J., KHAN G. C., FLETCHER D. R., SAUNDERS J. H. & DAVIES D. S. (1980) Mono-oxygenase activity of human liver in microsomal fractions of needle biopsy specimens. *Br. J. Clin. Pharmacol.* **9**, 11.
10. BORGA O. (1974) Lakemedels interaktion vid protein bindning och distribution. *Social styrelsens kommittee fur lakemedels information* **1**, 24.
11. BRODIE B. B., GILLETTE J. R. & LA DU B. N. (1958) Enzymatic metabolism of drugs and other foreign compounds. *Ann. Rev. Biochem.* **27**, 427.
12. BROTHERTON W. P. & MATTEO R. S. (1981) Pharmacokinetics and pharmacodynamics of metocurine in humans with and without renal failure. *Anesthesiology* **55**, 273.
13. BROWN B. R. & SIPES I. G. (1977) Biotransformation and hepatotoxicity of Halothane. *Biochem. Pharmacol.* **26**, 2091.
14. BURCH P. G. & STANSKI D. R. (1981) Pharmacokinetics of thiopental in renal failure. *Anesthesiology* **55**, A176.
15. CARLOS R., CALVO R. & BRILL S. (1979) Plasma protein binding of etomidate in patients with renal failure or hepatic cirrhosis. *Clin. Pharmacokin.* **4**, 144.
16. CASTLEDEN C. M., KAYE C. M. & PARSON R. L. (1975) The effect of age on plasma levels of propranolol and practolol in man. *Br. J. Clin. Pharmacol.* **2**, 303.
17. COOPER D. Y., LEVIN S., NARASIMHULA S., ROSENTHAL O. & ESTABROOK R. W. (1975) Photochemical action spectrum of

the terminal oxidase of mixed function oxidase systems. *Science* **147**, 400.

18. CRONNELLY R. & MORRIS R. B. (1982) Antagonism of neuromuscular blockade. *Br. J. Anaesth.* **54**, 183.

19. DARBY F. J., NEWNES W. & PRICE-EVANS D. A. (1970) Human liver microsomal drug metabolism. *Biochem. Pharmacol.* **19**, 1514.

20. DAVIES D. S., THORGEIRSSON S. S., BRECKENRIDGE A. & ORME M. (1973) Inter-individual differences in rates of drug oxidation in man. *Drug Metab. Dispos.* **1**, 411.

21. DRAYER D. E. (1977) Active drug metabolites and renal failure. *Am. J. Med.* **62**, 486.

22. DU CAILAR J. (1972) The effects in man of infusions of Althesin with particular regard to the cardiovascular system. *Postgrad. Med. J.* **48** (suppl. 2), 72.

23. DUVALDESTIN P., AGOSTON S., HENZEL D., KERSTEN U. W. & DESMONTS J. M. (1978) Pancuronium pharmacokinetics in patients with liver cirrhosis. *Br. J. Anaesth.* **50**, 1131.

24. DUVALDESTIN P., BERTRAND J. C., CONCINA D., HENZEL P., LARENG L. & DESMONTS J. M. (1979) Pharmacokinetics of fazadinium in patients with renal failure *Br. J. Anaesth.* **51**, 943.

25. DUVALDESTIN P. & HENZEL D. (1982) Binding of tubocurarine, fazadinium, pancuronium and ORG NC 45 to serum proteins in normal man and in patients with cirrhosis. *Br. J. Anaesth.* **54**, 513.

26. DUVALDESTIN P., SAADA J., HENZEL D. & SAUMON G. (1980) Fazadinium pharmacokinetics in patients with liver disease. *Br. J. Anaesth.* **52**, 789.

27. ESTABROOK R. W. & COHEN B. (1969) Organization of the microsomal electron transport system. In Gillette J. R. *et al.* (eds.) *Microsomes and Drug Oxidations.* Academic Press, New York.

28. FAHEY M. R., MORRIS R. B., MILLER R. D., NGUYEN T-L. & UPTON R. A. (1981) Pharmacokinetics of ORG NC 45 (Norcuron) in patients with and without renal disease. *Br. J. Anaesth.* **52**, 1049.

29. FARRELL G. C., COOKSLEY W. G. E. & POWELL L. W. (1979) Drug metabolism in liver disease: activity of hepatic metabolising enzymes. *Clin. Pharmacol. Ther.* **26**, 483.

30. GARFINKEL D. (1958) Studies on pig liver microsomes. I: enzymic and pigment composition of different microsomal fractions. *Arch. Biochem. Biophys.* **77**, 498.

31. GIBALDI M. (1977) Drug distribution in renal failure. *Am. J. Med.* **62**, 471.

32. GUENGERICH F. P. & COON M. J. (1975) Role of phospholipid in reconstituted liver microsomal enzyme system containing highly purified cytochrome P450. *Fed. Proc.* **34**, 622.

33. HILDEBRANDT A. G. & ESTABROOK R. W. (1971) Evidence for the participation of cytochrome b_5 in hepatic microsomal mixed-function oxidation reactions. *Arch. Biochem. Biophys.* **143**, 66.

34. HOLLY J. M. P., TRAFFORD D. J. H., SEAR J. W. & MAKIN H. L. J. (1981) *In vivo* metabolism of Althesin (alphaxalone and alphadolone acetate) in man. *J. Pharm. Pharmacol.* **33**, 427.

35. HOMEIDA M., JACKSON L., & ROBERTS C. J. C. (1978) Decreased first-pass metabolism of labetalol in chronic liver disease. *Br. Med. J.* **2**, 1048.

36. HOOPER W. D., BOCHNER F., EADIE M. J. & TYRER J. H. (1973) Plasma protein binding of diphenylhydantoin: Effects of sex hormones, renal and hepatic disease. *Clin. Pharmacol. Ther.* **15**, 276.

37. HUG C. C., ALDRETE J. A., SAMPSON J. F. & MURPHY M. R. (1979) Morphine anaesthesia in patients with liver failure. *Anesthesiology* **51**, S30.

38. HUG C. C., MURPHY M. R., SAMPSON J. R., TERBLANCHE J. & ALDRETE J. A. (1981) Biotransformation of morphine and fentanyl in anhepatic dogs. *Anesthesiology* **55**, A261.

39. HUGHES R. L., CAMPBELL D. & FITCH W. (1980) Effects of enflurane and halothane on liver blood flow and oxygen consumption in the greyhound. *Br. J. Anaesth.* **52**, 1079.

40. HUGHES R. L., MATHIE R. T., CAMPBELL D. & FITCH W. (1979) Effect of hypercarbia on hepatic blood flow and oxygen consumption in the greyhound. *Br. J. Anaesth.* **51**, 289.

41. HUGHES R. L., MATHIE R. T., FITCH W. & CAMPBELL D. (1979) Liver blood flow and oxygen consumption during hypocapnia and IPPV in the greyhound. *J. Applied Physiol.* **47**, 29.

42. IRESTEDT L. & ANDREEN M. (1979) Effects of neuroleptanaesthesia (NLA) on haemodynamics and oxygen consumption in the dog with spinal reference to the liver and preportal tissues. *Acta Anaesth. Scand.* **23**, 1.

43. IRESTEDT L. & ANDREEN M. (1979) Effects of enflurane on haemodynamics and oxygen consumption in the dog with special reference to the liver and preportal tissues. *Acta Anaesth. Scand.* **23**, 13.

44. ISHERWOOD C. N., MURRAY G. R., CHAN K., CALVEY T. N. & WILLIAMS N. E. (1982) The effect of liver disease on the metabolism and elimination of phenoperidine in man. *Br. J. Clin. Pharmacol.* **13**, 612P.

45. JORDO L., ATTMAN P. C., AURELL M., JOHANSSON L., JOHNSSON G. & REHARDH C. G. (1980) Pharmacokinetic and pharmacodynamic properties of metoprolol in patients with impaired renal function *Clin. Pharmacokin.* **5**, 169.

46. KANGAS L., KANTO J., FORSSTROM J. & ILISALO E. (1976) Protein binding of diazepam and N-demethyldiazapam in patients with poor renal function. *Clin. Nephrology* **4**, 114.

47. KLINGENBERG M. (1958) Pigments of rat liver microsomes. *Arch. Biochem. Biophys.* **75**, 376.

48. KLOTZ U. (1976) Pathophysiological and disease-induced changes in drug distribution volume: pharmacokinetic implications. *Clin. Pharmacokin.* **1**, 204.

49. KLOTZ U., AVANT G. R., HOYUMPA A., SCHENKER S. & WILKINSON G. R. (1975) The effects of age and liver disease on the disposition and elimination of diazepam in adult man. *J. Clin. Invest.* **55**, 347.

50. KLOTZ U., McHORSE T. S., WILKINSON G. R. & SCHENKER S. (1974) The effects of cirrhosis on the disposition and elimination of meperidine in man. *Clin. Pharmacol. Ther.* **16**, 667.

51. KNODELL R. G., FARLEIGH R. M., STEELE N. M. & BOND J. H. (1982) Effects of liver congestion on hepatic drug metabolism in the rat. *J. Pharmacol. Exp. Ther.* **222**, 52.

52. LU A. Y. H. (1976) Liver microsomal drug-metabolising enzyme system: functional components and their properties. *Fed. Proc.* **35**, 2460.

53. LU A. Y. & COON M. J. (1968) Role of hemoprotein P450 in fatty acid omega hydroxylation in a soluble enzyme system from liver microsomes. *J. Biol. Chem.* **243**, 1331.

54. McHORSE T. S., WILKINSON G. R., JOHNSON R. & SCHENKER S. (1975) Effect of acute viral hepatitis in man on the disposition and elimination of meperidine. *Gastroenterology* **68**, 775.

55. McLEOD K., WATSON M. J. & RAWLINS M. D. (1976) Pharmacokinetics of pancuronium in patients with normal and impaired renal function. *Br. J. Anaesth.* **48**, 341.

56. MASON H. S., YAMANO T., NORTH J. C., HASHIMOTO Y. & SAKAGISHI P. (1965) The structure and oxidase function of liver microsomes. In King T. E. *et al.* (eds.), *Symposium on oxidases and related oxidation reduction enzymes.* Academic Press, New York.

57. MAY B., HELMSTAEDT D., BUSTGENS L. & McLEAN A. (1974) The relation between cytochrome P450 in liver biopsies and drug metabolism in patients with

liver disease and in morphine addiction. *Clin. Sci. Mol. Med.* **46**, 11p.

58. MEFFIN P. J., WINKLE R. A., PETERS F. A. & HARRISON D. C. (1978) Dose-dependent acebutolol disposition after oral administration. *Clin. Pharmacol. Ther.* **24**, 542.

59. NIES A. S., SHAND D. G. & WILKINSON G. R. (1976) Altered hepatic blood flow and drug disposition. *Clin. Pharmacokin.* **1**, 135.

60. NOVELLI G. P., MARSILI M. & LORENZI (1975) Influence of liver metabolism on the actions of Althesin and thipentone. *Br. J. Anaesth.* **47**, 913.

61. OLSEN G. D., BENNETT W. M. & PORTER G. A. (1975) Morphine and phenytoin binding to plasma proteins in renal and hepatic failure. *Clin. Pharmacol. Ther.* **17**, 677.

62. OMURA T., SATO R., COOPER D. Y., ROSENTHAL O. & ESTABROOK R. W. (1965) Function of cytochrome P450 of microsomes. *Fed. Proc.* **24**, 1181.

63. PATWARDHAN R., JOHNSON R., SHEEHAN J., DESMOND P., WILKINSON G., HOYUMPA A., BRANCH R. & SCHENKER S. (1981) Morphine metabolism in cirrhosis. *Gastroenterology* **80**, 1344.

64. PELKONEN O., KALTIALA E. H., LARMI T. K. I. & KARKI N. T. (1974) Cytochrome P450 linked mono-oxygenase system and drug-induced spectral interactions in human liver microsomes. *Chem. Biol. Interactions* **9**, 205.

65. PENTIKAINEN P. J., NEUVONEN P. J., TARPILA S. & SYVALAHTI E. (1978) Effects of cirrhosis of the liver on the pharmacokinetics of chlormethiazole. *Br. Med. J.* **2**, 861.

66. PESSAYRE D., LEBREC D., DESCATOIRE V., PEIGNOUX M. & BENHAMOU J-P. (1978) Mechanism for reduced drug clearance in patients with cirrhosis. *Gastroenterology* **74**, 566.

67. POND S. M., TONG T., BENOWITZ N. L. & JACOB P. (1979) Bioavailability and clear-ance of meperidine in patients with chronic liver disease. *Clin. Pharmacol. Ther.* **25**, 242.

68. POPPER H. & SCHAFFNER F. (1970) Pathophysiology of cholestasis. *Human Pathol.* **1**, 1.

69. RAMZAN M. I., SHANKS C. A. & TRIGGS E. J. (1981) Gallamine disposition in surgical patients with chronic renal failure. *Br. J. Clin. Pharmacol.* **12**, 141.

70. RAMZEN I. M., SHANKS C. A. & TRIGGS E. J. (1981) Pharmacokinetics and phar-macodynamics of gallamine triethiodide in patients with total biliary obstruction. *Anesth. Analg.* **60**, 289.

71. REIDENBERG M. (1977) Biotransform-ation of drugs in renal failure. *Am. J. Med.* **62**, 482.

72. RIETBROCK I. & LAZARUS G. (1979) Leberfunktion unter Anästhesie—und Intensivbedingungen. *Med. Klin.* **74**, 1790.

73. SAIDMAN L. J. & EGER E. I. (1966) The effect of thiopental metabolism on dur-ation of anaesthesia. *Anesthesiology* **27**, 118.

74. SCHAFFNER F. & POPPER H. (1969) Cholestasis is the result of hypoactive hypertrophic smooth endoplasmic reti-culum in the hepatocyte. *Lancet* **2**, 355.

75. SCHOENE B., FLEISCHMANN R. A., REMMER H. & OLDERHAUSEN H. F. V. (1972) Determination of drug metabolis-ing enzymes in needle biopsies of human liver. *Eur. J. Clin. Pharmacol.* **4**, 65.

76. SCOTT D. B., BEAMISH D., HUDSON I. M. & JOSTELL K-G. (1980) Prolonged infu-sion of chlormethiazole in intensive care. *Br. J. Anaesth.* **52**, 541.

77. SEAR J. W. (1981) The metabolism of steroid intravenous anaesthetic agents and their modification by liver disease. PhD thesis; University of Bristol.

78. SEAR J. W., MAKIN H. L. J., STAFFORD M. A., TRAFFORD D. J. H. & PRYS-ROBERTS C. (1981) Disposition and meta-bolism of Althesin in patients with cirrho-tic liver disease. *Br. J. Anaesth.* **53**, 1093.

79. SEAR J. W. & PRYS-ROBERTS C. (1979) Plasma alphaxalone concentration during continuous infusion of Althesin. *Br. J. Anaesth.* **51**, 861.

80. SEAR J. W. & PRYS-ROBERTS C. (1982) Effect of anti-hypertensive therapy on the pharmacokinetics of Althesin by infusion to man. *Br. J. Anaesth* **54**, 1130.

81. SHULL H. J., WILKINSON G. R., JOHNSON R. & SCHENKER S. (1976) Normal disposition of oxazepam in acute viral hepatitis and cirrhosis. *Ann. Int. Med.* **84**, 420.

82. SJOQUIST F. & VON BAHR C. (1973) Interindividual differences in drug oxidation: clinical importance. *Drug Metab. Dispos.* **1**, 469.

83. SOMOGYI A., SHANKS C. A. & TRIGGS E. J. (1977) The effect of renal failure on the disposition and neuromuscular blocking action of pancuronium bromide. *Europ. J. Clin. Pharmacol.* **12**, 23.

84. SOMOGYI A. A., SHANKS C. A. & TRIGGS E. J. (1977) Disposition kinetics of pancuronium bromide in patients with total biliary obstruction. *Br. J. Anaesth.* **49**, 1103.

85. STROEBEL H. W., LU A. Y., HEIDEMA J. & COON M. J. (1970) Phosphatidyl choline requirement in the enzymatic reduction of hemoprotein P450, and in fatty acid, hydrocarbon and drug hydroxylation. *J. Biol. Chem.* **245**, 4851.

86. STRUNIN L., STRUNIN J. M., KNIGHTS K. M. & WARD M. E. (1977) Metabolism of ^{14}C labelled alphaxalone in man. *Br. J. Anaesth.* **49**, 609.

87. TERNER U. K., WIEBE L. I., NOUJAIM A. A., DOSSETOR J. B. & SANDERS E. J. (1978) The effects of acute and chronic uraemia in rats on their hepatic microsomal enzyme activity. *Clin. Biochem.* **11**, 156.

88. THIESSEN J. J., SELLERS E. M., DENBEIGH P. & DOLMAN L. (1976) Plasma protein binding of diazepam and tolbutamide in chronic alcoholics. *J. Clin. Pharmacol.* **16**, 345.

89. THOMPSON F. D., JOEKES A. M. & FOULKES D. M. (1972) Pharmacodynamics of propranolol in renal failure. *Br. Med. J.* **2**, 434.

90. THOMSON I. A., HUGHES R. L., FITCH W. & CAMPBELL D. (1982) Effect of nitrous oxide on liver haemodynamics and oxygen consumption in the greyhound. *Anaesthesia* **37**, 548.

91. THOMSON P. D., MELMON K. L., RICHARDSON J. A., COHN K., STEINBRUNN W., CUDIHEE R. & ROWLAND M. (1973) Lidocaine pharmacokinetics in advanced heart failure, liver disease and renal failure in humans. *Ann. Internal Med.* **78**, 499.

91a. VAN BEEM H. B. H., MANGER F. W., BOXTEL C. VAN & BENTEM N. VAN (1982) Pharmacokinetics of etomidate in patients with liver cirrhosis. *Anaesthesia:* volume of summaries, Sixth European Congress of Anesthesiology, London Abstract **426**, p. 233.

92. VERBEECK R. (1982) Glucuronidation and disposition of drug glucuronides in patients with renal failure. A review. *Drug Metab. Dispos.* **10**, 87.

93. VON BAHR C., GROTH C-G., JANSSON J., LUNDGREN G., LIND M. & GLAUMANN H. (1980) Drug metabolism in human liver *in vitro*: establishment of a human liver bank. *Clin. Pharmacol. Ther.* **27**, 711.

94. WARD S., JUDGE S. & CORALL I. (1982) Pharmacokinetics of pancuronium bromide in liver failure. *Br. J. Anaesth.* **54**, 227P.

95. WESTRA P., VERMEER H. A., DELANGE A. R., SCAF A. H. J., MEIJER D. F. K. & WESSELING H. (1981) Hepatic and renal disposition of pancuronium and galamine in patients with extra-hepatic cholestasis. *Br. J. Anaesth.* **53**, 331.

96. WILKINSON G. R. & SHAND D. G. (1975) A physiological approach to hepatic drug clearance. *Clin. Pharmacol. Ther.* **18**, 377.

97. WILLIAMS R. L., BLASCHKE T. F., MEFFIN P. J., MELMON K. L. & ROWLAND M. (1976) Influence of viral hepatitis on the disposition of two compounds with high hepatic clearance: lidocaine and indocyaine green. *Clin. Pharmacol. Ther.* **20**, 290.

98. WOOD A. J. J., KORNHAUSER D. M., WILKINSON G. R., SHAND D. G. & BRANCH R. A. (1978) The influence of cirrhosis on steady state blood concentrations of unbound propranolol after oral administration. *Clin. Pharmacokin.* **3**, 478.

5 Pharmacokinetics of Inhaled Anaesthetics

W. W. MAPLESON

The way in which inhaled anaesthetics are taken up, distributed and excreted from the body has been extensively studied both experimentally and theoretically, and good agreement obtained between experiment and theory. Unlike the empirical treatment found in some studies of the pharmacokinetics of injected agents, the theory for inhaled anaesthetics is derived directly from the physiology of the body and the physico-chemical properties of the anaesthetic. The theory is now sufficiently far advanced that, given the necessary physiological and physicochemical data, and given a computer to solve the mathematical equations, it can predict reliably what will happen, in pharmacokinetic terms, for almost any specified circumstance. However, although pages of computer-generated graphs may show what to expect in a wide range of circumstances, they do not help the anaesthetist to *understand* what is happening.

Fortunately, the mathematical equations which govern the uptake and distribution of inhaled anaesthetics in the body are, with some reservations, the same as those which govern the movement of water in a system of cylindrical containers interconnected by pipes. Consequently, such a system can be designed to be an analogue of the uptake of inhaled anaesthetics. Then the movement of water in the analogue mimics the movement of anaesthetic in the patient. Accordingiy, the water analogue can be used to visualise what happens to an anaesthetic when it is inhaled, and hence aid in understanding the pharmacokinetics of inhaled anaesthetics.

In this chapter the water analogue is first described and explained, and then used to deduce the general pattern of uptake and distribution and how this varies with time, with inspired tension, with different anaesthetics, with different patients (specifically children and obese patients) and with changes of ventilation and circulation. Normally it is assumed that the anaesthetic is administered from a non-rebreathing system, but the effects of a closed breathing system are also considered.

The water analogue

Fig. 5.1 shows a system of cylindrical containers interconnected by pipes and containing water. Given certain assumptions, the mathematical equations governing the movement of water in the system are identical to those governing the uptake, distribution and elimination of volatile and gaseous anaesthetics in the body. Therefore Fig. 5.1 is an analogue of the pharmacokinetics of such anaesthetics. The nature of the analogy is as follows.

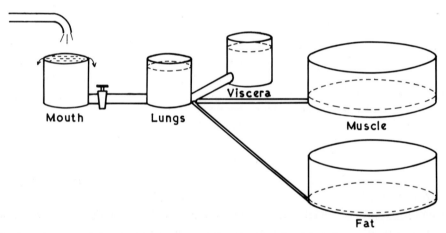

Fig. 5.1   A water analogue of the uptake and distribution of an inhaled anaesthetic from a non-rebreathing anaesthetic breathing system.

The water represents the anaesthetic itself: volume of water corresponding to quantity of anaesthetic vapour. The containers correspond to various groups of organs and tissues and represent the storage capacities of those groups for the anaesthetic. (The groups are often referred to as 'compartments'.) The pipes represent the ability of the ventilation to transport the anaesthetic between the mouth and the lungs and of the circulation to transport it between the lungs and the tissues. Thus the viscera (mainly heart, brain, liver, kidneys and gut) have a small total volume and therefore a small storage capacity, and so are represented by a small container. However, they have a rich blood supply, which is therefore represented by a large pipe. There is a large volume of muscle (and therefore a large container), but this has a poor blood supply at rest (a narrow pipe). There is a moderate volume of fat, but it has a large storage capacity because inhaled anaesthetics are more soluble in fat than in water (hence a large container) and it has a very poor blood supply (a very narrow pipe).

The depth of water in each container represents the partial pressure or tension of anaesthetic in the corresponding organs or tissues. The overflowing container at the mouth represents a constant inspired tension provided by a non-rebreathing anaesthetic breathing system. If the mouth container is imagined to have telescopic sides, it can represent an adjustable inspired tension.

The general pattern of uptake and distribution

When the tap is opened, water flows through the ventilation pipe into the lung container where the level begins to rise; when the vaporiser is turned on, or when the face mask is applied, anaesthetic is conducted by the ventilation to the lungs where the tension begins to rise. As it does so, anaesthetic is conducted on by the circulation to all the tissues of the body. In the case of the viscera the pipe is large and the container small so the tension rises rapidly and nearly keeps pace with the rising tension in the lungs. In the case of the muscle the pipe is small and the container large, so the tension rises slowly and lags far behind that in the lungs. In the case of the fat the latter is true, only more so. Eventually, in the absence of metabolism of the anaesthetic, all the tissues will finally come into equilibrium with the constant inspired tension.

The effect of metabolism

When there is metabolism, this can be represented by punching a hole of appropriate size in the container corresponding to the site of metabolism. Then the system will never reach equilibrium. In addition, the outflow of water from the site of metabolism should form the inflow to another version of the analogue (on a lower shelf) which would model the pharmacokinetics of the metabolite. However, except for trichloroethylene, these effects are small and, given time, the tissues will come very close to equilibrium.

Validation of the water analogue

So far, this account of the water analogue has been only qualitative. However, it should be stressed that, if the analogue was constructed with sufficient accuracy and in such a way as to ensure laminar flow in the pipes (so that the flow through each pipe is proportional to the pressure difference across it), then the analogue would form an accurate quantitative representation of one set of mathematical equations, i.e. of one mathematical model (work by Copperman reported by Kety[15]) of the pharmacokinetics of inhaled anaesthetics. That particular model was the best available in 1951 and the first to give a good fit to experimental data[17]. Subsequently, many refinements to the model have been introduced [3, 7, 8, 11, 13, 21, 23, 25, 27, 33, 35] and some of the refined models, quantified by carefully documented data [1, 4, 19, 23, 24], have been shown to give very close agreement with experimental results obtained in circumstances which severely tested the validity of the theory[2, 5, 25]. However, the refinements have all been in the nature of correction factors and none of them has made a great difference to the results, except perhaps in extreme circumstances. Therefore the water analogue provides a very good approximation to what happens in practice. In addition, it provides an easily understood means of visualising what is happening, and even of deducing what will happen, in various circumstances. Accordingly it is used here to expound the general principles of the pharmacokinetics of inhaled anaesthetics. The general pattern of distribution has already been deduced; now the effects, on that general pattern, of various changes of circumstance will be considered.

Effects of different inspired tensions

Suppose that the inspired tension were half that considered so far. To represent this in the water analogue the height of the 'mouth' container in Fig. 5.1 would need to be halved. Then, at equilibrium, the lung and tissue containers would be only half full. Therefore, only half as much anaesthetic has to be driven into the system; but only half the head of pressure is available to drive it in. Therefore it might be deduced that these two factors of a half would cancel, and that the time to reach equilibrium would be independent of the inspired tension. In fact, because of one of the refinements mentioned above (the 'concentration effect'[9] or 'uptake-ventilation effect'[20]) the approach to equilibrium is rather more rapid at high concentrations than at low, a phenomenon which is not reproduced by the analogue in Fig. 5.1. However, the effect is appreciable only above about 20 % volume/volume concentration and therefore, in modern anaesthetic practice, is virtually confined to nitrous oxide. Even then, the effect is not great and is difficult to explain, so its detailed consideration is deferred until the end of the chapter, where a more elaborate water analogue is described.

Effects of different anaesthetics

The way in which the analogue had to be changed to represent different inspired tensions was simple: the changes needed to represent different anaesthetics are more complex. These changes all stem from the differences in the solubility of different anaesthetics in blood and body tissues. Ostwald solubility coefficients for a range of anaesthetics are given in Table 5.1. They can be summarised qualitatively as follows. Solubility in blood is 'low' for xenon, ethylene, nitrous oxide and cyclopropane, and 'high' for the remainder—fairly high for isoflurane, enflurane and halothane, very high for chloroform, trichloroethylene, methoxyflurane and diethyl ether. Solubility in

Table 5.1 Ostwald solubility coefficients (λ) at 37°C (atm^{-1})[34].

	λ_{blood}
Xenon	0.14
Ethylene	0.15
Nitrous oxide	0.47
Cyclopropane	0.55
Isoflurane	1.4
Enflurane	1.9
Halothane	2.4
Chloroform	8
Trichloroethylene	9
Methoxyflurane	11
Diethyl ether	12

$\lambda_{aqueous\ tissue} = 1-3 \times \lambda_{blood}$
$\lambda_{adipose\ tissue} = 2-70 \times \lambda_{blood}$

aqueous tissues for any given anaesthetic is similar to or rather higher than its solubility in blood. Solubility in adipose tissue is commonly much higher than in blood. The way in which these solubility coefficients influence the shape and size of the water analogue is as follows.

From the quantitative theory of the water analogue[22] it emerges that the cross-sectional area of a container corresponds to the storage capacity of the tissues represented according to the anaesthetic represented. Therefore the cross-sectional area of each container must be proportional to volume of tissue multiplied by the solubility of the anaesthetic in that tissue. The effect of this is shown in Fig. 5.2 which contains two accurately scaled versions of the analogue drawn with the aid of a computer program and graph plotter (see the caption). One version is for nitrous oxide, a low-solubility anaesthetic, the other for halothane, an anaesthetic of fairly high solubility. It can be seen that, with halothane, all the tissue containers are much larger than with nitrous oxide because of the greater solubility of halothane, especially in fat, but that, with both agents, the viscera container is smaller than the one for muscle, because the volume of tissue is less. Moreover an anaesthetic which is more soluble in blood will be more effectively carried by a given blood supply: therefore 'transporting ability', represented by the size of the pipe, is proportional to blood flow multiplied by the solubility of the anaesthetic in the blood. Therefore the pipes representing the blood flow are all larger for the high-solubility halothane than for the low-solubility nitrous oxide; but in both cases the pipes to the viscera, muscle and fat are large, medium and small respectively, because the corresponding blood flows are large, medium and small.

Incidentally, it must be understood that the flow of water through the blood-flow pipes corresponds to the net flow of anaesthetic from lungs to tissues[22], i.e. the flow carried to the tissues in the arterial blood (which is assumed to be in equilibrium with

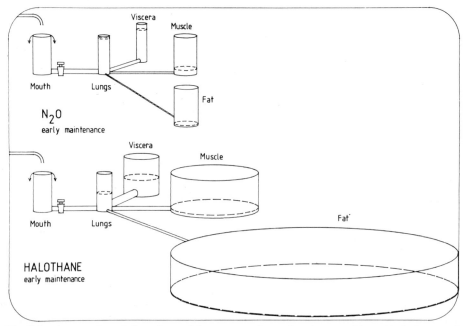

Fig. 5.2   Accurately scaled versions of the water analogue for nitrous oxide and halothane early in maintenance (after 6 min of 75 % nitrous oxide and 20 min of 1 % halothane, both at constant inspired tension). The diagrams were drawn by a graph plotter (Hewlett Packard 9862A) controlled by a minicomputer (Data General Nova 2) using a program written in Fortran by the author with Assembler subroutines by R. T. Chilcoat for driving the plotter. The dimensions are based on the 70 kg standard man[7] with alveolar ventilation and cardiac output slightly depressed by anaesthesia (3.2 and 6.0 litres min^{-1} respectively) and with preferred values for solubility coefficients[34]. The water levels were computed by a separate Fortran program, which corresponded to 'Model O'[23] with the 'concentration effect' included.

alveolar gas) *less* the flow of anaesthetic returned to the lungs from the tissues in the venous blood (which is assumed to be in equilibrium with the tissues drained). Similarly, the flow of water through the ventilation pipe represents the flow of anaesthetic inspired, less that expired.

If a *working*, quantitative analogue were to be constructed, the sizes of the pipes would need to be such that the fourth power of the bore of a pipe was proportional to transporting ability and all pipes would need to be the same length. However, the diagrams in this chapter have been drawn in such a way that the square of the bore is proportional to transporting ability, because this matches the visual differences in the pipe size to the visual differences in container size (where storage capacity is proportional to the square of the diameter). In addition, pipe lengths have been chosen purely on the basis of obtaining a clear, compact picture.

The height of the mouth container is the same in both versions of the analogue in Fig. 5.2 but, to the extent that the time to reach equilibrium is independent of inspired tension, these can represent quite different inspired tensions for the two agents. Bearing this in mind, it can be seen that, in order to achieve equilibrium in the low-solubility case, only a small quantity of anaesthetic (per unit inspired tension) has to go into the system, whereas, in the high-solubility case, a much larger quantity has to go in. The blood-flow pipes are larger (although only proportionately so), but the ventilation pipe is the same size in both cases. Therefore equilibrium takes longer with high-solubility anaesthetics.

However, anaesthetists are not normally concerned with complete equilibrium. They are much more interested in the tension of anaesthetics in the brain and other vital organs. For anaesthetics of both low and high solubility the blood-flow pipe to the viscera is large in relation to the size of the viscera container, therefore the brain tension always follows the lung tension closely. In the low-solubility case the pipes to the muscle and fat containers are small in relation to the ventilation pipe, so that drainage to these containers from the lungs is slow. Therefore the lung tension, and with it the brain tension, can get quite close to equilibrium with the inspired tension long before complete equilibrium has been achieved. This is because a small pressure difference from mouth to alveoli will provide all the inflow to the lungs, through the relatively large ventilation pipe, needed to balance the outflow from the lungs through the narrow pipes to muscle and fat, even in the face of maximal tension differences between the lungs and the muscle and fat. In the high-solubility case, on the other hand, not only is complete equilibrium slow, but also the pipes to the muscle and fat containers are together comparable in size with the ventilation pipe. Therefore the lung tension, and with it the brain tension, is held down, and cannot approach equilibrium until at least the muscle is nearly equilibrated. In other words, the alveolar and arterial tensions, and hence the brain tension, 'float' at about half way between inspired and muscle tensions. And, because the muscle tension takes many hours to approach equilibrium, the lung and brain tensions never approach closely to the inspired tension during any normal duration of anaesthesia.

In the case of an anaesthetic of very high solubility, such as methoxyflurane or ether, the same is even more true: the containers are so large (Fig. 5.3 for methoxyflurane) that equilibration is extremely slow—it takes days or weeks rather than hours[18]. Furthermore, the pipes to muscle and fat are together so large compared to the ventilation pipe that the lung tension remains far below the inspired tension throughout any ordinary duration of anaesthesia. Indeed, Fig. 5.3 may prompt the question of how anaesthesia can ever be induced with an agent of such high solubility? The answer is to use the 'overpressure' technique shown in Fig. 5.4; the inspired tension is made much higher initially than the tension required in the brain for anaesthesia. Having achieved the desired depth of anaesthesia the anaesthetist must, of course, reduce the inspired tension. Furthermore, to maintain a constant arterial and brain tension from then on, the inspired tension must be further and progressively reduced. (This argument also applies in lesser degree to the fairly high-solubility agents halothane and enflurane.)

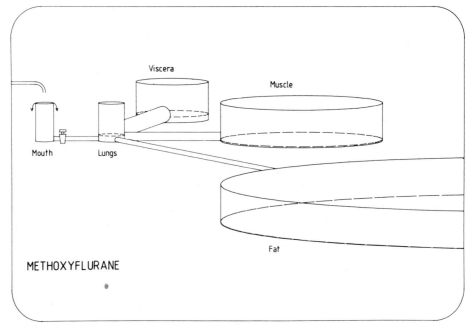

Fig. 5.3   Water analogue for methoxyflurane after 20 min of a constant inspired tension.

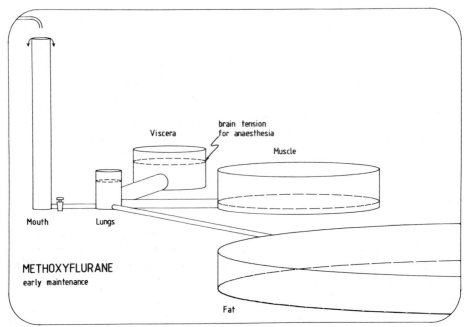

Fig. 5.4   Water analogue for methoxyflurane showing the use of a constant seven-fold 'overpressure' to obtain the desired tension in the brain in 20 min.

In the water analogue of any anaesthetic of very high solubility (chloroform to diethyl ether in Table 5.1) the muscle pipe alone is considerably larger than the ventilation pipe. Therefore, remembering that transporting ability is proportional to the square of the bore in the diagrams, it follows that the transporting ability of the muscle pipe is very much greater, and so the pressure drop from mouth to lungs must always be much more than that from lungs to muscle.

It then follows that quite large percentage changes in lung tension have only a small effect on the pressure difference from mouth to lungs and therefore only a small effect on the rate of inflow of anaesthetic to the body. Therefore inhalation anaesthesia with an agent of very high solubility is more akin pharmacokinetically to intravenous-infusion anaesthesia than to anaesthesia with N_2O or cyclopropane. Thus, it was shown above that, with a low-solubility agent, a change of inspired tension is rapidly followed by an almost equal change in lung and brain tension; in such circumstances the anaesthetist is near to having direct control of brain tension. However, with an agent of very high solubility, because of the 'inertia' of the system, a change of inspired tension produces only a very slow change of lung and brain tension: the only thing which is changed instantaneously is the rate at which anaesthetic is driven into the system—the 'rate of infusion' of the anaesthetic. In fact, with a non-rebreathing anaesthetic breathing system (closed systems are considered below), it is nearly true to say that the 'rate of infusion' of a very high solubility anaesthetic is proportional to inspired concentration multiplied by alveolar ventilation.

Effects of different patients

So far in this chapter it has been implicitly assumed that all patients are alike and unaffected by the anaesthetic. In this section the effects of different sizes and shapes of patients will be considered, in the next, the effects of changes in ventilation and perfusion. It will still be assumed that a non-rebreathing anaesthetic breathing system is used so that the anaesthetist does have direct control of the inspired tension, although not of the brain tension except with low-solubility anaesthetics.

Children

The versions of the water analogue in Figs. 5.2–5.4 and most subsequent figures, have been quantitatively matched to a standard 70 kg man[7]. To match the analogue to a child it must be scaled down in size. However, the containers must be scaled in proportion to body volume and hence to body mass; but the pipes must be scaled in proportion to ventilation and cardiac output, and therefore approximately in proportion to body surface area or to the two-thirds power of body mass. Therefore the pipes are scaled down less than the containers, thereby becoming increased in size relative to the containers. Accordingly it can be deduced that induction will be faster, recovery will be faster, and the response to any change of inspired tension will be faster. Although clinical experience usually accords with the last two of those deductions, many anaesthetists find that induction is slower in children than in adults. Assuming that the comparison is between pure inhalation inductions in both cases and that the premedications are equivalent, there are several possible reasons for this. Firstly, the anaesthetist may use a smaller inspired tension on the basis that the child 'needs less than the adult', but in fact the smaller ventilation and cardiac output will ensure that the child's uptake is less to the appropriate degree for any given inspired tension. Secondly, even if the anaesthetist does use the same inspired tension as in the adult, MAC[10, 26] for the child (effectively the brain tension, in per cent of a standard atmosphere, needed to produce surgical anaesthesia in 50 % of the population) is greater[14] than in the adult. Finally, other reasons may occur to the reader after studying the section below on the effect of changes of ventilation and circulation on induction.

Obese patients

The most obvious characteristic of obese patients is that they have more body fat than normal (Fig. 5.5 for halothane) but this, of itself, has remarkably little effect. This is because, even in the normal patient, the storage capacity of the fat compartment for high-solubility anaesthetics is already so large that fat tension is low throughout any ordinary duration of anaesthesia. However, the blood flow to fat is also increased, although less than in proportion to the volume of fat[16], and commonly ventilation is reduced. Therefore the inflow to the lungs is decreased, the outflow is increased, lung tension and brain tension rise more slowly, and induction is slower. Furthermore, during maintenance, the lung tension will 'float' at a smaller fraction of the inspired tension so that either anaesthesia will be lighter or a higher inspired tension must be used. Measurements in patients[31] showed that end-tidal tensions of halothane were a smaller fraction of inspired tension during maintenance in obese patients, although not to a statistically significant degree.

If the inspired tension is indeed adjusted to maintain the same lung tension as in a normal patient, then, at the end of two hours' anaesthesia, the lung, viscera and muscle tensions will be the same in both cases, but there will be a greater quantity (but somewhat lower tension) of anaesthetic in the fat compartment of the obese patient. Therefore recovery will start from essentially the same conditions in both cases, but in the obese patient the greater blood flow to fat will speed up recovery by aiding redistribution, while the reduced ventilation will slow it down. However, the increase in the size of the fat pipe is greater than the decrease in size of the ventilation pipe, so, at first, the speeding up effect can be expected to dominate. Later, as the lung tension falls and fat tension rises, the speeding up effect of the increased blood flow to fat will be dominated by the slowing down effect of the decreased ventilation and late stages of recovery will be prolonged. Qualitatively this is in agreement with the observations of

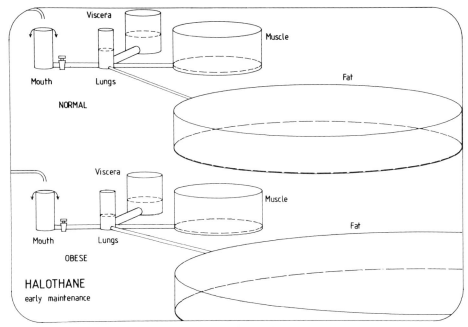

Fig. 5.5 Water analogue for halothane in the standard 70 kg ('normal') (as in all other versions of this chapter) and in a patient whose lean tissues are the same as in the standard man but whose adipose tissue is increased until it forms 45 % of the increased total body mass ('obese'). This leads to a consequent increase in cardiac output of 0.42 litre min^{-1}[16], increase in blood volume of 0.85 litre[7], and decrease in alveolar ventilation of 0.54 litre min^{-1}[31]. As a result, total body mass is 106.6 kg, cardiac output 6.42 litres min^{-1}, and alveolar ventilation 2.66 litres min^{-1}.

Saraiva *et al.*[31] but a quantitative comparison (unpublished work by the author) shows a discrepancy which could well be explained by direct diffusion of anaesthetic into fat from adjacent tissues[24, 29] independently of the blood supply to the fat.

Effects of changes of ventilation and circulation

Induction

During induction the objective is to raise the tension of anaesthetic in the brain to the desired level, usually as quickly as is conveniently possible. To understand how the attainment of this objective may be influenced by changes of ventilation and circulation, it is necessary to use a more elaborate version of the water analogue, with a separate compartment for the brain (Fig. 5.6 for nitrous oxide and halothane). From this it can be seen that, in order to deliver anaesthetic to the brain quickly, what is needed is a large ventilation and a large blood supply to the brain. Therefore anything which increases these will increase the speed of induction. This, of course, is the

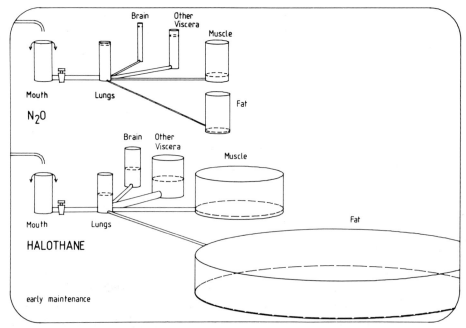

Fig. 5.6 Water analogues for nitrous oxide and halothane early in maintenance, as in Fig. 5.2 but with a separate compartment for the brain.

rationale of the classic teaching of administering CO_2 during an ether induction: this increases the arterial tension of CO_2, which in turn increases the ventilation and increases the blood flow to the brain. The need for this artificial acceleration of induction is probably greatest with ether because, not only does its very high solubility lead to an inherently slow rise in brain tension, but also this cannot be fully compensated by 'overpressure' because of the physical characteristics of diethyl ether. The mechanism of this acceleration of induction by CO_2 inhalation applies in some degree to anaesthetics of all solubilities; but those of lower solubility produce inherently more rapid induction, so that the incentive to accelerate it is usually lacking—especially since, in current clinical practice, the inhaled anaesthetic is normally required only to 'take over' as the intravenous induction agent wears off. Therefore it is particularly interesting to find as recently as 1975 [6] a recommendation to use CO_2 to accelerate induction with nitrous oxide and halothane in dental anaesthesia.

It can also be deduced from Fig. 5.6 that any reduction in the blood flow to compartments other than the brain will reduce the drainage of anaesthetic from the lungs, thereby allowing the tension there to rise more rapidly and the brain tension to follow it up. Therefore, if the patient is in a low-cardiac-output state, but the brain blood flow is preferentially maintained, induction will be faster. Conversely, in a high-cardiac-output state, induction may be prolonged. This argument, like that of CO_2 inhalation, applies to anaesthetics of all solubilities, although the effect is more marked the higher the solubility.

Maintenance

The effects of changes of ventilation and circulation during maintenance are much more dependent on solubility. Thus, with a low-solubility anaesthetic (e.g. N_2O, in Fig. 5.6) the pipes to muscle and fat are so small compared to the ventilation pipe that the lung, brain and other-viscera tensions are close to the inspired tension from early in maintenance onwards. Therefore even halving or doubling of the transporting abilities of these pipes would have little effect on brain tension. Complete respiratory arrest would lead to a slow fall in brain tension as the lung, brain and other-viscera containers slowly emptied into muscle and fat; but it seems unlikely that the patient would become aware before the anaesthetist restored ventilation.

On the other hand, in the case of agents of fairly high solubility (e.g. halothane, in the lower half of Fig. 5.6) or of very high solubility (e.g. methoxyflurane, Fig. 5.4) the lung and brain tensions float at a 'balance' level, somewhere between the inspired tension and the muscle and fat tensions, such that inflow of anaesthetic to the lungs from the mouth is equal to outflow to the tissues. Therefore any change in the sizes of the pipes concerned will alter inflow or outflow and upset the balance. For instance, if the ventilation increases, the inflow to the lungs is increased, so the lung tension rises until a new balance level is reached and the brain tension follows the lung tension upwards, so that anaesthesia is deepened. Conversely, if the ventilation decreases, the brain tension falls and anaesthesia is lightened. Thus, so long as the patient is breathing spontaneously, this operates as a negative-feedback or safety system, protecting the patient, to some extent, from inappropriate inspired tensions. However, if the patient's ventilation is controlled, this negative-feedback system is no longer operative; ventilation is unaffected by deepening anaesthesia. In these circumstances any reduction in cardiac output reduces the drainage from the lungs so that the lung tension rises towards the mouth tension. Usually the blood flow to the brain is well maintained in the face of falling cardiac output, but, even if it falls in the same proportion as cardiac output, immediately prior to the drop in cardiac output the brain tension would have been close to the lung tension. Therefore, when the lung tension rises the brain tension follows it upwards, even if more slowly than normally. Therefore, a reduction in cardiac output leads to a deepening of anaesthesia, and probably also to an increase in tension in the heart as well, and therefore quite possibly to a further fall in circulation and a further rise in tension. In other words, there is now a positive-feedback system or 'danger system' in which, in extreme circumstances, the condition of the patient may deteriorate to the point of cardiac arrest—unless the inspired tension is reduced.

Closed breathing systems

Throughout this chapter so far it has been assumed that the anaesthetic was administered from a non-rebreathing system. When a closed breathing system is used the process of uptake and distribution is greatly altered. To understand this the breathing system must be incorporated in the water analogue. One example will be considered here: a totally closed anaesthetic breathing system with the vaporiser outside the breathing system. The water analogue of this is shown in Fig. 5.7. The container which was previously labelled 'mouth' now corresponds to the breathing system, the tension in which depends on a balance of inflow and outflow. Since the system is totally closed, the only outflow is to the lungs, by virtue of the uptake by the patient. The inflow is the anaesthetic in the fresh-gas flow, and this inflow is equal to the vaporiser tension, represented by the constant head of pressure in the vaporiser container, multiplied by the fresh-gas flow, represented by the size of the very small 'basal fresh-gas flow' pipe. The analogue makes it clear that, in a totally closed system, the anaesthetist has no direct control even of inspired tension (let alone brain tension), indeed he does not even have any direct *knowledge* of the inspired tension unless he measures it or calculates it. In these circumstances, the rate of inflow is totally

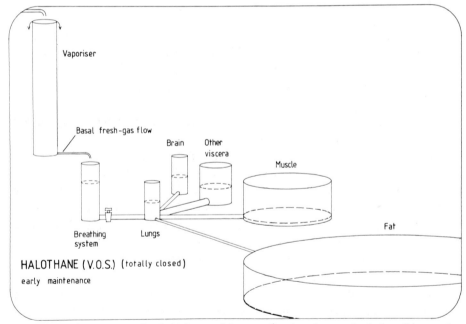

Fig. 5.7 Water analogue for halothane with a totally closed anaesthetic breathing system (vaporiser outside the breathing system) early in maintenance (i.e. after 20 min during which the vaporiser tension has been varied in such a way as to maintain the inspired tension constant). Note that all other versions of the water analogue in this chapter are for a non-rebreathing anaesthetic system.

unaffected by changes of lung or even inspired tension; therefore what the anaesthetist does control is the rate of inflow of anaesthetic and, apart from transient differences, the rate of uptake must equal this inflow, since there is nowhere else for it to go. Accordingly, a totally closed breathing system, with almost any anaesthetic, makes an even closer pharmacokinetic parallel to an intravenous infusion than does an anaesthetic of very high solubility in a non-rebreathing system.

In particular, if the ventilation decreases, there will be only a temporary drop in uptake, because anaesthetic will accumulate in the breathing system until the inspired tension is high enough to make outflow (uptake by the patient) again equal to inflow. Therefore changes of ventilation have no permanent effect on lung and brain tension and the 'safety mechanism' described above (of depressed ventilation with a non-rebreathing system leading to reduced lung and brain tension) no longer operates.

If the cardiac output falls, then again there can be only a transient fall in rate of uptake. The increase in lung tension which follows from the decrease in cardiac output leads in turn to a rise in inspired tension and hence a greater eventual rise in lung and brain tensions than with the fixed inspired tension of the non-rebreathing system. In other words, the 'danger mechanism' is even more active.

Recovery from anaesthesia

For recovery the inspired tension is reduced to zero. Then, with the low-solubility anaesthetics, just as the approach to equilibrium is rapid at induction, so it is in recovery, which is therefore rapid. Conversely, with the high-solubility anaesthetics, just as the approach is slow at induction, so it is in recovery, and recovery is slow. Furthermore, during recovery from a high-solubility anaesthetic there is no equivalent to raising the inspired tension to a high level—the best that can be done is to ensure that the inspired tension is reduced fully to zero.

If the process of elimination is examined more closely it is possible to distinguish two phases of recovery. For instance, in the case of halothane it was explained above how, during maintenance, the lung tension 'floated' about half way between the inspired and muscle tensions—such that inflow was equal to outflow. Fig. 5.8 (lower diagram) shows the water levels (upper pecked lines) after two hours of halothane anaesthesia: the muscle is about half way to equilibrium, so the lungs, brain and other viscera are about three-quarters of the way there—although the fat tension is still hardly distinguishable from zero.

During recovery the lung, brain and other-viscera tensions 'float' in exactly the same way: when the inspired tension is reduced to zero (the mouth container in Fig. 5.8 is removed) the lung tension falls fairly rapidly, and the brain and other viscera tensions follow it down, until a new 'floating' level (lower pecked lines) is reached somewhere between the new, zero, inspired tension and the muscle tension. Thus there is a first phase of recovery which is relatively rapid, but which is only partial.

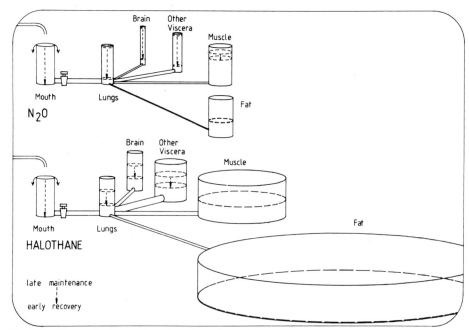

Fig. 5.8 Water analogues for nitrous oxide and for halothane, each from a non-rebreathing anaesthetic system. The upper water levels are for 'late maintenance', i.e. after the inspired tension has been constant for 1 hour in the case of nitrous oxide and 2 hours for halothane. The lower levels are for 'early recovery', i.e. after a further 10 min in both cases with zero inspired tension (mouth container removed).

Thereafter, any further fall in lung and brain tensions must wait on the slow fall in muscle tension; therefore the second phase, full recovery, is a much slower process.

With a low-solubility agent the lung, brain and other-viscera tensions can still be thought of as 'floating' but always close to the inspired tension. Thus, after one hour of nitrous oxide anaesthesia, (Fig. 5.8, upper diagram, upper water levels) they are very close to the inspired tension, because the muscle is then nearly equilibrated, and even the fat is almost half way to equilibrium; during recovery (Fig. 5.8, lower water levels in the upper diagram, mouth container removed) the lung tension falls rapidly to a level very close to zero and the brain tension follows it down rapidly, so that even the first, rapid phase of recovery is almost complete, even though there is still a high tension of anaesthetic in the muscle and fat.

At the other extreme, with an agent of very high solubility (Fig. 5.9, methoxyflurane) the lung, brain and other-viscera tensions are closely 'tied' to the muscle tension by the large muscle–blood-flow pipe. Therefore when, after two hours' maintenance at constant lung tension (upper water levels), the inspired tension is reduced to zero (mouth container removed), the lung, brain and other viscera tensions fall only from a little above the muscle tension to a little below (lower water levels). In

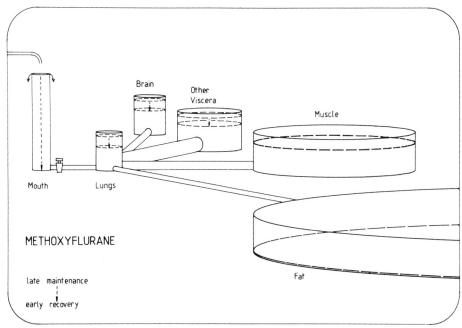

Fig. 5.9 Water analogue for methoxyflurane in late maintenance (upper water levels), i.e. after 2 hours in which the inspired tension has been controlled in such a way as to maintain an approximately constant lung tension, and in early recovery (lower water levels), i.e. after a further 10 min, with zero inspired tension.

other words, the initial rapid phase of recovery is only very small in extent; the second phase, full recovery, with the brain tension almost down to zero, must wait on the emptying of the muscle compartment which, with agents of very high solubility, is a very slow process indeed.

The remedy usually proposed for hastening recovery is hyperventilation: increasing the size of the ventilation pipe in Figs 5.8 and 5.9 after the inspired tension has been reduced to zero. This will undoubtedly accelerate the first phase of recovery, but if recovery is slow and this is not expected, hyperventilation may not be instituted until some minutes have passed. By that time the lung and brain tensions may have nearly reached their new 'floating' levels. If so, by increasing outflow from the lungs, hyperventilation will certainly reduce the 'floating' levels of the lung and brain tensions for as long as it is maintained, and anaesthesia will certainly lighten. However, if the hyperventilation is maintained for only a few minutes, this is too short a time to have any appreciable effect on the muscle tension and the long-term progress of recovery will hardly be affected. Therefore, when the hyperventilation is stopped (the ventilation pipe diminishes in size again) the lung and brain tensions will, at the very least, fall more slowly than otherwise, perhaps cease to fall altogether for a while and, in extreme cases, may actually rise again—particularly if the hyperventilation has reduced arterial CO_2 tension, and subsequent spontaneous ventilation is less than before. (These conclusions, derived qualitatively from the water analogue, have been checked quantitatively by computation.) Thus, with all high-solubility anaesthetics there is some risk of reanaesthetisation after hyperventilation.

The concentration effect and second-gas effect

Finally, the difficult question of why the approach to equilibrium is rather more rapid at high volume/volume inspired concentrations than at low, i.e. the question of how the 'concentration effect' arises, must be considered. The reason why the water analogue does not faithfully represent the concentration effect lies in the fact that there are two aspects to uptake from the lungs into the blood. One aspect is the removal of molecules of anaesthetic from the lungs by solution: this is faithfully reproduced in the water analogue by the flow of water away from the lung container into the tissue containers, thereby slowing down the rise of the water level in the lung container compared to that for a totally insoluble agent. The other aspect of uptake is the removal of *gas volume* from the lungs (which is an inseparable corollary of the removal of molecules of anaesthetic) and this is not represented in the water analogue.

At low concentrations the rate of gas volume removal is only a few tens of millilitres per minute, but with nitrous oxide inspired at 80 volumes per cent, it can be of the order of $1\,l\,min^{-1}$ in the first few minutes. Then, by the law of conservation of matter, one of three things must happen. One possibility is that the functional residual capacity (FRC) of the lungs decreases. In the water analogue this would be represented by the cross-sectional area of the lung container diminishing without any change in the volume of water in it and therefore with an increase in the *depth* of water (anaesthetic tension) within it, and hence a more rapid uptake into the tissues, but less rapid inflow from the mouth. The net result would be a slightly more rapid approach to equilibrium because, in the end, less anaesthetic would be stored in the lungs. However, although FRC commonly does decrease during induction this occurs with many different anaesthetics, including even non-inhaled ones[28]. Therefore, although a fall in FRC will accelerate the approach to equilibrium, there is no sound reason to expect the rate of fall, and hence the degree of acceleration, to be closely associated with inspired concentration—as it would be if the fall in FRC were solely *due* to the removal of gas volume. One study[32] appeared to give support to such an association, although an alternative explanation of the results has been given[30]. Of course, an FRC of 3 litres cannot decrease at the rate of $1\,l\,min^{-1}$ for long!

The second possibility is that the patient will expire less volume in each breath, so as to maintain the FRC constant. The third possibility is that the patient will inspire more volume in each breath in order both to maintain the FRC and to maintain a normal expired ventilation, so that CO_2 washout is not diminished. The second possibility is equivalent to the third coupled with a reduction in ventilation, so only the third possibility will be considered here.

In the water analogue the flow of water through the ventilation pipe represents the net effect of the flow of anaesthetic from mouth to lungs in the inspired ventilation, less the flow out in the expired ventilation, the inspired and expired ventilations being assumed equal. Make these equal inspired and expired ventilations, represented by the pipe, equal to the normal ventilation that would occur with a low inspired concentration. Then, at high concentrations, there is an additional inspired-only ventilation which brings anaesthetic into the lungs at the inspired tension, but which does not go back out of the lungs. This can be represented (Fig. 5.10) by a second constant-head device, producing the same tension as at the mouth, but set on a higher plane than the rest of the analogue (like the vaporiser container in the analogue of the closed breathing system) and discharging through a narrow pipe directly into the lung container. The transporting ability of this pipe (representing the inspired-only ventilation) would need to be continuously matched to the rate of gas volume removal from the lungs, which would be proportional to the rate of flow of water from the lungs to the tissues. However, it must be remembered that the water flow represents millilitres of anaesthetic vapour per minute *per unit inspired tension of anaesthetic*, whereas the

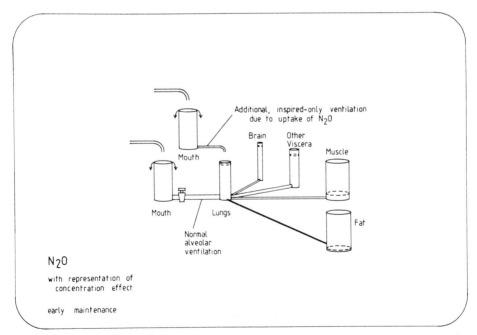

Fig. 5.10 Water analogue of nitrous oxide, incorporating a representation of the concentration effect, after 5 min of 75 %: rate of uptake by solution, and therefore excess of inspired ventilation over expired ventilation ('additional, inspired-only ventilation'), is then equal to 0.5 litre min^{-1}.

transporting ability of the inspired-only ventilation pipe must be proportional to absolute uptake in ml min^{-1}.

Such a model, with an automatically adjusting pipe diameter, would be complex to construct, but its action is relatively easy to imagine, at least qualitatively. Thus, it was shown in the main part of this chapter that a single height of mouth container could correspond to any inspired tension and that this appeared to lead to the conclusion that the rate of approach to equilibrium was independent of the inspired tension. However, it can now be seen that, as the inspired volume/volume concentration is increased (comparing one induction with another), the volume uptake increases and therefore the size of inspired-only ventilation pipe increases—from a negligible size to one which, for 75 % nitrous oxide, represents about a quarter of the transporting ability of that of the main ventilation pipe (which strictly represents the *alveolar* ventilation of about 4 l min^{-1}). From this it is clear that the approach to equilibrium will be appreciably faster at high concentration than at low. In the limit, with 100 % nitrous oxide inspired, the gas volume which was removed from the lungs by solution, would be replaced by pure nitrous oxide, i.e. it would be fully replaced. Therefore the lung tension would rise in the same way as if it were purely a matter of lung washout, with no loss by solution in the blood, i.e. as if (so far as lung tension is concerned) the nitrous oxide were completely insoluble in blood.

The magnitude of the concentration effect can be minimised by saying that, according to computation for a standard man [21], the alveolar tension of nitrous oxide is 15 % closer to equilibrium (95 % as against 80 %) after 5 min of 75 % than after 5 min of 1 %; or it can be maximised by saying that it takes three times as long to reach 80 % of equilibrium with 1 % instead of 75 % nitrous oxide (5 min instead of 1.5 min). However, to the clinical anaesthetist, the striking difference would be that one patient would be anaesthetised and the other wide-awake. The one type of comparison which is of clinical importance in induction is that, if 80 % nitrous oxide is used for induction at normal atmospheric pressure, then 40 % nitrous oxide in a pressure chamber at 2 atmospheres, although it would give the same inspired tension of about 80 kPa, would give a slightly slower induction because of the lesser degree of concentration effect.

An interesting corollary of the concentration effect arises when two anaesthetics are administered together, say halothane and nitrous oxide. To represent this circumstance two water analogues would be required, one for each agent, and each with an additional overflowing 'mouth' container and inspiration-only ventilation pipe, discharging directly into the lungs container. The height of the additional container would be the same as the main mouth container in each case, i.e. proportional to the inspired tension of the agent represented, but the size of the inspired-only ventilation pipe must be proportional to the *total* rate of gas volume uptake (nitrous oxide plus halothane) and therefore would be the same in both cases. Since the volume rate of uptake of nitrous oxide is much greater than that of halothane at clinical concentrations, the effect essentially is that the uptake of nitrous oxide engenders an additional inflow of inspired mixture, containing halothane and nitrous oxide, enhancing the uptake of halothane. This effect of the uptake of one agent, which itself is subject to a noticeable concentration effect on the uptake of another, which is not, has been called the 'second gas effect'[12]. As with the concentration effect, its magnitude[21] can be minimised by saying that after 5 min of halothane the alveolar tension will be 6% closer (40% against 34%) to equilibrium with the inspired tension, if it is carried in 75% nitrous oxide, than if it is carried in oxygen or air; or it can be maximised by saying that it takes more than twice as long (5 min against 2.3 min) to reach 30% of equilibrium if the halothane is carried in air or oxygen rather than 75% nitrous oxide. However, in terms of induction of anaesthesia, this small difference in speed of approach to equilibrium would be swamped by the difference between the presence and absence of 75% nitrous oxide.

Conclusions

This chapter has shown that the water analogue is a help in understanding the pharmacokinetics of inhaled anaesthetics and in making qualitative deductions for a wide variety of circumstances. However, a warning must be given that, when qualitative deduction reveals two mechanisms acting in opposite directions, it may be impossible to deduce even the direction of the net effect. Then quantitative theory, or experiment, or clinical observation is essential.

REFERENCES

1. ALLOTT P. R., STEWARD A., FLOOK V. & MAPLESON W. W. (1973) Variation with temperature of the solubilities of inhaled anaesthetics in water, oil and biological media. *Br. J. Anaesth.* **45**, 294–300.
2. ALLOTT P. R., STEWARD A. & MAPLESON W. W. (1976) Pharmacokinetics of halothane in the dog; comparison of theory and measurement in individuals. *Br. J. Anaesth.* **48**, 279–95.
3. ASHMAN M. N., BLESSER W. B. & EPSTEIN R. M. (1970) A nonlinear model for the uptake and distribution of halothane in man. *Anesthesiology* **33**, 419–29.
4. COWLES A. L., BORGSTEDT H. H. & GILLIES A. J. (1971) Tissue weights and rates of blood flow in man for the prediction of anesthetic uptake and distribution. *Anesthesiology* **35**, 523–6.

5. COWLES A. L., BORGSTEDT H. H. & GILLIES A. J. (1972) The uptake and distribution of four inhalation anesthetics in dogs. *Anesthesiology* **36**, 558–70.
6. DAVIES J., BURNS T. H. S. & BRACKEN A. (1975) Use of Entonox plus carbon dioxide in the dental surgery. *Br. J. Anaesth.* **47**, 603–6.
7. DAVIS N. R. & MAPLESON W. W. (1981) Structure and quantification of a physiological model of the distribution of injected agents and inhaled anaesthetics. *Br. J. Anaesth.* **53**, 399–405.
8. EGER E. I., II (1963a) A mathematical model of uptake and distribution. In Papper E. M. & Kitz R. J. (eds.), *Uptake and Distribution of Anesthetic Agents*, pp. 72–87. McGraw-Hill, New York.

9. EGER E. I., II (1963b) Applications of a mathematical model of gas uptake. In Papper E. M. & Kitz R. J. (eds.), *Uptake and Distribution of Anesthetic Agents*, pp. 88–103. McGraw-Hill, New York.

10. EGER E. I., II (1974) *Anesthetic Uptake and Action*, p. 1. Williams and Wilkins, Baltimore, Maryland.

11. EPSTEIN R. M. (1968) Theoretical analysis of the effect of concentration-dependent solubility upon the uptake of anesthetic agents. *Anesthesiology* **29**, 187–8.

12. EPSTEIN R. M., RACKOW H., SALANITRE E. & WOLF G. L. (1964) Influence of the concentration effect on the uptake of anesthetic mixtures: the second gas effect. *Anesthesiology* **25**, 364–71.

13. FUKUI Y. & SMITH N. T. (1981) Interactions among ventilation, the circulation, and the uptake and distribution of halothane – use of a hybrid computer multiple model. *Anesthesiology* **54**, 107–24.

14. GREGORY G. A., EGER E. I., II & MUNSON E. S. (1969) The relationship between age and halothane requirement in man. *Anesthesiology* **30**, 488–91.

15. KETY S. S. (1951) Theory and applications of the exchange of inert gas at the lungs and tissues. *Pharmacol. Rev.* **3**, 1–41.

16. LESSER G. T. & DEUTSCH S. (1967) Measurement of adipose tissue blood flow and perfusion in man by uptake of ^{85}Kr. *J. Appl. Physiol.* **23**, 621–30.

17. MAPLESON W. W. (1962) The rate of uptake of halothane vapour in man. *Br. J. Anaesth.* **34**, 11–18.

18. MAPLESON W. W. (1963a) Quantitative prediction of anesthetic concentrations. In Papper E. M. & Kitz R. J. (eds.), *Uptake and Distribution of Anesthetic Agents*, pp. 104–19. McGraw-Hill, New York.

19. MAPLESON W. W. (1963b) An electric analogue for uptake and exchange of inert gases and other agents. *J. Appl. Physiol.* **18**, 197–204.

20. MAPLESON W. W. (1964a) Mathematical aspects of the uptake, distribution and elimination of inhaled gases and vapours. *Br. J. Anaesth.* **36**, 129–39.

21. MAPLESON W. W. (1964b) Inert gas-exchange theory using an electric analogue. *J. Appl. Physiol.* **19**, 1193–99.

22. MAPLESON W. W. (1972) Kinetics. In Chenoweth M. B. (ed.), *Modern Inhalation Anesthetics* (Vol 30 of the *Handbook of Experimental Pharmacology*), pp. 326–44. Springer-Verlag, Berlin.

23. MAPLESON W. W. (1973) Circulation-time models of the uptake of inhaled anaesthetics and data for quantifying them. *Br. J. Anaesth.* **45**, 319–34 and **50** (1978) 731.

24. MAPLESON W. W. (1977) Diffusion in relation to the distribution of inhaled anaesthetics in the body. *Bull. Inst. Math. Appl.* **13**, 8–12.

25. MAPLESON W. W., SMITH W. D. A., SIEBOLD K., HARGREAVES M. D. & CLARKE G. M. (1974) Nitrous oxide anaesthesia induced at atmospheric and hyperbaric pressures. Part II: Comparison of measured and theoretical pharmacokinetic data. *Br. J. Anaesth.* **46**, 13–28.

26. MERKEL G. & EGER E. I., II (1963) A comparative study of halothane and halopropane anesthesia. *Anesthesiology* **24**, 346–57.

27. MUNSON E. S., EGER E. I., II & BOWERS D. L. (1973) Effects of anesthetic-depressed ventilation and cardiac output on anesthetic uptake: a computer non-linear simulation. *Anesthesiology* **38**, 251–9.

28. NUNN J. F. (1977) *Applied Respiratory Physiology*, 2nd edition, p. 66. Butterworths, London.

29. PERL W. (1963) Large-scale diffusion between body compartments. In Papper E. M. & Kitz R. J. (eds.), *Uptake and Distribution of Anesthetic Agents*, pp. 224–7. McGraw-Hill, New York.

30. REHDER K., SESSLER A. D. & MARSH H. M. (1975) General anesthesia and the lung. *Am. Rev. Resp. Dis.* **112**, 541–63.
31. SARAIVA R. A., LUNN J. N., MAPLESON W. W., WILLIS B. A. & FRANCE J. M. (1977) Adiposity and the pharmacokinetics of halothane. *Anaesthesia* **32**, 240–6.
32. SHAH J., JONES J. G., GALVIN J. & TOMLIN P. J. (1971) Pulmonary gas exchange during induction of anaesthesia with nitrous oxide in seated subjects. *Br. J. Anaesth.* **43**, 1013–21.
33. SMITH N. T., ZWART A. & BENEKEN J. E. W. (1972) Interaction between the circulatory effects and the uptake and distribution of halothane: use of a multiple model. *Anesthesiology* **37**, 47–58.
34. STEWARD A., ALLOTT P. R., COWLES A. L. & MAPLESON W. W. (1973) Solubility coefficients for inhaled anaesthetics for water, oil and biological media. *Br. J. Anaesth.* **45**, 282–93.
35. ZWART A., SMITH N. T. & BENEKEN J. E. W. (1972) Multiple model approach to uptake and distribution of halothane: the use of an analog computer. *Computers and Biomedical Res.* **5**, 228–38.

6 Pharmacokinetics of Barbiturates

DONALD R. STANSKI

THIOPENTONE PHARMACOKINETICS AND PHARMACODYNAMICS
Thiopentone pharmacokinetics
Thiopentone pharmacodynamics
Thiopentone pharmacokinetics in disease states

METHOHEXITONE PHARMACOKINETICS

HEXOBARBITONE PHARMACOKINETICS

PENTOBARBITONE PHARMACOKINETICS

GLOSSARY

Of the numerous barbiturates that are available, only thiopentone, thiamylal, methohexitone, hexobarbitone and pentobarbitone have significant use in clinical anaesthesia. Because the pharmacological properties of thiamylal are virtually identical to those of thiopentone and there is minimal pharmacokinetic data for it, thiamylal will not be discussed in this chapter. Thiopentone, methohexitone and hexobarbitone are extensively used to induce and to maintain anaesthesia. Although pentobarbitone is not useful to induce anaesthesia, it is a pharmacologically active metabolite of thiopentone and it has been used for premedication and as an anaesthetic supplement. Thiopentone, methohexitone, and pentobarbitone represent a spectrum of pharmacokinetic properties that will be compared and contrasted in this chapter. The pharmacokinetics of these barbiturates will be related to their clinical effects in anaesthesia. The small amount of pharmacokinetic data available for hexobarbitone will be included.

THIOPENTONE PHARMACOKINETICS AND DYNAMICS

Thiopentone pharmacokinetics

Distribution kinetics and terminal elimination half-life

From the introduction of thiopentone into clinical anaesthesia in 1936 until 1950, the short duration of thiopentone's anaesthetic effect was attributed to its rapid elimination from the body[27]. With the development of a specific spectrophotometric assay, Brodie *et al.*[12] found the elimination half-life after an intravenous bolus dose to be 4.6 h, much too long to account for the short effect. These same investigators later demonstrated that high cerebral blood flow and lipid solubility resulted in rapid thiopentone penetration into the central nervous system[11]. Rapid recovery from thiopentone was attributed to redistribution from the brain to body fat, which has a high capacity to store thiopentone, but a much lower blood flow than the central nervous system[9]. Thiopentone was one of the first drugs for which a redistribution mechanism for termination of the pharmacological effect was demonstrated. Thus pharmacokinetic analysis was instrumental in understanding the clinical behaviour of the drug.

While Brodie *et al.*[12] were correct in determining the relatively long elimination half-life of thiopentone, the limitations of their assay sensitivity and sampling duration prevented them from gathering data accurate enough to form a complete picture of thiopentone's distribution and elimination. Subsequent pharmacokinetic research with more sensitive assays and frequent sampling has allowed a more complete understanding of thiopentone kinetics[14, 24, 36].

Fig. 6.1 displays the thiopentone plasma concentration vs. time relationship obtained after an intravenous injection of thiopentone. The plasma decay curve of

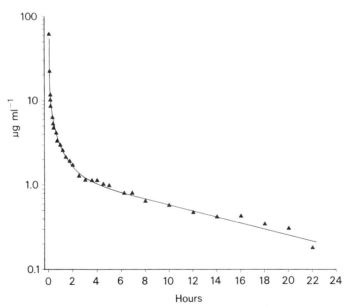

Fig. 6.1 The log plasma concentration vs. time data from a single patient given thiopentone $6.4\,\mathrm{mg\,kg^{-1}}$ as a two minute infusion. Solid line represents the triexponential equation determined by nonlinear regression. The triangles represent the measured thiopentone plasma concentrations in plasma. Adapted with permission of the publisher and authors[47].

thiopentone can be characterised by a triexponential equation interpreted as a three-compartment pharmacokinetic model. Table 6.1 details the available thiopentone pharmacokinetic studies obtained in healthy surgical patients or volunteers. The induction of anaesthesia within seconds of administering a bolus intravenous injection of thiopentone suggests that the brain is most likely within or extremely close to the central compartment. This is expected because the central compartment is composed of the vessel-rich tissues, such as the brain.

Peak plasma concentrations of thiopentone are achieved within one circulation time after a bolus intravenous injection. Two distribution phases commence simultaneously. The rapid distribution half-life ranges from 2 to 4 min, while the slow distribution half-life is 45–60 min. The rapid distribution phase most likely represents equilibration of the vessel-rich tissues of the central compartment, with a less rapidly equilibrating, shallow compartment (possibly skeletal muscle or lean tissues). It is during this phase that awakening from the thiopentone anaesthesia will occur after a single dose of moderate size.

After 4–5 rapid distribution half-lives (12–17 min), the slow distribution phase becomes predominant. This phase represents the equilibration of the central and shallow compartment with a deeper, more slowly equilibrating compartment (possibly fat). Equilibration of tissues equilibrating slowly with plasma requires 2–4 h before the terminal elimination phase becomes obvious. It is possible to speculate on the tissues that make up the peripheral compartments only because of our extensive understanding of the tissue distribution of thiopentone obtained from the physiological models of thiopentone disposition. These will be discussed later.

In order to determine the terminal elimination half-life of thiopentone, accurately blood samples must be taken for at least 24 h. Two studies with this sampling duration have found the terminal elimination half-life to be 10–12 h[14, 36]. The less extensive blood sampling study performed by Brodie *et al.*[10] and Ghoneim and Van Hamme[24] led them to underestimate the thiopentone terminal elimination half-life at 4–6 h.

The terminal elimination half-life of 10–12 h is only applicable to thiopentone doses up to 2 g. As will be discussed later, a larger dose of thiopentone may result in dose-dependent elimination. In dose-dependent kinetics, as the thiopentone dose increases the terminal elimination half-life also increases. Thiopentone's elimination half-life is larger than methohexitone's and smaller than that of pentobarbitone (Table 6.1).

Clearance

The terminal elimination half-life of a drug is determined by the two primary pharmacokinetic variables, clearance and volume of distribution at steady state. Thiopentone clearance from the body is almost exclusively due to hepatic metabolism.

Table 6.1 Barbiturate pharmacokinetics.

Drug	Distribution half-lives (min)	Elimination half-life (h)	Clearance (ml kg^{-1} min^{-1})	V_D^{ss}* (1 kg^{-1})	Data source
Thiopentone	2.4–3.3 (rapid) 47.0 (slow)	5.1–11.5	1.6 – 4.3	1.5 –3.3	[13, 24, 36]
Methohexitone	4.8–6.2 (rapid) 60.0 (slow)	1.5– 4.0	9.9–12.1	1.13–2.1	[6, 28]
Hexobarbitone		4.3– 5.5	3.3 –3.6	1.07–1.25	[7, 8, 41, 49]
Pentobarbitone	240.0 (slow)	17.2–50.0	0.36–0.48	0.99–1.94	[10, 20, 40, 44]

*V_D^{ss} = Volume of distribution at steady state.
The values for each pharmacokinetic parameter represent the range of mean values reported in the individual studies indicated under 'data source'.

The high lipid solubility of thiopentone results in extensive renal tubular reabsorption, and therefore minimal renal elimination of the unchanged drug. The total body clearance of thiopentone ranges from 1.6 to 4.3 ml kg^{-1} min^{-1}. Assuming that hepatic blood flow is 21 ml kg^{-1} min^{-1}, the calculated range of thiopentone's hepatic extraction ratio is 0.08–0.20. This low hepatic extraction ratio indicates that thiopentone has capacity-limited, binding-sensitive elimination[4]. Changes in protein binding and hepatic enzyme activity will affect thiopentone clearance.

Significant biotransformation of thiopentone occurs in the liver. The predominant route of its metabolism in man is omega-oxidation, resulting in the production of thiopentone carboxylic acid, which is pharmacologically inactive[12]. To a minor extent, thiopentone undergoes desulphuration to form the pharmacologically active metabolite, pentobarbitone, which is further metabolised to inactive products. Only low plasma concentrations of pentobarbitone were measured in patients 15 min after intravenous administration of thiopentone in total doses of 450–1275 mg[21]. In contrast, more recent studies[45] have shown that infusions of large doses of thiopentone, used clinically for cerebral resuscitation (300–500 mg/kg, administered over 2–3 days), resulted in pharmacologically significant plasma concentrations of pentobarbitone (3–7 μg ml^{-1}). This suggests that the rate of formation of pentobarbitone is slow, and it does not contribute to the anaesthetic effect of a single dose of thiopentone.

Thiopentone's clearance (due to metabolism) is smaller than methohexitone's and larger than that of pentobarbitone (Table 6.1). Because the volume of distribution at steady state for these three barbiturates is similar, differences in the terminal elimination half-life are entirely due to differences in hepatic clearance (i.e. biotransformation). The contribution of metabolism to the termination of thiopentone's anaesthetic effect has recently been re-examined by a pharmacokinetic characterisation of the distribution and elimination phases[14]. Because of thiopentone's relatively low clearance, it was postulated that metabolism contributes very little to the termination of the anesthetic effect of a single intravenous bolus dose. In these studies, the brain was considered the anatomical equivalent of the central compartment. One minute after thiopentone administration, metabolism accounted for only 14% of the drug eliminated from the central compartment. Fifteen minutes after administration, when the central nervous system effects of thiopentone were mostly dissipated, the metabolic clearance had increased to only 18%. Therefore, the decline of thiopentone concentration in the brain and the termination of its effects during the first 15 minutes after a single intravenous injection result primarily from redistribution of the drug to muscle and fat tissues.

Volume of distribution at steady state

The other pharmacokinetic variable that determines thiopentone's terminal elimination half-life is the volume of distribution at steady state. Because thiopentone is highly lipid soluble it undergoes extensive distribution to tissues, especially fat. Thiopentone's volume of distribution at steady state ranges from 1.3 to 3.3 l kg^{-1} and is similar to that of methohexitone and pentobarbitone. While high lipid solubility allows rapid penetration of all biological membranes it is not the sole factor in determining the volume of distribution of a drug. Numerous other drugs used in anesthesia have a large volume of distribution at steady state. These include ketamine (3 l kg^{-1}) [17, 48] and the narcotic analgesics (fentanyl, pethidine and morphine at 3–5 l kg^{-1}) [34, 35, 46]. The low clearance and large volume of distribution at steady state result in thiopentone's moderately long terminal elimination half-life. The suggestion that the rate-limiting step for thiopentone elimination from the body is its slow return from fat to plasma is analogous to stating that it has a large distribution volume where most of the drug is not in the plasma or central compartment and is thus unavailable for elimination [24].

Protein binding

Thiopentone is moderately bound to plasma proteins, specifically albumin [23]. In healthy surgical patients, the free fraction ranges from 15 to 25 %. If the free fraction of thiopental is increased secondary to disease or to the presence of another drug, a greater fraction of the thiopentone present in the cerebral circulation will be available for penetration into the brain. This will be most prominent when the plasma thiopental concentration is high relative to the brain concentration, as would be the case immediately after a bolus intravenous injection. Thus, a greater pharmacological effect will occur for a given dose of thiopentone when less drug is bound to plasma proteins. The same phenomena would also increase the incidence of thiopentone adverse effects, specifically cardiovascular depression. Higher concentrations of unbound thiopentone in plasma could heighten levels in the heart and vasculature, predisposing to greater myocardial depression and hypotension [22]. The increased thiopentone-free fraction will also enhance its redistribution from brain to other tissues, and thereby shorten the duration of anaesthesia.

An elevated thiopentone-free fraction can occur if a second drug has a greater affinity than thiopentone for binding sites on albumin. Studies *in vitro* have shown that aspirin, indomethacin, mefenamic acid, phenylbutazone, and naproxen can increase the thiopentone-free fraction [15]. Generally, very high concentrations of these drugs are required before significant displacement of thiopentone occurs. Their effect on thiopentone protein binding after the usual therapeutic doses are unknown. Csögör and Kerek [18] have shown that in patients pretreated with sulphafurazole, the thiopentone dose necessary to induce anaesthesia was reduced and the recovery time was more rapid when compared with normal controls. They attribute this to an increased thiopentone-free fraction in the presence of the sulpha drug.

Thiopental pharmacodynamics

The termination of thiopentone's effects was initially attributed to redistribution from brain to fat stores[9]. In 1966, Price *et al.*[38, 39] developed a physiological model that simulated thiopentone distribution throughout the body. This model predicted that lean tissues (muscle, skin) were more important than body fat in the redistribution of thiopentone from the central nervous system. While the partition coefficient of thiopentone between plasma and muscle was less than that of fat, the large mass of muscle tissues (one-half of the body mass compared to the one-fifth of the body mass represented by fat) enhanced the role of this lean tissue in the immediate termination of the thiopentone's effect. Goldstein and Aronow[26] arrived at a similar conclusion after examining the tissue distribution of thiopentone and pentobarbitone in the rat. Other investigators have also developed more complicated physiological models that characterise thiopentone disposition in man[3, 25]. These models all reinforce the suggestion of Price *et al.*[39] that thiopentone redistribution is initially more to muscle than to fat. Dissenting arguments about this concept have been presented[31].

While the termination of thiopentone's anaesthetic effect after a single intravenous dose has been generally attributed to its redistribution from brain to muscle and fat, there has been little scientific study of this mechanism in man or animals. The necessity of tissue sampling to characterise the tissue redistribution precludes meaningful research in man. Because pharmacokinetic data for thiopentone in man is limited to plasma concentration vs. time data, we are limited to speculating on the relationship of thiopentone's rapid and slow distribution phases relative to the tissue redistribution pattern. Accurate characterisation of the rapid and slow distribution phases is very dependent on the site of sampling (arterial vs. venous), frequency of sampling, time for sample collection, and the methods of nonlinear regression analysis of the data. Speculation about the relationship of the pharmacokinetic distribution phases of thiopentone to the true physiological redistribution mechanism should be done cautiously.

The relationship of thiopentone concentration in plasma to the degree of central nervous system depression has not been evaluated extensively. Becker[2] studied this relationship by first administering an intravenous bolus dose of thiopentone (2.5 mg kg^{-1}), and then rapidly infusing 1.5 mg kg^{-1} min^{-1} to healthy surgical patients. The total and free thiopentone plasma concentrations at which there was no movement in response to a noxious stimulus (squeezing of the trapezius muscle) were measured. Becker demonstrated that lack of movement to a squeezing of the trapezius muscle was analogous to lack of movement to a surgical incision. The latter is the standard stimulus in the measurement of **MAC** for inhalation anaesthetics. At a total thiopentone concentration of 42.2 ± 2.8 $\mu g/ml^{-1}$ (SD) and a free concentration of 6.3 ± 0.6 μg ml^{-1}, patients did not respond to this noxious stimulus. It must be noted that the thiopentone plasma concentrations in Becker's study were not obtained at steady state and there is an unknown degree of disequilibrium between brain and plasma thiopentone concentrations.

Thiopentone pharmacokinetics in disease states

In chronic renal failure, the dose of thiopentone necessary to induce anaesthesia is reduced by one-half[19]. This may be related to a change in protein binding. The thiopentone-free fraction in plasma increased from 22 % in normal patients to 53 % in patients with chronic renal failure[22]. The increased thiopentone-free fraction results in higher brain concentrations for any given dose and may account for the lower dosage requirement. An alternative explanation may be an increased brain sensitivity to thiopentone in chronic renal failure. Burch and Stanski[13] have examined thiopentone pharmacokinetics in patients with renal failure. In their study, the thiopentone-free fraction increased significantly from $15.7 \pm 2.4 \%$ (SD) in the normal patients, to $28.0 \pm 6.5 \%$ in those with impaired function. Using the total drug concentration (bound + free) in plasma, they estimated that the increased free drug concentration in chronic renal failure resulted in a larger total drug clearance $(4.5 \pm 1.1 \text{ ml kg}^{-1} \text{ min}^{-1}$ in renal failure vs. $3.2 \pm 0.6 \text{ ml kg}^{-1} \text{ min}^{-1}$ in normals) since thiopentone elimination by the liver is proportional to the free drug concentration. The volume of distribution at steady state also increased ($3.0 \pm 1.0 \text{ l kg}^{-1}$ in renal failure vs. $1.9 \pm 0.5 \text{ l kg}^{-1}$ in normals), due to the increased free fraction of thiopentone in plasma; that is, more of the plasma thiopentone was available for diffusion into tissues. Because the changes in clearance and volume of distribution were approximately equal in magnitude, the terminal elimination half-life was unaffected (10.2 ± 2.0 h in renal failure vs. 9.7 ± 2.6 h with normal kidneys). When the pharmacokinetic variables were calculated using only the free drug concentration, the free drug clearance (intrinsic clearance) and volume of distribution of the unbound drug at steady state were unchanged in renal failure compared to the normal state. Also, the calculated estimates of thiopentone binding to tissues were unaffected by chronic renal failure. Thus, the extent of thiopentone metabolism (intrinsic clearance) and distribution (volume of distribution at steady state) are unchanged in chronic renal disease. The pharmaco-kinetic changes seen in renal failure using the total drug concentrations are due solely to the alterations in thiopental binding to plasma proteins. These data suggest that it is prudent to reduce the rate of thiopentone administration in renal failure. A slower rate of administration in the presence of the decreased protein binding will prevent the transient occurrence of excessive thiopentone concentrations (and toxicity) in the central nervous system and cardiovascular system. The total dose required for the induction and maintenance of anesthesia will be unaltered in the presence of renal failure, assuming that the central nervous system sensitivity to thiopental is unaltered.

In chronic hepatic dysfunction, Shideman *et al.*[43] observed a decreased thiopentone dose requirement and longer duration of effect. The pharmacokinetic fate of thiopentone in hepatic dysfunction remains unknown; however, an increased free thiopentone fraction has been demonstrated[22]. The pharmacokinetic basis of an altered response to thiopentone in hepatic dysfunction patients may be similar to that of chronic renal failure patients.

Morgan *et al.*[37] have examined the pharmacokinetics of thiopentone in pregnant females undergoing Caesarean section. The elimination half-life of thiopentone increased significantly (26.1 ± 12.6 h in pregnancy vs. 11.5 ± 1.0 h in nonpregnant patients) because of a larger volume of distribution at steady state (3.8 ± 2.3 l kg^{-1} in pregnancy vs. 1.6 ± 0.66 l kg^{-1} in nonpregnant patients). Thiopentone binding to plasma proteins and clearance were not significantly altered in the pregnant patient. The basis for the increased volume of distribution and elimination half-life at the end of pregnancy are unknown and the significance of these changes for the mother and fetus has not been demonstrated.

Dose-response studies have shown that the thiopentone dosage requirement decreases with increasing age[16]. Jung *et al.*[29] examined the pharmacokinetics of thiopentone in the aged. The elimination half-life increased from 5 to 9 h in patients 20–30 years of age, to 13 to 20 h in patients 60–80 years of age. This was caused by an age-related increase in the volume of distribution at steady state; thiopentone clearance was not affected. The increased volume of distribution is most likely due to the age-related decline of muscle mass and increased proportion of body fat. This pharmacokinetic study does not explain the altered thiopentone dosage requirement with increasing age. Either the redistribution of thiopentone to muscle and fat could be slower, or the central nervous system is more sensitive to thiopentone in the elderly patient. Further research is necessary to eludicate the basis of the altered dosage requirements in the elderly.

When very high doses are used over prolonged periods of time, the pharmacokinetics of thiopentone elimination change from first order to zero order (nonlinear)[45]. For example, a thiopentone dose of 500 mg kg^{-1} given over a 24 hour period for cerebral resuscitation of anoxic encephalopathy resulted in the plasma decay curve shown in Fig. 6.2. At thiopentone plasma concentrations above 60 μg ml^{-1} in plasma, zero order pharmacokinetics were evident and the elimination half-life was markedly prolonged, approaching 70 h. At lower concentrations the elimination half-life became closer to the first order value of 6–12 h. Saturation of the hepatic enzymes biotransforming thiopentone is the probable mechanism of the nonlinear kinetics.

The nonlinear elimination of high doses of thiopentone has some important clinical implications. During a continuous infusion of thiopentone, it is necessary to measure the plasma concentration every 4–6 h. As the thiopentone plasma concentrations approach the levels of saturation (30–50 μg ml^{-1}), it is necessary to reduce the infusion rate to prevent excessively high thiopentone concentrations. If saturation occurs, the long elimination half-life associated with zero order kinetics will prolong the time between termination of the infusion and the opportunity to assess cerebral function.

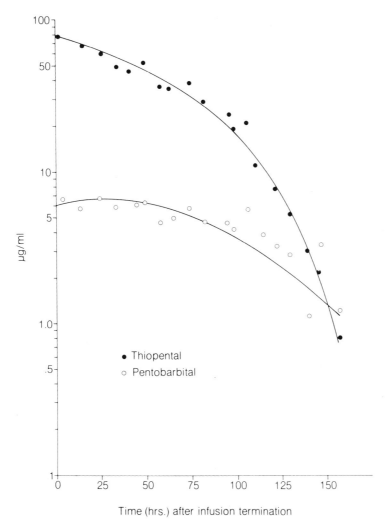

Fig. 6.2 Plasma concentrations of thiopentone and pentobarbitone in a patient who received thiopentone in a total dose of 502 mg kg^{-1} as an infusion over 42 h for cerebral resuscitation. The solid line if the nonlinear regression characterisation of the data fit to a Michaelis–Menten pharmacokinetic model. Adapted with permission of the publisher and authors[45].

METHOHEXITONE PHARMACOKINETICS

Methohexitone is an oxybarbiturate that is 2–3 times more potent than thiopentone. It does not enjoy the clinical popularity of thiopentone, due in part to a higher incidence of undesirable side-effects such as spontaneous movement, hiccups, and occasionally seizure activity[1, 42].

Methohexitone has a pharmacokinetic profile that is distinctly different from thiopentone. Fig. 6.3 compares the plasma decay curves of thiopentone and methohexitone in surgical patients[28]. After intravenous injection and frequent arterial blood sampling, both drugs exhibit a triexponential decay in plasma. The numerical value of the rapid and slow distribution phases are similar. While tissue redistribution studies for methohexitone are not as extensive as those for thiopentone, there is no reason to expect that the tissue redistribution mechanism differs.

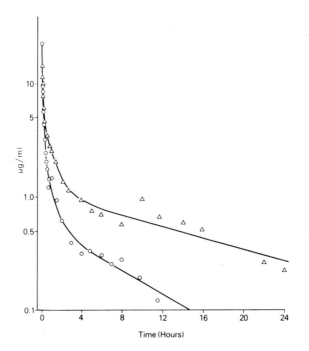

Fig. 6.3 A comparison of the pharmacokinetic profile of thiopentone and methohexitone both used for the induction of surgical anaesthesia. The solid line represents the triexponential equation determined by nonlinear regression. Note the significantly shorter methohexitone terminal elimination half-life.
$\triangle$ = thiopentone
6.1 mg kg^{-1};
$\bigcirc$ = methohexitone
2.9 mg kg^{-1}.

The terminal elimination half-time for methohexitone is approximately one-half the value for thiopentone (Table 6.1). The longer terminal elimination half-time of 4.0 ± 2.5 h was obtained in patients undergoing surgery[28]. This contrasts with the value of 1.6 ± 0.7 h obtained for normal volunteers by Breimer[6]. Because the volume of distribution at steady state is similar for thiopentone and methohexitone, methohexitone's shorter terminal elimination half-life is due exclusively to its higher clearance. Methohexitone clearance is estimated to be 12.1 ± 2.3 ml kg^{-1} min^{-1} in volunteers and 9.9 ± 2.9 ml kg^{-1} min^{-1} in surgical patients. This increased clearance relative to thiopental indicates a greater ability of the liver to metabolise methohexitone. Methohexitone's hepatic extraction ratio is approximately 0.4–0.6, two to four times higher than that of thiopentone. Thus, methohexitone's intermediate hepatic extraction ratio and clearance will be sensitive to alterations in hepatic blood flow. This may explain the lower clearance found in surgical patients relative to volunteers where surgery and anaesthesia with the inhalational anaesthetics will decrease hepatic blood flow[30]. Methohexitone has a similar degee of protein binding to thiopentone[5]. Its biotransformation has not been studied in man.

While methohexitone does have a higher clearance than thiopentone, redistribution from brain to muscle and fat during the first 15–30 min after a single intravenous injection is similar and is the predominant mechanism of terminating the anaesthetic effect[28]. However, if multiple doses of either drug are given over time so that the redistribution mechanism becomes less efficient, recovery from methohexitone should be more rapid than from thiopentone due to the higher clearance and shorter elimination half-life of methohexitone. Unfortunately there are no studies to support this speculation. Also there is no information on the relationship of methohexitone concentration in plasma to the depth of anaesthesia, and the effects of age or disease states on methohexitone pharmacokinetics are unknown.

HEXOBARBITONE PHARMACOKINETICS

Hexobarbitone is used as an intravenous anaesthetic supplement and hypnotic. It is of interest pharmacokinetically because (a) its elimination half-time is intermediate between those of methohexitone and thiopentone, and (b) it has been used as a model substrate in studies of hepatic drug metabolism which is responsible for its elimination from the body[7, 8, 41, 49]. The pharmacokinetics in normal human volunteers are summarised in Table 6.1. As expected, the clearance of hexobarbitone is reduced and the elimination half-time prolonged in the presence of impaired liver function (e.g., acute hepatitis cirrhosis)[7, 49]. Conversely, enhancement of hepatic microsomal drug metabolising activity increases its clearance and shortens its elimination half-time. The latter may be of particular interest to anaesthesiologists participating in the intensive care of critically ill patients, because it has been shown that the elimination of hexobarbitone (sometimes used by continuous intravenous for sedation of such patients) increases with the duration of the patient's care, especially with the development of septicaemia[41]. The individual factors responsible for these changes in its elimination have not been positively identified, but the likely ones include correction of impaired hepatic oxygenation, hyperthermia, induction of drug metabolising enzyme function by hormones and by drugs. Fluctuations in the distribution volumes of hexobarbitone are also likely to contribute to both pharmacodynamic and pharmacokinetic variability among patients and in the same patient under different conditions[41].

PENTOBARBITONE PHARMACOKINETICS

The use of pentobarbitone as a premedication for clinical anaesthesia has declined as the use of the benzodiazepines has increased. As noted above, pentobarbitone is an active metabolite of thiopentone. Pentobarbitone differs from thiopentone in having an oxygen rather than a sulphur atom on the barbiturate ring; this imparts significantly different pharmacokinetic and physiochemical properties. The most obvious physio-chemical difference is lipid solubility: the sulphur atom in thiopentone increases its lipid solubility by a factor of 66 times relative to pentobarbitone. Fig. 6.4 shows the pentobarbitone plasma decay curve of Smith *et al.*[44]. The decay curve is biexpo-nential with a distribution half-life of approximately 4 h. This prolonged distribution phase relative to thiopentone or methohexitone may be secondary to the decreased lipid solubility and a correspondingly slow rate of penetration of biological mem-branes. The decreased lipid solubility also delays its penetration of the blood–brain barrier, thus slowing the brain accumulation of pentobarbitone after a bolus intravenous injection. The onset of central nervous system depression is slow, and this limits the usefulness of pentobarbitone as an agent for induction of anaesthesia[26].

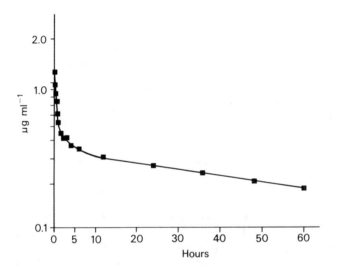

Fig. 6.4 The plasma decay curve for pentobar-bitone drawn from the data of Smith *et al.*[44].

Estimates of pentobarbitone's terminal elimination half-life vary from 17 to 50 h[10, 20, 40, 44]. Given the similar volume of distribution at steady state, the long elimination phase is due solely to a very low hepatic clearance. Pentobarbitone's clearance of $0.3–0.5 \, ml \, kg^{-1} \, min^{-1}$ is about one-tenth the clearance of thiopentone. Thus the elimination of pentobarbitone is capacity-dependent and sensitive to changes in its binding to plasma proteins. An increase in the free fraction of pentobarbitone in plasma or the induction of hepatic enzyme activity will increase the clearance of pentobarbitone. Pentobarbitone with a free fraction of 65–70% is less protein-bound than thiopentone. Pentobarbitone's clearance from the body is due almost exclusively to hepatic biotransformation. Its main metabolite in man is the alcohol, hydroxy-pentobarbitone, which is eliminated in the urine[32]. The slow rate of pentobarbitone biotransformation relative to thiopentone and methohexitone may be due to its low lipid solubility which limits its rate of penetration into the lipid environment of the hepatic smooth endoplasmic reticulum, the site of pentobarbitone biotransformation.

As with methohexitone, there is limited data concerning the relationship of pentobarbitone concentration in plasma and the degree of central nervous system depression. Pentobarbitone plasma concentrations of $35-45\,\mu g$ ml^{-1} have been achieved during its continuous infusion for control of elevated intracranial pressure in patients with acute head injuries[33]. Unfortunately, the optimal therapeutic concentrations of pentobarbitone in plasma have not been determined for purposes of 'cerebral resuscitation'.

GLOSSARY

Generic name		Trade name
British	American	
Thiopentone	Thiopental	Pentothal
Methohexitone	Methohexital	Brevital
Hexobarbitone	Hexobarbital	—
Pentobarbitone	Pentobarbital	Nembutal

REFERENCES

1. BARRY C. T., GUY J., GOAT V. & BUCHAN A. S. (1971) Methohexitone and thiopentone: Response to stimuli and incidence of some side effects. *Br. J. Anaesth.* **43**, 963–71.
2. BECKER K. E. (1978) Plasma levels of thiopental necessary for anesthesia. *Anesthesiology* **49**, 192–6.
3. BISCHOFF K. B. & DEDRICK R. L. (1968) Thiopental pharmacokinetics. *J. Pharm. Sci.* **57**, 1346–51.
4. BLASCHKE T. F. (1977) Protein binding and kinetics of drugs in liver disease. *Clin. Pharmacokinet.* **2**, 32–44.
5. BRAND L., MARK L. C. & SNELL M. (1963) Physiological disposition of methohexital in man. *Anesthesiology* **24**, 331–6.
6. BREIMER D. D. (1976) Pharmacokinetics of methohexitone following intravenous infusion in humans. *Br. J. Anaesth.* **48**, 643–9.
7. BREIMER D. D., ZILLY W. & RICHTER E. (1975) Pharmacokinetics of hexobarbital in acute hepatitis and after apparent recovery. *Clin. Pharm. Ther.* **18**, 43–50.
8. BREIMER D. D., ZILLY W. & RICHTER E. (1978) Influence of corticosteroid on hexobarbital and tolbutamide disposition. *Clin. Pharm. Ther.* **24**, 208–12.
9. BRODIE B. B., BERNSTEIN E. & MARK L. C. (1952) The role of body fat in limiting the duration of action of thiopental. *J. Pharmacol. Exp. Ther.* **105**, 421–6.
10. BRODIE B. B., BURNS J. J., MARK L. C., *et al.* (1953) The fate of pentobarbital in man and dog and a method for its estimation in biological material. *J. Pharmacol. Exp. Ther.* **109**, 26–34.

11. BRODIE B. B., KURZ H. & SCHANKER L. S. (1960) The importance of dissociation constant and lipid solubility in influencing the passage of drugs into the CSF. *J. Pharmacol. Exp. Ther.* **130**, 20–5.

12. BRODIE B. B., MARK L. C., PAPPER E. M., *et al.* (1950) The fate of thiopental in man and a method for its estimation in biological material. *J. Pharmacol. Exp. Ther.* **98**, 85–96.

13. BURCH P. G. & STANSKI D. R. (1982) The role of decreased protein binding in thiopental pharmacokinetics. *Clin. Pharmacol. Ther.* **32**, 212–17.

14. BURCH P. G. & STANSKI D. R. (1983) The role of metabolism and protein binding in thiopental anesthesia. *Anesthesiology* **58**, 146–52.

15. CHAPLIN M. D., ROSZKOWSKI A. P. & RICHARDS R. K. (1973) Displacement of thiopental from plasma proteins by nonsteroidol anti-inflammatory agents. *Proc. Soc. Exp. Biol. Med.* **143**, 667–71.

16. CHRISTENSEN J. H. & ANDREASEN F. (1978) Individual variation in response to thiopental. *Acta Anaesth. Scand.* **22**, 303–13.

17. CLEMENTS J. A. & NIMMO W. S. (1981) Pharmacokinetics and analgesic effect of ketamine in man. *Br. J. Anaesth.* **53**, 27–30.

18. CSÖGÖR S. I. & KEREK S. F. (1970) Enhancement of thiopentone anesthesia by sulphafurazole. *Br. J. Anaesth.* **42**, 988–90.

19. DUNDEE J. W. & RICHARDS R. K. (1954) Effect of azotemia upon the action of intravenous barbiturate anesthesia. *Anesthesiology* **15**, 333–46.

20. EHRNEBO M. (1974) Pharmacokinetics and distribution properties of pentobarbital in humans following oral and intravenous administration. *J. Pharm. Sci.* **63**, 1114–18.

21. FURANO E. S. & GREENE N. M. (1963) Metabolic breakdown of thiopental in man determined by gas chromatographic analysis of serum barbiturate levels. *Anesthesiology* **24**, 796–800.

22. GHONEIM M. M. & PANDYA H. (1975) Plasma protein binding of thiopental in patients with impaired renal or hepatic function. *Anesthesiology* **42**, 545–9.

23. GHONEIM M. M., PANDYA H. B., KELLEY S. E., FISHER L. J. & CORRY R. J. (1976) Binding of thiopental to plasma proteins. *Anesthesiology* **45**, 635–9.

24. GHONEIM M. M. & VAN HAMME M. J. (1978) Pharmacokinetics of thiopentone: Effects of enflurane and nitrous oxide anesthesia and surgery. *Br. J. Anaesth.* **50**, 1237–41.

25. GILLIS P. P., DEANGELIS R. J. & WYNN R. L. (1976) Nonlinear pharmacokinetic model of intravenous anesthesia. *J. Pharm. Sci.* **65**, 1001–6.

26. GOLDSTEIN A. & ARONOW L. (1960) The durations of action of thiopental and pentobarbital. *J. Pharmacol. Exp. Ther.* **128**, 1–6.

27. GOODMAN L. S. & GILLMAN A. (1942) *The pharmacological basis of therapeutics*, p. 137. MacMillan, New York.

28. HUDSON R. J., STANSKI D. R. & BURCH P. G. (1982) Comparative pharmacokinetics of methohexital and thiopental. *Anesthesiology* **57**, A240.

29. JUNG D., MAYERSOHN M., PERRIER D., CALKINS J. & SAUNDERS R. (1982) Thiopental disposition as a function of age in female patients undergoing surgery. *Anesthesiology* **56**, 263–8.

30. LARSON C. P., MAZZE R. I., COOPERMANN L. H. & WOLLMAN H. (1974) Effects of anesthetics on cerebral, renal and splanchic circulation. *Anesthesiology* **41**, 169–81.

31. MARK L. C. (1971) Translocation of drugs and other exogenous chemicals into adipose tissue. In Brodie B. B. & Gillette J. J. (eds.), *Concepts in Biochemical Pharmacology, Part I*, pp. 258–75. Springer-Verlag, Berlin.

32. MARK L. C. (1963) Metabolism of barbiturates in man. *Clin. Pharmacol. Ther.* **4**, 504–30.

33. MARSHALL L. F., SMITH R. W. & SHAPIRO H. M. (1979) The outcome with aggressive treatment in severe head injuries. II. Acute and chronic barbiturate administration in the management of head injury. *J. Neurosurg.* **50**, 26–30.

34. MATHER L. E., TUCKER G. T., PFLUGER A. E., LINDOP M. J. & WILKERSON C. (1975) Meperidine kinetics in man – intravenous injection in surgical patients and volunteers. *Clin. Pharmacol. Ther.* **17**, 21–30.

35. MCCLAIN D. A. & HUG C. C. (1980) Intravenous fentanyl kinetics. *Clin. Pharmacol. Ther.* **28**, 106–14.

36. MORGAN D. J., BLACKMAN G. L., PAULL J. D. & WOLF L. J. (1981) Pharmacokinetics and plasma binding of thiopental: I. Studies in surgical patients. *Anesthesiology* **54**, 468–73.

37. MORGAN D. J., BLACKMAN G. L., PAULL J. D. & WOLF L. J. (1981) Pharmacokinetics and plasma binding of thiopental: II. Studies at Caesarean section. *Anesthesiology* **54**, 474–80.

38. PRICE H. L. (1960) A dynamic concept of the distribution of thiopental in the human body. *Anesthesiology* **21**, 40–5.

39. PRICE H. L., KOVNAT P. J., SAFER J. H., CONNER E. H. & PRICE M. L. (1960) The uptake of thiopental by body tissues and its relation to the duration of narcosis. *Clin. Pharmacol. Ther.* **1**, 16–22.

40. REIDENBERG M. M., LOWENTHAL P. T., BRIGGS W. & GASPARO M. (1976) Pentobarbital elimination in patients with poor renal function. *Clin. Pharmacol. Ther.* **20**, 67–71.

41. RIETBROCK I., LAZARUS G., RICHTER E. & BREIMER D. D. (1981) Hexobarbitone disposition at different stages of intensive care treatment. *Br. J. Anaesth.* **53**, 283–93.

42. ROCKHOFF M. & GOUDSOUZIAN N. G. (1981) Seizures induced by methohexital. *Anesthesiology* **54**, 333–5.

43. SHIDEMAN F. E., KELLEY A. R., LEE L. E., *et al.* (1949) The role of the liver in the detoxification of thiopental (pentothal) by man. *Anesthesiology* **10**, 421–8.

44. SMITH R. B., DITTERT L. W., GRIFFEN W. O., *et al.* (1973) Pharmacokinetics of pentobarbital after intravenous and oral administration. *J. Pharmacokinet. Biopharm.* **1**, 5–16.

45. STANSKI D. R., MIHM F. G., ROSENTHAL M. H. & KALMAN S. M. (1980) Pharmacokinetics of high dose thiopental used for cerebral resuscitation. *Anesthesiology* **53**, 169–71.

46. STANSKI D. R., PAALZOW L. & EDLUND P. (1982) Morphine pharmacokinetics – radioimmunoassay vs. gas liquid chromatography. *J. Pharm. Sci.* **71**, 314–17.

47. STANSKI D. R. & WATKINS W. D. (1982) *Drug Disposition in Anesthesia.* Grune and Stratton, New York.

48. WIEBER J., GUGLER R., HENGSTMANN J. H., *et al.* (1975) Pharmacokinetics of ketamine in man. *Anaesthestist* **24**, 260–3.

49. ZILLY W., BREIMER D. D. & RICHTER E. (1978) Hexobarbitone disposition in compensated and decompensated cirrhosis of the liver. *Clin. Pharmacol. Ther.* **23**, 525–34.

7 Non-barbiturate Intravenous Anaesthetics and Continuous Infusion Anaesthesia

C. PRYS-ROBERTS and J. W. SEAR

ADMINISTRATION OF A SINGLE DOSE
Steroid anaesthetics
Eugenol derivatives
Hindered phenols
Imidazoles

ANAESTHESIA BY CONTINUOUS INTRAVENOUS INFUSION
Minimum infusion rate
Infusions of steroid anaesthetics
Infusions of propanidid
Infusions of etomidate
Infusions of di-isopropyl phenol
Barbiturates by infusion

GLOSSARY

Despite the initial and continuing success of barbiturate anaesthetics there has been a persistent search for new intravenous anaesthetics, starting with the discovery of steroid anaesthetics by Selye[89]. This has continued to the present day with the recent discoveries of new steroid compounds[5] and the development of etomidate and di-isopropyl phenol. These short-acting anaesthetics were introduced initially as alternatives to thiopentone, methohexitone and other barbiturates for the induction of anaesthesia. More recently much attention has been focussed on the use of repeated incremental doses to supplement nitrous oxide anaesthesia for short surgical procedures[81], and subsequently the use of continuous infusions, either as the sole anaesthetic agent or in combination with nitrous oxide or other intravenous drugs. In this chapter we will consider the pharmacokinetics of these non-barbiturate anaesthetics when used as a single dose for the induction of anaesthesia, and secondly the pharmacokinetics of barbiturates and non-barbiturates as a continuous infusion.

ADMINISTRATION OF A SINGLE DOSE

Steroid anaesthetics

Althesin

Although hydroxydione[60] was used over a period of ten years after its introduction, the main steroid in common use has been Althesin; a mixture of two steroids, alphaxalone (9 mg/ml) and alphadolone acetate (3 mg/ml) in an oily vehicle, Cremophor EL (see Chapter 15), to give a solution containing 12 mg ml^{-1} of total steroid anaesthetic (Fig 7.1).

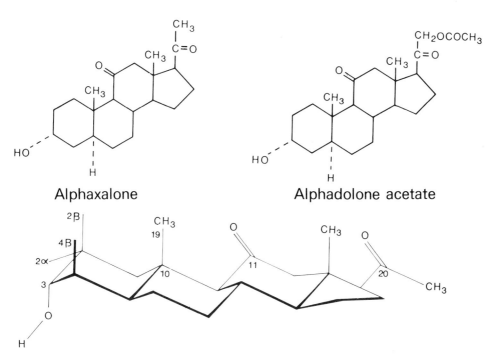

Fig. 7.1 Structures of alphaxalone and alphadolone acetate showing position of the hydroxyl group in the 3α position and the dione group in the 11 position. Compare the chemical representation of the steroid molecule with the spatial representation of alphaxalone (below) in which the hydroxyl group is shown in the 3α position below the plane of the steroid molecule (associated with anaesthetic action), as opposed to the 3β position above the plane of the rings (not associated with anaesthetic action).

Alphaxalone (3α-hydroxy-5α-pregnane-11,20-dione) is an odourless white crystalline powder with a melting point of 165–171°C. It is virtually insoluble in water, but freely soluble in chloroform and acetone.

Alphadolone acetate (21-acetoxy-3α hydroxy-5α pregnane-11,20-dione) is a similar crystalline powder with a higher melting point (175–181°C). It is wholly insoluble in water. Both steroids possess anaesthetic activity, but the potency of alphaxalone is twice that of alphadolone acetate. The latter is present solely to increase the solubility of alphaxalone. Because of their low aqueous solubility, the anaesthetic agents are retained in solution by the polyoxyethylated castor oil derivative, Cremophor EL, which also acts as the solubilising agent to form a clear aqueous solution with a low viscosity and neutral pH.

Althesin is an effective anaesthetic agent in most species of animals, except in the dog, where the solvent Cremophor EL often causes marked hypotension due to histamine release[17]. It may be administered either as an induction agent, or by continuous infusion.

In man, the duration of anaesthesia following a single dose of Althesin is dose-dependent and recovery from anaesthesia is faster following Althesin compared with thiopentone[19, 39, 93]. This is probably related to differences in the disposition of the two drugs. Althesin is rapidly inactivated by hepatic conjuguation while thiopentone undergoes a slower redistribution and metabolism (see Chapters 4 and 6).

Pharmacokinetics of Althesin

The initial studies on the pharmacokinetics of Althesin in man were reported by Dubois[27]. After induction with a bolus dose of $549 \, \mu g \, kg^{-1}$ alphaxalone, plasma was sampled for 90 min, and drug concentrations assayed by gas liquid chromatography. The elimination half-life of alphaxalone was 29 min. However, there were several technical problems associated with the analysis of the plasma alphaxalone concentrations when less than about $0.1 \, \mu g \, ml^{-1}$. Nevertheless the half-life was not significantly different from that subsequently determined by Simpson[90], also following a single bolus intravenous injection. Simpson sampled for 120 min after injection, and determined the systemic clearance of alphaxalone ($21.1 \, ml \, kg^{-1} \, min^{-1}$) to be similar to that of lignocaine (Table 7.1). The volumes of distribution (V_1 and V_D^{ss}) were $0.18 \, l \, kg^{-1}$ and $0.79 \, l \, kg^{-1}$ respectively.

Recovery after short-duration anaesthesia with Althesin

In two groups of patients given Althesin or minaxolone to supplement nitrous oxide for short surgical procedures[81], recollection of date of birth as an index of recovery occurred more rapidly after Althesin (5.7 min) compared to minaxolone (20.7 min). Similar short recovery periods have been observed following methohexitone or Althesin, with or without fentanyl[21].

Table 7.1   Pharmacokinetics of Althesin, minaxolone and methohexitone.

Patients (n)	$T_{\frac{1}{2}}^{\alpha}$ (min)	$T_{\frac{1}{2}}^{\beta}$ (min)	V_1 (l kg^{-1})	V_D^{β} (l kg^{-1})	Cl_p (ml kg^{-1}min^{-1})	Duration of sampling min	Source
Althesin							
Bolus (6)	1.62	34.3	0.18	1.38	21.1	120	[90]
Infusion							
Healthy (9)	2.84	90.9	1.49	2.22	16.9	240	[83, 86]
Treated HT (9)	6.63	112.0	0.46	1.19	7.7	240	[86]
Minaxolone							
Bolus (9)	2.1	47.2	0.36	1.59	26.0	180	[29]
Infusion (9)	3.12	87.3	1.23	2.17	17.4	240	[87]
Infusion (5)	16.0	104.0	1.80	4.10^b	42.0^a	240	[53, 54]
Methohexitone							
Bolus (9)	4.8 50.0	240.0		2.10^b	9.9	720	[43]
Infusion (4)	6.2	97.0	0.29	1.13	12.1	420	[10]

(a) whole blood clearance; (b) V_D^{ss}

Metabolism of Althesin

The uptake and body distribution of Althesin in the rat is similar to that of other non-anaesthetic steroid compounds. Alphaxalone and alphadolone acetate labelled with ^{14}C were shown, by autoradiography[15], to be rapidly localised within the central nervous system following intravenous injection. By the third minute, there was concentration of the drug within the liver and subsequently excretion into the bile duct and duodenum. After the first hour, appreciable quantities of the drug were found within the caecum and colon, and very little in other tissues of the body. Although small quantities of Althesin are also distributed to other tissues within the body, its duration of action in the mouse has been found to be inversely related to both the total and dry body masses. Accordingly, the duration of anaesthesia is prolonged in animals that are undernourished, when compared to a matched well-fed group. This is probably related to the higher liver metabolic enzyme activity in the latter group of animals[74]. Subsequent studies in the rat confirmed the relationship between the mixed-function oxidase enzymes, and cytochrome P450, and the duration of anaesthesia following intraperitoneal Althesin[80].

Studies in the rat showed that alphaxalone is degraded in the liver and excreted in the bile, urine and faeces. The main metabolites detected were 2α-hydroxy, 16α-hydroxy, and 2α, 16α-di-hydroxy alphaxalone[18].

Initial studies in man were carried out using ^{14}C$_{21}$ labelled alphaxalone. A high urinary clearance of the isotope was seen, with greater than 59 % of the administered radioactivity appearing in the urine over the first 24 hours[92]. In patients with chronic renal failure, the systemic clearance of radioactivity was not significantly slower.

More recent studies have used GC–MS (see Chapter 3) as the method of detecting and measuring the concentrations of the Althesin steroids and their metabolites in blood, bile and urine. Alphaxalone, alphadolone acetate, alphadolone and 20α-reduced alphaxalone have all been detected[42]. The kinetics of systemic clearance of alphaxalone and alphadolone were similar in patients with normal hepatic function and those with compensated primary biliary cirrhosis[82]. The plasma concentration of unconjugated 20α-reduced alphaxalone remained low throughout a continuous infusion of Althesin despite changes in the plasma alphaxalone concentration.

In the pooled urine collected over 24 hours after operation, the main metabolites (90–95 %) were detected in the glucuronide fraction of the urine (Fig. 7.2). The major chromatographic peak was 20α-reduced alphaxalone. In some of the patients studied,

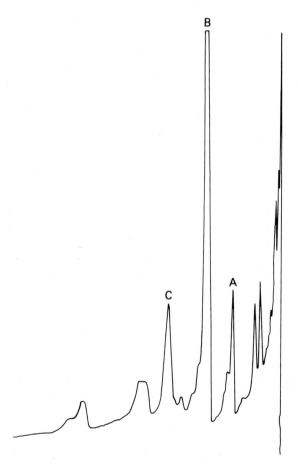

Fig. 7.2 Total Ion Current trace obtained after extraction of the urine as described by Edwards R. W. H., Kellie A. E. and Wade A. P. (1953) *Mem. Soc. Endocrinol.* No. 2, 53. The glucuronide fraction of the urine was derivatised to form trimethylsilyl ethers, and run on OV1 at 250°C. The peaks were identified by mass fragmentography as follows: A alphaxalone; B 20-reduced alphaxalone; and C alphadolone. Reproduced by permission of the authors and the publishers.

the relative amounts of alphaxalone and its metabolite were altered—indicating biovariability in the extent of degradation of the steroids. The presence of a higher urinary concentration of 20α-reduced alphaxalone, mainly as the glucuronide, and the low plasma metabolite concentration is similar to that seen with other endogenous steroids. The high metabolic clearance rate (MCR) of glucuronide conjugates, which approximates to the glomerular filtration rate (GFR) may offer an explanation of these findings.

Alphadolone, as its glucuronide, was the other urinary metabolite; no alphadolone acetate, as free steroid or glucuronide, was detected in any of the urine samples using the technique of selective ion monitoring (SIM). No 11-reduced compounds (derived through keto-reduction of either alphaxalone or alphadolone acetate) or 20-reduced alphadolone was detected in the urine. Similarly no metabolites with additional hydroxyl groups, which would tend to increase hydrophilicity, were found in samples of plasma, urine or bile.

Samples of bile were collected, from indwelling bile duct T-tube, over the 24 hour period post-operation, and assayed in a similar fashion to that described for urine[31]. Holly and his colleagues[42] failed to reveal the presence of alphaxalone, alphadolone acetate, or any of their metabolites, in any of the extracted fractions.

This is in contrast to the findings of Strunin *et al.*[92], who found radioactivity in the bile within 10 min of a single dose of 10–20 μC ^{14}C alphaxalone. The disparity between these papers may be due to radiochemical impurities of the labelled alphaxalone, or to a failure of extraction of the Althesin steroids or their metabolites by the method used by Holly. However, it is more likely that the activity recorded by Strunin was not due to the presence of alphaxalone or its 20α-reduced metabolite, but rather due to other hydrophilic metabolites or molecules not extracted by ethyl acetate.

Desmet *et al.*[23], using gas liquid chromatography, studied the rate of excretion of alphaxalone in the urine of patients given a bolus dose of 110 μl kg^{-1} Althesin (990 μg kg^{-1} alphaxalone) followed by an infusion of Althesin for 90 min (130 μg kg^{-1} min^{-1} alphaxalone). The total dose of alphaxalone was 25.2 mg kg^{-1}. Urine was collected in 6-hourly aliquots and hydrolysed with β-glucuronidase from *Helix pomata*. Thus, the total urinary alphaxalone (free unconjugated and glucuronide of alphaxalone) were measured. The urinary excretion varied from 680 to 1380 μg alphaxalone over the first 24–30 hours; so accounting for less than 1 % of the injected dose.

Althesin by infusion has also been used to sedate for controlled ventilation of a single patient with acute hepatic necrosis following ingestion of paracetamol and salicylates. The urinary metabolites of Althesin in this patient showed evidence of impaired glucuronidation. Approximately 50 % of the parent steroids and their metabolites were excreted in the free, unconjugated urinary fraction, compared with 90–95 % as the glucuronide conjugates in the healthy individual (Table 7.2)[82].

Table 7.2 Metabolism of Althesin in patients with normal hepatic function, proven primary biliary cirrhosis, and acute hepatic necrosis [80, 82].

Patient group	Conjugated steroids		Unconjugated steroids	
Healthy patients and patients with cirrhosis	>95%	Alphaxalone 20α-reduced alphaxalone Alphadolone	<5%	
Patient with acute hepatic necrosis	50%	Alphaxalone 20α-reduced alphaxalone	50%	Alphadolone (mainly) Alphaxalone 20α-reduced alphaxalone (trace)

Extra-hepatic metabolism of Althesin

Until recently, the possible metabolic effect of passage of intravenous anaesthetic agents through the lung has been ignored. However, Nicholas and his colleagues[61] have recently demonstrated the *in vitro* metabolism of alphaxalone. The rate of metabolism in lung tissue shows different enzyme kinetics to those previously reported for the rat liver *in vitro*. There is also evidence of a difference in the metabolic end products—the rat lung metabolising alphaxalone to 3α, 11-dihydroxy-5α-pregnane-20-one, and 5α-pregnane, 3α, 11, 20-triol. The former of these metabolites has an anaesthetic activity of about 25% that of the parent molecule, while reduction of the 20-carbonyl group leads to compounds with little anaesthetic potency. The lung does not, however, appear to have a major role in glucuronidation. In the event of human lung tissue having a steroid dehydrogenase enzyme with similar kinetic constants to the liver, the role of pulmonary metabolism may possibly affect induction of anaesthesia. Other studies in the rat have suggested that the lung may have a storage role for lipophilic drugs[49]. This is seen with alphaxalone after infusion for 10 minutes, where the efflux from the lung does not follow that of dextran, a drug that remains solely in the vascular compartment. If pulmonary storage occurs to any extent in man, there may be considerable build up, especially after prolonged infusion. The release of drug, after cessation of the infusion, may lead to the production of secondary peaks during the elimination phase. These have been observed in both man and experimental animals.

Hypersensitivity to Althesin

Althesin has been shown to cause hypersensitivity reactions both on first and especially subsequent injections in a low proportion of patients, variously estimated between 1:900[33] and 1:10000[97]. The nature of this hypersensitivity has been shown to be due to induction of the alternate pathway of complement activation[70, 103], whereas after a previous administration of the drug the hypersensitivity shows the characteristics of an antigen–antibody mediated response involving the classical pathway of complement activation[70, 103]. The probable cause of these hypersensitivity reactions is believed to be the vehicle Cremophor EL[35]. To overcome these disadvantages of Althesin, two alternatives have been sought: an alternative formulation of the Althesin steroids, and the development of an alternative water-soluble steroid anaesthetic.

Minaxolone

The introduction of an 11α-dimethyl amino group and a 2β-ethoxy group, whilst still preserving the 3α-hydroxy group in the A ring of the steroid molecule, resulted in the water soluble compound, minaxolone (Fig. 7.3), which was marketed as the citrate[22]. This can be formulated into solutions of 0.5% or greater concentration at pH 4 or above. Heating to 100°C results in the slow formation of the 17β-epimer, which is anaesthetically inactive. It is probable that the combination of water solubility and high pharmacological activity may be associated with the unusual steric arrangement at the C_{11} position of the 11α-dimethylamino group. In animals, minaxolone citrate has very similar chracteristics to Althesin, as well as the advantage of being able to be given to the dog. However, initial studies in man using bolus doses of minaxolone and a comparison with both Althesin and methohexitone, showed recovery to be more prolonged[67, 81, 87]. This delayed recovery is probably related to the hydrophilicity of the agent, which must have a different spatial volume of distribution to the lipid soluble Althesin, and to a different partition coefficient between neural tissue and plasma.

   The decay kinetics after a bolus dose of minaxolone fitted to an open two-compartment pharmacokinetic model[29, 53, 54]. Although the elimination half-life of

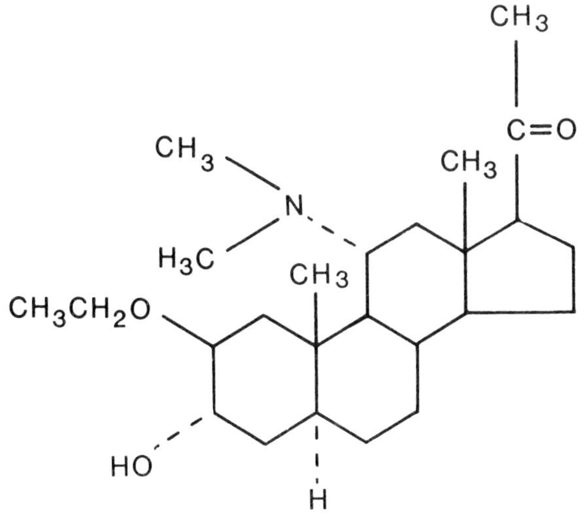

Fig. 7.3 Chemical structure of minaxolone. Note the presence of the hydroxyl group in the 3α position (associated with anaesthetic action), the 2β ethoxy group (associated with increased potency compared with alpha-xalone) and the dimethyl amino group replacing the dione group at the 11 position on ring C (conferring water solubility).

minaxolone was similar to that following an infusion of Althesin, there was an apparently different volume of distribution reflecting the hydrophilicity of minaxolone compared with the hydrophobicity of alphaxalone (Table 7.1). In the investigations of Mather and his colleagues[53, 54], pharmacokinetic profiles were obtained in volunteers following the administration of two different infusion regimes and separate bolus injections. All of these studies indicated an elimination half-life of 51–158 min, and a total body clearance of 1.8–3.2 l min^{-1}. This was 2 or 3 times that of indocynanine green clearance in the same subjects. Renal clearance was uniformly low, and accounted for only 0.5 % of the total body clearance. The mean values for the distribution volumes for minaxolone from these different studies were 1.7 l kg^{-1} for the initial volume (V_1) and 3.1 l kg^{-1} for the volume distribution at steady-state conditions. The onset of anaesthesia occurred at a mean blood concentration of 0.24 μg ml^{-1} minaxolone, with the subjects being able to give their correct date of birth at a mean concentration of 0.16 μg ml^{-1}. Thus, the pharmacokinetic characteristics of minaxolone in these studies in volunteers showed a total body clearance several times greater than that found for Althesin by Simpson[90] and Sear *et al.*[87], and for etomidate by Van Hamme[99]. The high total body clearance of minaxolone, coupled with the low renal clearance, indicates a significant role of the liver in metabolism. Whether other organs or tissues of the body are also involved in the clearance of minaxolone is uncertain. In the sheep, the hepatic extraction ratio was approximately 0.98 with an extraction ratio of 0.09 for the kidney and negligible metabolism of minaxolone by the lungs[37]. In a separate series of studies in the sheep, a linear relationship was found between steady-state blood concentration at various sequential constant rates of infusion of minaxolone. The high body-clearance in sheep (3–4 l min^{-1}) was independent of the dose; and so further confirms the linearity of minaxolone kinetics during infusion. Recovery from anaesthesia, where minaxolone has supplemented 66 % nitrous oxide in oxygen, occurred at similar plasma drug concentrations following bolus and infusion studies (0.27 μg ml^{-1} and 0.19 μg ml^{-1} respectively[80]).

Metabolism of minaxolone

In contrast to Althesin, the higher water solubility of minaxolone citrate results in the excretion of a higher percentage (50 %) of the drug as unconjugated steroid. The other main metabolites are the N-desmethyl O-desethyl and N-desmethyl, O-desethyl compounds, which have little or no anaesthetic activity. Table 7.3 shows data obtained, following analysis of aliquots of urine collected over 24 hours post-operation, from patients who received minaxolone citrate either as a single bolus dose or by continuous infusion. The urinary excretion of minaxolone also appears to be pH-dependent, with increased elimination under acidic conditions.

There are no data available to indicate whether biliary excretion of minaxolone citrate occurs in man; although it is present in rat bile as 16α-hydroxy minaxolone. In

Table 7.3   Metabolism of minaxolone citrate in man[80].

Plasma	Urine	
	Glucuronides (50%)	Free sterioids (50%)
N-desmethyl, O-desethyl minaxolone	+ +	0
↑		
N-desmethyl minaxolone	±	0
↑		
Minaxolone	±	+ +
↓		
O-desethyl minaxolone	+	+

There are no data available to indicate whether biliary excretion of minaxolone occurs in man, although it is seen in the rat.

the rabbit, analysis of the acidic fraction of bile shows the metabolism of minaxolone to be similar to progesterone with C_{21} oxidation to the corresponding carboxylic acid. Of the biliary excreted products, about 30% are finally eliminated in the urine following enterohepatic reabsorption.

Eugenol derivatives

Propanidid

This compound is another water-insoluble agent derived from eugenols and has to be formulated in Cremophor EL. The rapidity of recovery, following single doses or infusions of the drug, is due to its destruction by the enzyme plasma pseudocholinesterase to acid metabolites with no anaesthetic activity. There is little evidence that redistribution plays a significant role in the termination of activity of the agent.

Studies by Putter[68] suggested a biphasic decline of serum drug concentration after a single dose of 500 mg (Fig. 7.4). Blood concentrations decreased more sharply after a rapid injection (and hence greater peak concentrations) compared with a slower injection[25]. This would agree with the Michaelis–Menten kinetics of the esterase enzyme *in vitro*[94]. The peak concentration found after doses of 7 mg kg^{-1} are approximately 90 μmol l^{-1} while the concentration at the assumed V_{max} rate will be in excess of 166 μmol l^{-1}. Thus, the rate of degradation will be directly proportional to the drug concentration.

Studies in the dog[7] have shown the serum profile to be monophasic with a half-life of 4.8 min (dose 25 mg kg^{-1}). However, administration of the plasma esterase inhibitor BNPP, (Bis-(p-nitrophenyl)-phosphate) caused both a prolongation of

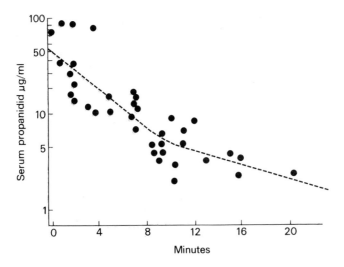

Fig. 7.4 Decay of serum propanidid concentrations after a single 500 mg dose of the drug. After Putter[68].

anaesthetic activity and a change in the pharmacokinetics of the drug. The decline in the drug concentration assumed a biphasic pattern, with a terminal phase half-life of 16.6 min. Other mechanisms for drug elimination must, therefore, exist. These may include redistribution to muscle and fat, the existence of alternative metabolic pathways, or the excretion of large amounts of unchanged active drug.

Hindered phenols

Di-isopropyl phenol (disoprofol)

The location of two isopropyl radicals in the 2 and 6 positions on a phenol molecule confers two important changes of property to phenol (Fig. 7.5). First the molecule becomes chemically inert but pharmacologically active as an anaesthetic[47]. Like Althesin and propanidid, di-isopropyl phenol is poorly soluble in water and is, therefore, formulated in Cremophor EL. Early studies of its effects in man[51] indicated two possible roles in human anaesthesia, firstly as an alternative to the barbiturates and Althesin for induction of anaesthesia[72, 73] and secondly as an agent for continuous infusion to maintain anaesthesia[64, 66]. Induction of anaesthesia can

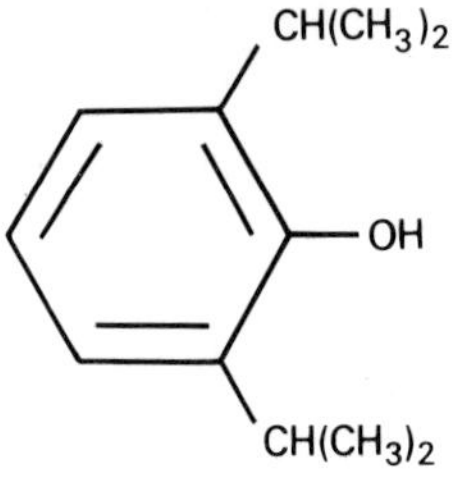

Fig. 7.5 Chemical structure of 2,6 di-isopropyl phenol (disoprofol).

be achieved with doses between 1 and $3 \, mg \, kg^{-1}$[4], the recovery times being respectively 3, 6 and 8 minutes after doses of 1, 2 and $3 \, mg \, kg^{-1}$. The whole blood concentrations at waking were 0.99, 1.00 and 1.13 $\mu g \, ml^{-1}$ respectively. These are all similar to the blood concentrations found at waking in patients who had received an infusion (see p. 149).

Recent clinical studies, using di-isophenol formulated as a solution of $10 \, mg \, ml^{-1}$ in an aqueous emulsion, have shown the drug to have similar induction characteristics to the formulation made up in Cremophor EL.

Pharmacokinetics

Data from experimental animals[3] have shown that di-isopropyl phenol has a very short distribution half-life and that during this phase there is a tenfold decrease of blood concentration. The elimination of the drug is also rapid in animals, values for the terminal half-life ranging from 16 to 55 min. Preliminary estimates in man indicate a terminal elimination half-life of about 55 min and a total body clearance of $3000–3500 \, ml \, min^{-1}$ [1, 4, 64].

Imidazoles

Etomidate

Etomidate (R(+)-ethyl-l-(α-methyl-benzyl)-imidazole-5-carboxylate) is a non-barbiturate, short acting anaesthetic agent introduced into clinical use in 1972[24] (Fig. 7.6). It is currently marketed as a preparation containing 20 mg in 10 ml of a 35% solution of propylene glycol (pH of this solution is between 4 and 7) for induction of anaesthesia.

Induction of anaesthesia may be achieved with the recommended dose of $0.3 \, mg \, kg^{-1}$, and this dose produces an equal duration of sleep to methohexitone

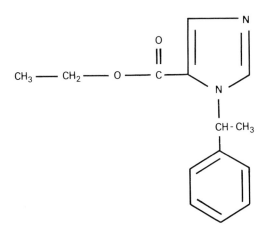

Fig. 7.6 Chemical structure of etomidate (hypnomidate).

1.5 mg kg^{-1} body weight[50]. The duration of sleep is dose-dependent and there is little evidence of cumulation of the drug even with repeated dosage. The speed of onset and short duration of action is the result of rapid uptake and elimination by the brain, and a fast redistribution of the drug from the plasma to other tissues. Whether metabolism occurs at a similarly rapid rate or whether storage of the drug within metabolic organs such as the liver and kidney occurs is not known. Etomidate is metabolised mainly in the liver by ether hydrolysis to pharmacologically inactive metabolites. The main metabolite in man is the corresponding carboxylic acid of etomidate. In man, approximately 75 % of the administered dose is excreted in the urine during the first 24 hours after administration, mainly as the inert metabolites. Only 2 % of the etomidate is excreted unchanged.

Using a tritium-labelled etomidate, Heykants *et al.*[41] were able to further characterise the urinary metabolites. Prior to glucuronide hydrolysis with β-glucuronidase (EC 2.4.6), basic or neutral compounds accounted for only 2.4 % of the radioactivity in pooled urine samples. The largest fraction of activity (67 %) were the polar acidic compounds, extractable with n-butanol. About 24 % radioactivity was excreted as hydrophillic substances. Following glucuronide hydrolysis, there were increases of about 5 % in total radioactivity of the neutral fraction, and 12 % of polar acidic compounds. As a result, the % hydrophilic compounds decreased from 24 to 9.

In vitro protein binding of etomidate has been studied by equilibrium dialysis using radiolabelled etomidate and its major metabolite, the corresponding carboxylic acid[52]. A 4 % solution of human serum albumen was found to bind 78.5 % etomidate and 60.5 % of the metabolite. A 1.5 % solution of human gamma-globulin bound not more than 3 % etomidate and none of the metabolite. Total plasma protein binding of etomidate was 76.5 % in man, the distribution percentages for blood cells, plasma proteins and plasma water being 37.7 %, 47.6 % and 14.7 % respectively. The major metabolite of etomidate was distributed to the same components in the fraction 26.3 %, 47.7 % and 26.2 % respectively. Total protein binding of the metabolite was 64.3 %.

Pharmacokinetics

After intravenous injection in man, Heykants *et al.*[40] showed the plasma concentration of unchanged etomidate to decay in a biphasic manner, with an elimination half-life of 75 min. The plasma concentration of metabolites increases over the first 30 min after administration, and then decrease with a slower half-life of 160 min. During transport in the blood, about 76 % of etomidate is bound to plasma proteins. The distribution of both optical isomers of etomidate (R (+) and S (−)) does not differ substantially in blood, brain or liver. However, the S (−) form has considerably less hypnotic effect, suggesting a stereospecificity of the 'receptor' area in the brain. Kinetic studies have shown wide variations in the clearance of etomidate after both single doses and continuous infusions. Early investigations by Van Hamme *et al.*[99] followed the plasma concentration of etomidate in 8 patients receiving an induction dose of 0.3 mg kg^{-1}. Anaesthesia in these patients was maintained with $1\frac{1}{2}$–2% enflurane in nitrous oxide–oxygen anaesthesia for an average duration of $3\frac{1}{2}$ hours. Plasma samples were taken over a 10-hour period following the induction dose, and analysed for plasma etomidate concentrations by gas chromatography–mass spectrometry. The results were consistent with those from a drug showing a three-compartment distribution model, the individual plasma half-lives being 2.6 min, 28.7 min, and 275.4 min respectively. The apparent volume of distribution was 4.51 l kg^{-1}, and the systemic or plasma clearance rate 11.7 ml kg^{-1} min^{-1}.

Subsequent studies by Schuttler *et al.*[79] in 1980 also looked at the kinetics after a single dose of 20 mg etomidate. As in the study described by Van Hamme, the patients received enflurane in nitrous oxide–oxygen for the maintenance of anaesthesia. However, Schuttler's data was best fitted to a two-compartment model, with an elimination half-life of 67.5 min, an apparent distribution volume of 2.2 l kg^{-1} and systemic clearance of 23.8 ml kg^{-1}. The differences between these two studies are not readily accountable.

More recent work from Schüttler and his colleagues[77] has shown that, in the presence of a steady-state concentration of fentanyl (10 ng ml^{-1}) the clearance of 20 mg etomidate was reduced from about 1600 to 400 ml min^{-1}, with little alteration of the elimination half-life. However, the initial volume of distribution (V_1) decreased from 21 l, to 5 l, and V_D^β from 160 l to about 40 l. The exact nature of this kinetic drug interaction is not known, but may possibly involve saturation of the enzymes responsible for the metabolism of etomidate. The clinical implications of such interactions are a prolongation of recovery after fentanyl-etomidate anaesthesia.

Studies by other workers[48] who infused fentanyl to a steady-state concentration of 20 ng ml^{-1}, have shown no change in the clearance of etomidate following its use as a continuous infusion for the maintenance of anaesthesia in patients undergoing elective abdominopelvic surgery.

ANAESTHESIA BY CONTINUOUS INTRAVENOUS INFUSION

The concept of anaesthetic potency, as defined by the amount of drug required to anaesthetise the average patient, has been developed primarily for the inhalation agents. The minimum alveolar concentration (MAC) was first described by Merkel and Eger[32, 55] and is the alveolar concentration of an anaesthetic in oxygen needed to produce a lack of reflex response to the initial surgical skin incision in 50% patients (ED_{50} or AD_{50}). Thus, MAC is a median response in an assumed normal distribution of values in a study population. This concept has allowed the construction of dose-response curves for the volatile and gaseous anaesthetics; allowing comparisons between the agents and investigation of the interaction of other drugs at equipotent concentrations[69]. An important feature of the concept is the constant relationship between the alveolar concentration of the gas or vapour, and the partial pressure of the agent in the blood. This depends on the agent's partition coefficient between the gaseous and blood phases. Thus, at a constant alveolar concentration of the agent, the concentration in arterial blood will remain constant. If the alveolar concentration is doubled or trebled, the blood concentration will similarly increase.

Minimum infusion rate

While MAC is now accepted as the standard index of equipotency for gaseous and volatile anaesthetics, no comparable index for intravenous agents was available at the time continuous intravenous infusion anaesthesia was developing. Prys-Roberts proposed[62, 63, 83, 84] that the infusion rate of an intravenous anaesthetic, which would prevent movement in response to an initial surgical skin incision in 50% of patients, should be adopted as a comparable standard ED_{50} for intravenous agents. This minimum infusion rate (MIR) would allow comparisons of equipotency to be made, not only between intravenous agents, but also between intravenous agents and their volatile and gaseous counterparts. As the same endpoint is used, the MIR for an intravenous agent should be equivalent to the MAC value for a volatile or gaseous anaesthetic. By the same token, proportional 50% mixtures of intravenous and gaseous anaesthetics should provide an equipotent anaesthetic combination comparable to 1 MIR of an intravenous agent, or 1 MAC of a volatile or gaseous anaesthetic.

Clearly, in both cases, the true index of equipotency would be the plasma concentration of the anaesthetic which, *in a steady-state*, would suppress movement in response to an initial surgical stimulus in 50% of patients. In the case of the volatile and gaseous agents, the plasma partial pressure is directly related to the mean alveolar concentration of the agent by the partition coefficient (λ) for the individual agent (see Chapter 5). In the case of the intravenous agents no such simple relationship exists. The plasma concentration of an intravenous anaesthetic under steady-state conditions of infusion is primarily determined by the ratio of the steady-state infusion rate to the plasma clearance of the drug (see Chapter 1). Therefore all the factors which determine the clearance of the drug will influence the relationship between infusion rate and plasma concentration of the intravenous anaesthetic. Despite these differences the use of an infusion rate as an index of equipotency has considerable merit when viewed in the context of clinical anaesthesia.

Dose-response curves

In order to determine the infusion rate appropriate to maintain surgical anaesthesia in 100% of patients, a dose-response curve for that agent must be determined under specific conditions. To give an example, the minimum infusion rate for Althesin used to supplement 66% nitrous oxide can be determined in the following way. Groups of 8–10 patients are randomly allocated to receive a bolus induction dose followed by a high infusion rate for 10 minutes, and one of 5–8 predetermined infusion rates for the subsequent anaesthesia[88]. After a period of not less than 25 minutes[O. G. W. Bastard, pers. commun.] the stable plasma concentrations will have been achieved[58, 71, 98, 100, 101] and the plasma concentration of the intravenous anaesthetic will have reached a plateau value within 5% of the long-term steady-state value. The response of each patient in each group to the initial surgical incision is then determined, and the percentage of the patients in each group responding to incision by movement, or no movement, can be plotted against the infusion rate (Fig. 7.7) on a Probit plot (see Chapter 2). In this way, the effect of other influences such as premedication, age, pre-existing disease or drug therapy, and the use of nitrous oxide, can be graphically represented in such a way as to allow determination of both the ED_{50} (MIR) or ED_{95} for each intravenous anaesthetic under a wide variety of conditions[88].

When considering the use of an intravenous anaesthetic as a supplement to 66% nitrous oxide, the question must be considered as to what proportion of the anaesthetic effect is contributed by the nitrous oxide, and how much by the intravenous anaesthetic. If one assumes that under steady-state conditions an inspired N_2O concentration of 66% results in an alveolar concentration of about 45–50%, which represents approximately 0.4 MAC based on the value of MAC for nitrous oxide as 105% equivalent to a partial pressure of 800mmHg[69]. One can then consider the infusion rate of an intravenous agent used together with 66% nitrous oxide as representing 0.6 of the true MIR for that agent.

Infusions of steroid anaesthetics

Althesin

First reports of the administration of Althesin by infusion were given by du Cailar[14] and Savege *et al.*[76]. The first attempts to determine dose-response relationships for Althesin were based on early attempts to define MIR by a different approach to that defined above (C. Prys-Roberts, unpub. obs. 1976), in which the infusion rate which just abolished movement in response to a continuing surgical stimulus was determined. At that time, and on the basis of the small numbers of patients studied, it was assumed that a number of such infusion rates would be normally distributed and that the mean value would be equivalent to MIR in that 50% of the values would be above and 50% below the mean. The value for the MIR for Althesin in combination with nitrous oxide (66%) in patients premedicated with morphine 0.15 mg kg^{-1} was 18 µg kg^{-1} min^{-1} as total Althesin steroids, equivalent to 13.5 µg kg^{-1} min^{-1} as alphaxalone[83]. Recent studies have indicated that the distribution of values of MIR is non-Gaussian[88], but the median value for the MIR as alphaxalone (13.6 μg kg^{-1} min^{-1}: 95% tolerance limits 10.2 and 18.2 μg kg^{-1} min^{-1}) was very close to the earlier figure. After 30–40 min at an alphaxalone infusion rate of 18 μg kg^{-1} min^{-1} the mean plasma concentration of alphaxalone was 1.91 $\pm$ 0.09 μg ml^{-1}[83, 84]. The variation (range 1.05 to 3.08 μg ml^{-1}) was not related to patient sex, body build or age. One explanation may be that different degrees of protein and tissue binding, and especially liver blood flow, may have contributed to the variation. The plasma clearance for these patients (Table 7.1) was of the same order as that found for single dose administrations[90] in normal patients.

In normal patients, increasing the infusion rates by multiples of MIR was related to a linear increase of plasma concentration, though at 5 × MIR (67.5 μg kg^{-1} min^{-1} alphaxalone) the mean plasma concentration was only just over twice the plasma concentration at 1 MIR (3.93 $\pm$ 0.28 μg ml^{-1}).

In a series of hypertensive patients, treated with β-adrenoceptor antagonists and/or guanethidine analogues, we found a significant decrease of plasma clearance (Table 7.1) compatible with the measured decrease of cardiac output and a presumed decrease of splanchnic blood flow[86]. Comparable decreased clearance of lignocaine has been observed in patients receiving β-adrenoceptor antagonists[9], in contrast to the higher values for lignocaine clearance[8] in normal patients, comparable with the values for clearance of alphaxalone, minaxolone, methohexitone and di-isopropyl phenol.

Hepatic dysfunction has been considered in Chapter 4 as a major factor influencing the pharmacokinetic profile of drugs which are flow-limited in their hepatic bio-transformation. By comparison with the normal patients described above, the infusion of alphaxalone at 15.1 and 70.0 μg kg^{-1} min^{-1} respectively in 15 patients with cirrhotic liver disease undergoing portocaval anastomosis, resulted in plasma concentrations of 0.72 $\pm$ 0.13 and 1.61 $\pm$ 0.35 μg ml^{-1}[80, 82].

Effects of premedication on MIR for Althesin

Fig. 7.7 indicates the differences in drug requirement, estimated by the ED$_{50}$ and ED$_{95}$ values for both Althesin and methohexitone, in patients premedicated with diazepam rather than morphine[88]. Other data in the literature, reviewed by Towler *et al.*[97] are more difficult to reconcile with our own results for a number of reasons because of major differences in the design of the various studies.

Minaxolone

During infusion of minaxolone to supplement nitrous oxide (66%) there was marked cardiovascular stability both in normotensive and hypertensive patients[87]. There was no evidence of drug accumulation over periods of infusion up to 260 min. After induction with 0.5 mg kg^{-1} minaxolone and maintenance with an infusion of mean

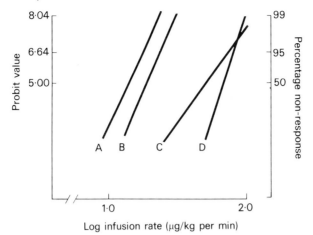

Fig. 7.7   Dose-response plots of four intravenous hypnotic drugs given by continuous infusion. The response is recorded as a quantal all-or-none response to the initial surgical incision, and then plotted as the probit value. Groups A and C were patients premedicated with morphine 0.15 mg kg^{-1} pre-operatively, and receiving infusions of Althesin or methohexitone respectively to supplement 67% nitrous oxide in oxygen; while Groups B and D were premedicated with diazepam 10 mg orally pre-operatively, and receiving infusions of Althesin or methohexitone respectively to supplement 67% nitrous oxide in oxygen. (Reproduced by permission of the Editor and Publishers of *Anaesthesia*.)

rate 11.0 μg kg^{-1} min^{-1}, the plasma minaxolone concentration after 60 min infusion was 0.62 μg ml^{-1}; and 0.63 μg ml^{-1} immediately prior to cessation of the infusion (mean time 155 min). The pharmacokinetic data for minaxolone infusion are shown in Table 7.1 and show a difference between the two studies described in the literature. Although pharmacokinetic profiles are usually believed to be dose-independent, the data from Mather and colleagues[53] were obtained with sub-anaesthetic doses in volunteers, whereas our results were obtained in fully anaesthetised patients receiving nitrous oxide, in whom the cardiac output values were 30% below those obtained in the awake patient.

Recovery after infusions of Althesin or Minaxolone

Following infusions of either of these drugs at 1–1.5 MIR lasting between 80 and 260 min, the decay of plasma concentrations followed a biphasic exponential pattern similar to that found after single dose administration of either drug[85] (Table 7.1). The relationship between recovery times, responding to command and recalling the correct data of birth, and the plasma concentration of the drugs are shown in Table 7.4, where they are compared with the results from studies of di-isopropyl phenol infusions[64]. It is interesting that the ratio between the plasma concentration at awakening (C_P^{aw}) and that during the previous steady-state infusion (C_P^{ss}) was very similar for each of the three anaesthetics, despite the wide difference in the times of recovery. This indicates a slower elimination of minaxolone, a hydrophilic steroid, from the brain by comparison with either alphaxalone (Althesin) or di-isopropyl phenol, both lipophilic drugs (Table 7.5).

Infusions of propanidid

There are several reports of propanidid being used by continuous infusion for the maintenance of anaesthesia in general anaesthetic practice, in children, and in the obstetric patient[57, 75]. The rate of administration for the maintenance of anaesthesia varied from about $1.5 \, mg \, kg^{-1} \, min^{-1}$ in children aged up to 8 years, to $50–100 \, mg \, min^{-1}$ in adults. No pharmacokinetic data are available. The use of propanidid, either by bolus injection or by infusion, may be associated with the release of histamine[26], with an incidence of reaction varying between 1 in 170[38] to 1 in 10 000[26].

Infusions of etomidate

The rapid metabolism and clearance of etomidate has allowed the drug to be used as part of a continuous intravenous anaesthetic technique by several authors. No information is currently available which would allow a dose-response curve to be constructed for infusions of etomidate, either alone or in combination with nitrous oxide. Attempts by the authors to construct such curves were hampered by the occurrence of spontaneous muscular movement on the part of the patient at low infusion rates, precluding the definition of an unequivocal end-point for the response to initial surgical incision. Schuttler and his colleagues[78] induced anaesthesia with an infusion of etomidate $8.0 \, mg \, min^{-1}$ for 10 min, and then maintained anaesthesia with a slower rate of $0.8 \, mg \, min^{-1}$. The mean etomidate plasma concentration at the end of a 60 min infusion period was $0.52 \, \mu g \, ml^{-1}$. Prompt recovery of consciousness followed cessation of the infusion (mean time 11.9 min), and the elimination half-life approximated to 46 min. This corresponds to a systemic clearance of $25.8 \, ml \, kg^{-1} \, min^{-1}$. Similar results were described by Walters and his colleagues[102] who studied the intra-operative kinetics of etomidate during a two-stage infusion programme in patients undergoing peripheral neurosurgical procedures. After an initial fast infusion of $100 \, \mu g \, kg^{-1} \, min^{-1}$, anaesthesia was maintained with an infusion of 10 μg etomidate kg^{-1} to supplement either 67% nitrous oxide in oxygen, or oxygen-enriched air. Additional analgesia was provided by increments of fentanyl $(5–12 \, \mu g \, kg^{-1}$ total dose).

Two notable features of this regimen were the achievement of stable concentrations of etomidate by approximately 40 min after commencement of the infusion, and the absence of any evidence of drug accumulation during the maintenance infusion phase (mean duration: 124 min). However, use of the fast infusion rate for the induction

Table 7.4 Relationships between plasma concentrations during steady-state infusion (C_P^{ss}) and at awakening (C_P^{aw}), and the times to recovery of response to command (T_{rc}) and recall of date of birth (T_{dob}), for Althesin (alphaxalone), minaxolone, and di-isopropyl phenol[64, 87].

	n	C_P^{ss} (μg ml^{-1})	C_P^{aw} (μg ml^{-1})	C_P^{aw}/C_P^{ss}	T_{rc}^* (min)	T_{dob}^* (min)
Althesin	11	1.91$\pm$0.1	0.90$\pm$0.1	0.48	12.2	26.3
Minaxolone	9	0.63$\pm$0.05	0.30$\pm$0.05	0.48	34.0	—
Di-isopropyl phenol	11	1.55$\pm$0.14	0.72$\pm$0.1	0.46	5.0	6.5

* T_{rc} and T_{dob} are geometric means.

Table 7.5 Correlations between time to recovery (T_{dob}) of recall of date of birth, total dose of drug administered, and duration of infusion, for infusions of Althesin, minaxolone, methohexitone, and di-isopropyl phenol. All data were derived from studies [65, 83, 87, 88] of patients premedicated with morphine 0.15 mg kg^{-1}, in whom the infusions were used to supplement nitrous oxide (67%) anaesthesia. Values quoted are for the correlation coefficient (r) and its significance derived from the equation $t = r\sqrt{\dfrac{n-2}{1-r^2}}$.

	Infusion rate (μg kg^{-1} min^{-1})	n	Duration of infusion (range) (min)	Total dose (range) (mg)	T_{dob} vs. duration (r)	T_{dob} vs. total dose (r)
Althesin (alphaxalone)	13–15*	25	36–289	43– 400*	0.33 n.s.	0.41 n.s.
Minaxolone	11–13	22	26–258	62– 226	0.45 p < 0.05	0.56 p < 0.01
Methohexitone	50–65	27	26–264	166–1300	0.72 p < 0.001	0.73 p < 0.001
Di-isopropyl phenol	50–60	8	54–124	160– 624	0 n.s.	0 n.s.

* infusion rates are quoted as rates for alphaxalone and total dose of alphaxalone.

Probit dose response curves for infusions of hypnotic agents with various premedication regimes[88]. All patients breathed 66% nitrous oxide in oxygen. A Althesin with morphine premedication; B Althesin with diazepam; C Methohexitone with morphine; D Methohexitone with diazepam.

	ED_{50} (MIR)	ED_{95}	ED_{95}/ED_{50}
A	13.73 (12.49–15.10)	18.34 (16.64–20.23)	1.34
B	18.47 (16.63–20.51)	24.18 (21.68–26.96)	1.31
C	48.79 (38.69–61.52)	75.72 (59.64–96.18)	1.55
D	66.01 (62.84–69.33)	80.72 (76.87–84.81)	1.22

Values quoted are expressed in μg kg^{-1} min^{-1}; with the rates for Althesin as alphaxalone (Mean and limits of 1 SEM).

of anaesthesia results in a C_p^{max}/C_p^{ss} ratio in excess of 5. There appeared to be no significant differences in the systemic clearance rates between those patients receiving etomidate to supplement 67 % nitrous oxide in oxygen (20.9 ml kg^{-1} min^{-1}; SEM 2.6) and those breathing oxygen-enriched air (26.7 ml kg^{-1} min^{-1}; SEM 3.6). However, for the same infusion regimen, the plasma etomidate concentrations were higher at all sampling points in those patients receiving nitrous oxide. Whether this may indicate a small decrease in the systemic clearance of etomidate due to the nitrous oxide is uncertain. However, an effect of anaesthetic concentrations of nitrous oxide in oxygen on the total hepatic blood flow of the greyhound has been found by Thomson and his colleagues[44, 96]. Despite the lack of difference in the pharmacokinetics of etomidate of these groups of patients, there was a marked pharmacodynamic difference with respect to the time to recovery to giving correct date of birth, geometric means: 15.1 min in patients receiving oxygen-enriched air; 59.1 min in the patients who received nitrous oxide in oxygen (p < 0.01).

Use in Intensive Care Unit—sedation

A technique of etomidate by infusion for sedation in the I.C.U. has been described by Edbrooke and colleagues[30]. The rate of infusion required varied between 2 and 40 μg kg^{-1} min^{-1}. In a separate kinetic study in 6 patients[105] the mean infusion rate of etomidate was 3.4 μg kg^{-1} min^{-1}, supplemented by fentanyl 0.034 μg kg^{-1} min^{-1}. An adequate level of sedation was achieved with a mean plasma etomidate concentration of 230 ng ml^{-1}. At steady-state conditions, there was a linear relationship between the infusion rate and the plasma etomidate concentration. The mean systemic clearance from the steady-state data approximated to 24 ml kg^{-1} min^{-1}.

Recent correspondence in the Lancet[106–8], has cast doubts over the efficacy and safety of etomidate by infusion for the maintenance of anaesthesia or sedation in the intensive care unit due to possible inhibition of adrenocortical response. The nature of the inhibition is unclear, but there does not appear to be suppression of some other indices of the stress response, such as the rise in blood sugar levels (J. Sear, pers. commun.).

Infusions of di-isopropyl phenol

Di-isopropyl phenol may be given as a continuous infusion, either alone or to supplement nitrous oxide for surgical anaesthesia. Under the latter conditions, in patients premedicated with morphine 0.15 mg kg^{-1}, the minimum infusion rate of di-isopropyl phenol was found to be 51.3 ± 3.8 μg kg^{-1} min^{-1} following induction with a single bolus dose of 1.5 mg kg^{-1} [64]. Under steady-state infusion conditions, at least 45 min after starting the infusion, the mean whole blood concentration of di-isopropyl phenol was 1.55 ± 0.14 μg ml^{-1}[66]. Di-isopropyl phenol is equally distributed between plasma and red cells[2]. At double the minimum infusion rate

(100 μg kg^{-1} min^{-1}) the mean whole blood concentration was 3.26 ± 0.54 μg ml^{-1} indicating a rather different relationship to that found for Althesin. The values for pharmacokinetic parameters were derived for patients by following the decay of whole blood concentration for 240 min after the end of infusions lasting between 75 and 184 min (Table 7.1). Recovery from anaesthesia with di-isopropyl phenol to supplement nitrous oxide was rapid and pleasant for the patient. Patients responded to command at 5.0 min (geometric mean; range 4.25–7.5 min) and recalled their date of birth at 6.5 min (geometric mean; range 5.0–9.0 min). The latter event was achieved at a mean whole blood concentration of 0.72 ± 0.1 μg ml^{-1}. No correlation was found between the recovery times and either the duration of infusion or total dose (Table 7.5).

Barbiturates by infusion

Thiopentone

Although there are reports of intraoperative use of thiopentone by infusion[6, 45] the main use of infusions are in the management of cerebral hypoxia after cardiorespiratory arrest[56, 91], and as a technique to sedate patients being artificially ventilated[13]. By inference, the thiopentone infusion rate needed to supplement 66 % N_2O in O_2 anaesthesia is 160–280 μg kg^{-1} min^{-1}. One of the main reasons for the lack of interest in the thiopentone infusions is the prolonged dose-dependent recovery; a reflection of the role of redistribution rather than metabolism in the elimination of drug from the vascular compartment.

Following prolonged infusion of thiopentone in doses of 300–500 mg kg^{-1} given over 2 days, its elimination rate fitted best to a Michaelis–Menten, rather than a first-order kinetic model; indicating that the pharmacokinetics of thiopentone may be influenced by either the total dose of drug or the duration of its administration. Thus, as the thiopentone dose increases, so does its elimination half-life. At concentrations greater than 60 μg ml^{-1} thiopentone, the elimination half-life approached 60–70 hours. However, at lower plasma concentrations, the half life was reduced and became closer to the first order value of 6–12 hours[11, 12, 33, 49].

During infusions of thiopentone, there is a plasma drug accumulation up to concentrations of 30–50 μg ml^{-1}. If saturation occurs, the long elimination half-life of the zero-order kinetic decay will also affect the time course of the pharmacodynamic effects observed[91]. In a separate haemodynamic study, where thiopentone was infused at a rate of about 150 mg hr^{-1} to 30 patients being ventilated for respiratory insufficiency, there was a slower build-up of the plasma thiopentone concentration. At 24–36 hours, the plasma thiopentone concentration was 8.8 ± 0.7 μg ml^{-1}, increasing to 18.5 ± 1.0 μg ml^{-1} at 48 hours. At these rates of infusion, there was only minimal cardiovascular depression. The elimination half-life on stopping the infusion was approximately 9 hours[13]. Whether this is similarly true for the pharmacokinetics of other agents when given at high doses by infusion remains to be determined.

Methohexitone

In contrast, the use of methohexitone by infusion to supplement N_2O or to maintain anaesthesia alone has been described by several authors[20, 28, 36, 46, 95, 104]. The rate of infusion varied between 30–90 $\mu g\,kg^{-1}\,min^{-1}$, dependent on the chosen premedication, inspired gas composition, and use or not of other analgesic drugs. More recently the haemodynamic effects of methohexitone infusions have been compared with those of the other infusion agents[65, 67]. For this purpose the MIR for methohexitone was determined, for patients breathing nitrous oxide (67%), to be 48.8 (range 38.7–61.5) $\mu g\,kg^{-1}\,min^{-1}$ (Fig. 7.1).

The pharmacokinetics of methohexitone have recently been described by Hudson and his colleagues in nine patients undergoing anaesthesia[43]. When given as a single bolus dose of 2.4 $mg\,kg^{-1}$, with arterial sampling for up to 12 hours after injection, the elimination half-life of methohexitone was 240 min. In contrast, Breimer[10] described the pharmacokinetics of methohexitone after infusion of a subanaesthetic dose (50 $\mu g\,kg^{-1}\,min^{-1}$) over 60 min to 4 volunteers. The elimination half-life in this set of studies was considerably shorter (97 min), although the systemic clearance was comparable in the two groups of subjects. It is probable that the longer half-life, in the patients of Hudson *et al.* was due to the decreased hepatic blood flow as a result of anaesthesia and surgery. Although methohexitone is more rapidly cleared and metabolised than thiopentone, redistribution is still important in the termination of the pharmacodynamic effects of a single dose of both drugs. If the tissue stores become saturated, by either repeated doses or an infusion of the drug, redistribution cannot continue and then recovery from methohexitone would be more rapid than from thiopentone because of the shorter elimination half-life.

Studies performed in the authors' departments have shown that infusions of methohexitone (60 $\mu g\,kg^{-1}\,min^{-1}$) to supplement 67% N_2O in the spontaneously breathing patient was associated with recovery to the recollection of the correct date of birth was dose-dependent for patients premedicated with either diazepam or morphine[88] (Table 7.5). Thus, the apparent increasing cumulative effects of methohexitone, after a total dose of about 500–600 mg, may limit the use of this agent to operations of less than 2 hours.

GLOSSARY

Generic name	Approved name and (Trade name)	North American Trade name
Alphaxalone and Alphadolone acetate in Cremophor EL	(Althesin)	Alfathesin (Canada)
Minaxolone	Minaxolone*	—
Propanidid in Cremophor EL	Propanidid (Epontol)	—
Etomidate in propylene glycol or absolute alcohol	Etomidate (Hypnomidate)	—
Di-isopropyl phenol in Cremophor EL	Disoprofol (Diprivan)*	—
Thiopentone sodium Methohexitone sodium	Thiopentone (Pentothal) Brietal	Thiopental Methohexital

* under review by the Committee for Safety of Medicines (UK).

REFERENCES

1. ADAM H. K., BRIGGS L. P., BAHAR M., DOUGLAS E. J. & DUNDEE J. W. (1983) Pharmacokinetic evaluation of ICI 35868 in man. *Br. J. Anaesth.* **55**, 97.
2. ADAM H. K., DOUGLAS E. J., PLUMMER G. F. & COSGROVE M. B. (1981) Estimation of ICI 35868 (Diprivan) in blood by high performance liquid chromatography, following coupling with Gibb's reagent. *J. Chromatography* **223** (Biomedical applications 12), 232–7.
3. ADAM H. K., GLEN J. B. & HOYLE P. A. (1980) Pharmacokinetics in laboratory animals of ICI 35868, a new i.v. anaesthetic agent. *Br. J. Anaesth.* **52**, 743–6.
4. ADAM H. K., KAY B. & DOUGLAS E. J. (1982) Blood disoprofol levels in anaesthetised patients. *Anaesthesia* **37**, 536–40.
5. AVELING W., SEAR J. W., FITCH W., CHANG H., WATERS A., COOPER G. M., SIMPSON P., SAVEGE T. M., PRYS-ROBERTS C. & CAMPBELL D. (1979) Early clinical evaluation of Minaxolone: a new intravenous steroid anaesthetic agent. *Lancet* **ii**, 71–73.
6. BLUNNIE W. P., ZACHARIAS M., DUNDEE J. W., DOGGART J. R. & MCILROY (1981) Liver enzyme studies with continuous intravenous anaesthesia. *Anaesthesia* **36**, 152.
7. BOYCE J. R., WRIGHT F. J., CERVENKO F. W., PIETAK S. P. & FAULKNER S. (1976) Prolongation of anesthetic action by BNPP (Bis-(P-nitrophenyl) phosphate) *Anesthesiology* **45**, 629.
8. BOYES R. N., SCOTT D. B., JEPSON R. J., GOODMAN M. J. & JULIAN D. G. (1971) Pharmacokinetics of lidocaine in man. *Clin. Pharmacol. Ther.* **12**, 105.
9. BRANCH R. A., SHAND D.G., WILKINSON G. R. & NIES A. S. (1973) The reduction of lidocaine clearance by dl-propranolol. An example of hemodynamic drug interaction. *J. Pharmacol. Exp. Ther.* **184**, 515.

10. BREIMER D. D. (1976) Pharmacokinetics of methohexitone following intravenous infusion in man. *Br. J. Anaesth.* **48**, 643.

11. BURCH P. G. & STANSKI D. R. (1981) Pharmacokinetics of thiopental in renal failure. *Anesthesiology* **55A**, 176.

12. BURCH P. G. & STANSKI D. R. (1981) Thiopental protein binding. *Anesthesiology* **55A**, 253.

13. CARLON G. C., KAHN R. C., GOLDINER P. L., HOWLAND W. S. & TURNBULL A. (1978) Long-term infusion of sodium thiopental—hemodynamic and respiratory effect. *Crit. Care Med.* **6**, 311.

14. Du CAILAR J. (1972) The effects in man of infusions of Althesin, with particular regard to the cardiovascular system. *Postgrad. Med. J.* **48** (suppl. 2), 72.

15. CARD B., McCULLOUGH R. J. & PRATT D. A. H. (1972) Tissue distribution of CT 1341 in the rat: An autoradiographic study. *Postgrad. Med. J.* **48** (suppl. 2), 34.

16. CHILD K. J., CURRIE J. P., DAVIS B., DODDS M. G., PEARCE D. R. & TWISSELL D. J. (1971) The pharmacological properties in animals of CT 1341—a new steroid anaesthetic agent. *Br. J. Anaesth.* **43**, 2.

17. CHILD K.J., DAVIS B., DODDS M. G. & TWISSELL D. J. (1972) Anaesthetic, cardiovascular and respiratory effects of a new steroidal agent CT 1341—a comparison with other intravenous anaesthetic drugs in the unrestrained cat. *Br. J. Pharmacol.* **46**, 189.

18. CHILD K. J., GIBSON W., HARNBY G. & HART J. W. (1972) Metabolism and excretion of Althesin (CT 1341) in the rat. *Postgrad. Med. J.* **48** (suppl. 2), 37.

19. CLARKE R. S. J., DUNDEE J. W. & CARSON I. W. (1972) Some aspects of the clinical pharmacology of Althesin. *Postgrad. Med. J.* **48** (suppl. 2), 62.

20. COLEMAN D. J. & DE VILLIERS J. C. (1964) Anaesthesia and stereotactic surgery. *Anaesthesia* **19**, 60.

21. CRAIG J., COOPER G. M. & SEAR J. W. (1982) Recovery from anaesthesia. Comparison between methohexitone, Althesin and etomidate. *Br. J. Anaesth.* **54**, 447.

22. DAVIS B., DODDS M. G., DOLAMORE P. G., GARDNER C. J., SAWYER P. R., TWISSELL D. J. & VALLANCE D. K. (1979) Minaxolone: a new water-soluble steroid anaesthetic. *Br. J. Anaesth.* **51**, 564.

23. DESMET G., NEMITZ B., BOITIEUX J. L., AGHA B. E. & MUIR J. F. (1979) Dosage de l'alphaxalone dans le sérum et les urines par chromatographie gaz-liquide. *Ann. Biol. Clin. (Paris)* **37**, 83.

24. DOENICKE A. (1974) Etomidate, a new intravenous hypnotic. *Acta Anaesthesiol. Belgica* **25**, 307.

25. DOENICKE A., KRUMEY I., KUGLER J. & KLEMPA J. (1968) Experimental studies of the breakdown of Epontol determination of propanidid in human serum. *Br. J. Anaesth.* **40**, 415–29.

26. DOENICKE A., LORENZ W., BEIGL R., BEZECNY H., UHLIG G., KALMAR L., PRAETORIUS B. & MANN G. (1973) Histamine release after intravenous application of short acting hypnotics: a comparison of etomidate, Althesin (CT 1341) and propanidid. *Br. J. Anaesth.* **45**, 1097–104.

27. DUBOIS M., ALLISON J. & GEDDES I. C. (1975) Determination of alphaxalone in human blood by gas liquid chromatography. *Br. J. Anaesth.* **47**, 902.

28. DUNKIN L. (1972) Methohexitone in the management of a disturbed patient: case report. *Br. J. Anaesth.* **44**, 971.

29. DUNN G. L., MORISON D. H., McCHESNEY J., PINE W., KUMANA C. R. & GUPTA R. N. (1980) The pharmacokinetics and pharmacodynamics of minaxolone. *Anesthesiology* **53s**, 48.

30. EDBROOKE D. L., MATHER S. J., DIXON A. M. & HEBRON B. S. (1982) Safer sedation for ventilated patients. A new application for etomidate. *Anaesthesia* **37**, 765.

31. EDWARDS R. W. H., KELLIE A. E. & WADE A. P. (1953) The extraction and

oxidation of urinary steroid conjugates. *Mem. Soc. Endocrinol.* No. **2**, 53.

32. EGER E. I., SAIDMAN L. J. & BRANDSTATER B. (1965) Minimum alveolar anesthetic concentrations: a standard of anesthetic potency. *Anesthesiology* **26**, 756.

33. EVANS J. M. & KEOGH J. A. M. (1977) Adverse reactions to intravenous anaesthetic induction agents. *Br. Med. J.* **2**, 735–6.

34. GHONEIM M. M. & VAN HAMME M. J. (1978) Pharmacokinetics of thiopentone: effects of enflurane and nitrous oxide anaesthesia and surgery. *Br. J. Anaesth.* **50**, 1237.

35. GLEN J. B., HUNTER S. C. & THOMSON D. S. (1982) The role of cremophor EL in anaphylactoid reactions to i.v. anaesthetics. *Br. J. Anaesth.* **54**, 231P.

36. GOLDIE L., FRIED Y., GOULD T. & PEDERSON T. M. (1968) Electroencephalographs in the subnormal and the mentally ill child. *Anaesthesia* **23**, 364.

37. GOURLAY G. K., MATHER L. E. & PARKING K. S. (1980) Minaxolone, a new steroidal anesthetic. Pharmacokinetics and organ extraction in sheep. *Drug. Metab. Dispos.* **8**, 452.

38. HARRFELDT H. P. (1973) 10 Jahre Kurznarkosen mit propanidid. In Zindler M., Yamamura H. & Wirth W. (eds.), *Intravenose narkose mit Propanidid*, pp. 234–42. Springer-Verlag, Berlin.

39. HEINONEN J., RIITTA O. & LOUHIJA A. (1973) Anaesthesia for cardioversion.: a comparison of Althesin and thiopentone. *Br. J. Anaesth.* **45**, 49.

40. HEYKANTS J., BRUGMANS J. & DOENICKE A. (1973) Pharmacokinetics of etomidate (R 26490) in human volunteers: plasma levels, metabolism and excretion. *Janssen Research Products Information Service. Clinical Research Report* R 26490/1.

41. HEYKANTS J. J. P., MEULDERMANS W. E. G., MICHIELS L. J. M., LEWI P. J. & JANSSEN P. A. J. (1975) Distribution, metabolism and excretion of etomidate, a

short-acting hypnotic drug, in the rat. Comparative study of (R)-(+) and (S)-(−) etomidate. (1975) reprinted from *Arch. Int. Pharmacodynamie Thér.* **216**, 113.

42. HOLLY J. M. P., TRAFFORD D. J. H., SEAR J. W. & MAKIN H. L. J. (1981) The *in vivo* metabolism of Althesin (alphaxalone and alphadolone acetate) in man. *J. Pharm. Pharmacol.* **33**, 427.

43. HUDSON R. J., STANSKI D. R. & BURCH P. A. (1982) Comparative pharmacokinetics of methohexital and thiopental. *Anesthesiology* **57**, A240.

44. HUGHES R. L., CAMPBELL D. & FITCH W. (1980) Effects of enflurane and halothane on liver blood flow and oxygen consumption in the greyhound. *Br. J. Anaesth.* **52**, 1079.

45. HUNTER A. R. (1972) Thiopentone supplemented anaesthesia for intracranial surgery. *Br. J. Anaesth.* **44**, 506.

46. HUNTER A. R. (1972) Methohexitone as a supplement to nitrous oxide during intracranial surgery. *Br. J. Anaesth.* **44**, 1188.

47. JAMES R. & GLEN J. B. (1980) Synthesis, biological evaluation and preliminary structure activity considerations of a series of alkylphenols as intravenous anesthetic agents. *J. Med. Chemistry.* **23**, 1350–7.

48. JONES D. & LAURENCE A. S. (1982) Fentanyl and etomidate plasma concentrations in a total i.v. anaesthetic technique to 6 hours after operation. *Br. J. Anaesth.* **54**, 1130.

49. JONES M. E. & NICHOLAS T. I. (1981) The pharmacokinetics of the intravenous steroid anesthetic Alphaxalone in the isolated perfused rat lung. *J. Pharmacokin. Biopharm.* **9**, 343.

50. KAY B. (1976) A dose-response relationship for etomidate, with some observations on cumulation. *Br. J. Anaesth.* **48**, 213.

51. KAY B. & ROLLY G. (1977) ICI 35868, a new intravenous induction agent. *Acta. Anaesth. Belg.* **28**, 303–17.

52. MANNES G. A. & DOENICKE A. (1977) Protein binding of etomidate. *Anaesthesiol. Resusc.* **106**, 6.

53. MATHER L. E., GOURLAY G. K., PARKIN K. S. & ROBERTS J. G. (1981) Pharmacodynamics of minaxolone, a new steroidal anesthetic. *J. Pharmacol. Exp. Ther.* **217**, 481.

54. MATHER L. E., SEOW L. T., ROBERTS J. G., GOURLAY G. K. & COUSINS M. J. (1981) Development of a model for integrated pharmacokinetic and pharmacodynamic studies of intravenous anaesthetic agents: application to minaxolone. *Eur. J. Clin. Pharmacol.* **19**, 371.

55. MERKEL G. & EGER E. I. (1963) A comparative study of halothane and halopropane anesthesia. Including method for determining equipotency. *Anesthesiology* **24**, 346.

56. MICHENFELDER J. D. & THEYE R. A. (1973) Cerebral protection by thiopental during hypoxia. *Anesthesiology* **39**, 510.

57. MILLET J. P. (1977) Le propanidide (Épontol) en perfusion veineuse prolongée pour l'opération césarienne. À propos de 41 observations. *Ann. Anesth. Franc.* **18**, 723–9.

58. MITENKO P. A. & OGILVIE R. I. (1972) Rapidly achieved plasma concentration plateaus with observations on theophylline kinetics. *Clin. Pharmacol. Ther.* **13**, 329.

59. MORGAN D. J., BLACKMAN G. L., PAULL J. D. & WOLF L. J. (1981) Pharmacokinetics and plasma binding of thiopental. I: Studies in surgical patients. *Anesthesiology* **54**, 468.

60. MURPHY F. J., GUADAGNI N. P. & DeBON F. (1955) Use of steroid anesthesia in surgery. *J. Am. Med. Assoc.* **158**, 1412.

61. NICHOLAS T. E., JONES M. E., JOHNSON D. W. & PHILLIPPI G. (1981) Metabolism of the steroid anaesthetic Alphaxalone by the isolated perfused rat lung. *J. Steroid Biochem.* **14**, 45.

62. PRYS-ROBERTS C. (1980) Practical and pharmacological implications of continuous intravenous anesthesia. *Acta. Anaesth. Belg.* **31**, 225–30.

63. PRYS-ROBERTS C. (1982) Cardiovascular effects of continuous intravenous anaesthesia compared with those of inhalational anaesthesia. *Acta. Anaesth. Scand.* **26** (Suppl. 75). 10–17.

64. PRYS-ROBERTS C., SEAR J. & ADAM H. K. (1981) Pharmacokinetics of continuous infusions of Althesin, minaxolone and ICI 35868 to supplement nitrous oxide anaesthesia in man. *Br. J. Anaesth.* **53**, 115P.

65. PRYS-ROBERTS C., SEAR J. W., LOW J. M., PHILLIPS K. C. & DAGNINO J. (1983) Hemodynamic and hepatic effects of methohexital infusion during nitrous oxide anesthesia in man. *Anesth. Analg.* **62**, 317.

66. PRYS-ROBERTS C., DAVIES J. R., CALVERLEY R. K. & GOODMAN N. W. (1983) Haemodynamic effects of infusions of di-isopropyl phenol (ICI 35868) during nitrous oxide anaesthesia in man. *Br. J. Anaesth.* **55**, 105.

67. PUNCHIHEWA V. G., ·MORGAN M., LUMLEY J. & WHITWAM J. G. (1980) Initial experience with minaxolone; a water-soluble steroid intravenous anaesthetic agent. *Anaesthesia* **35**, 214.

68. PUTTER J. (1970) Métabolisme et pharmacocinétique du propanidide. *Symposium consacré à l'Épontol et à sa place en Anesthésiologie*, pp. 13–25. Édition Théraplix, Paris.

69. QUASHA A. L., EGER E. I. & TINKER J. H. (1980) Determination and applications of MAC. *Anesthesiology* **53**, 315–34.

70. RADFORD S. G., LOCKYER J. A. & SIMPSON P. J. (1982) Immunological aspects of adverse reactions to Althesin. *Br. J. Anaesth.* **54**, 859–63.

71. RIGG J. R. A. & WONG T. Y. (1981) A method for achieving rapidly steady-state blood concentrations of i.v. drugs. *Br. J. Anaesth.* **53**, 1247–57.

72. ROGERS K. M., DEWAR K. M. S., McCUBBIN T. D. & SPENCE A. A. (1980) preliminary experience with ICI 35868 as an i.v. induction agent: comparison with Althesin. *Anaesthesia* **35**, 1182–7.

73. RUTTER D. V., MORGAN M., LUMLEY J. & OWEN R. (1980) ICI 35868 (Diprivan): a new intravenous induction agent. A comparison with methohexitone. *Anaesthesia* **35**, 1188–92.

74. SARAIVA R. A., NAGUNUMA L. I. & SETE M. (1978) Effect of undernutrition on the uptake and distribution of i.v. anaesthetic agents. A study in mice. *Br. J. Anaesth.* **50**, 365.

75. SAUVAGE M. R., KRIVOSIC R., CALMES M. O., ZIMMER R. & GAUTHIER LAFAYE J. P. (1974) Utilisation du propanidide en perfusion chez l'enfant de 0 à 8 ans. *Anesthesie Analgesie Réanimation* **31**, 237–47.

76. SAVEGE T. M., RAMSAY M. A. E., CURRAN J. P., COTTER J., WALLING P. T. & SIMPSON B. R. (1975) Intravenous anaesthesia by infusion: a technique using alphaxalone/alphadolone (Althesin). *Anaesthesia* **30**, 757–64.

77. SCHÜTTLER J., LAUVEN P. M., SCHWILDEN H. & STOECKEL H. (1982) Alterations of the pharmacokinetics of etomidate caused by fentanyl. *Anaesthesia:* Volume of Summaries, VIth European Congress of Anaesthesiology, London, Abstract 700, p 368.

78. SCHÜTTLER J., STOECKEL H., WILMS M., SCHWILDEN H. & LAUVEN P. M. (1980) Ein pharmakokinetisch begründetes Infusionsmodell für etomidat zur Aufrechterhaltung von steady state-Plasmaspiegeln. *Anaesthesist* **29**, 662.

79. SCHÜTTLER J., WILMS M., LAUVEN P. M., STOECKEL H. & KOENIG A. (1980) Pharmakokinetische Unter-suchungen über Etomidat beim Menschen. *Anaesthesist* **29**, 658.

80. SEAR J. W. (1981) The metabolism of steroid intravenous anaesthetic agents and their modification by liver disease. Ph. D. thesis; University of Bristol.

81. SEAR J. W., COOPER G. M., WILLIAMS N.B., SIMPSON P. J. & PRYS-ROBERTS C. (1980) Minaxolone or Althesin supplemented by nitrous oxide. A study in anaesthesia for short operative procedures. *Anaesthesia* **35**, 169.

82. SEAR J. W., MAKIN H. L. J., STAFFORD M. A., TRAFFORD D. J. H. & PRYS-ROBERTS C. (1981) Disposition and metabolism of Althesin in patients with cirrhotic liver disease. *Br. J. Anaesth.* **53**, 1093.

83. SEAR J. W. & PRYS-ROBERTS C. (1979) Plasma alphaxalone concentrations during continuous infusions of Althesin. *Br. J. Anaesth.* **51**, 861.

84. SEAR J. W. & PRYS-ROBERTS C. (1979) Dose related haemodynamic effects of continuous infusions of Althesin in man. *Br. J. Anaesth.* **51**, 867.

85. SEAR J. W. & PRYS-ROBERTS C. (1981) Alphadione and minaxolone pharmacokinetics. *Ann. Anesth. Franc.* **22**, 142–8.

86. SEAR J. W. & PRYS-ROBERTS C. (1982) Effects of anti-hypertensive therapy on the pharmacokinetics of Althesin by infusion to man . *Br. J. Anaes.* **54**, 1130–1.

87. SEAR J. W., PRYS-ROBERTS C., GRAY A. J. G., WALSH E. M., CURNOW J. S. H & DYE J. (1981) Infusions of minaxolone to supplement nitrous oxide-oxygen anaesthesia. A comparison with Althesin. *Br. J. Anaesth.* **53**, 339.

88. SEAR J. W., PHILLIPS K. C., ANDREWS C. J. H. & PRYS-ROBERTS C. (1983) Dose-response relationships for infusions of Althesin or Methohexitone. *Anaesthesia*, in press.

89. SELYE H. (1941) Anaesthetic effect of steroid hormones. *Proc. Soc. Exp. Biol. Med.* **46**, 116.

90. SIMPSON M. E. (1978) Pharmacokinetics of Althesin—comparison with ligno-caine. *Br. J. Anaesth.* **50**, 1231.

91. STANSKI D. R., MIMH F. G., ROSENTHAL M. H. & KALMAN S. M. (1980) Pharmacokinetics of high dose thiopental used in cerebral resuscitation. *Anesthesiology* **53**, 169.

92. STRUNIN L., STRUNIN J. M., KNIGHTS K. M. & WARD M. E. (1977) Metabolism of ¹⁴C-labelled alphaxalone in man. *Br. J. Anaesth.* **49**, 609.

93. SWERDLOW M., CHAKRABARTY S. K. & ZAHANGIR M. A. H. M. (1971) A trial of CT-1231. *Br. J. Anaesth.* **43**, 1075.

94. TAUSSIG P. E., BENNETT N. R. & STOJAK H. E. (1979) Interaction of propanidid and suxamethonium with human plasma cholinesterase *in vitro*. *Br. J. Anaesth.* **51**, 62P.

95. TEPFER M., DRYDEN G. E. & CREGGER I. (1964) Methohexital sodium drip intravenously for head and neck surgery. *J. Oral Surgery, Anesthesia and Hospital Dental Service* **22**, 215.

96. THOMSON I. A., HUGHES R. L., FITCH W. & CAMPBELL D. (1982) Effects of nitrous oxide on liver haemodynamics and oxygen consumption in the greyhound. *Anaesthesia* **37**, 548.

97. TOWLER C. M., GARRETT R. T. & SEAR J. W. (1982) Althesin infusions for maintenance of anaesthesia. *Anaesthesia* **37**, 428.

98. TSUEI S. E., NATION R. L. & THOMAS J. (1980) Design of infusion regimens to achieve and maintain a predetermined plasma drug level range. *Clin. Pharmacol. Ther.* **28**, 289.

99. VAN HAMME M. J., GHONEIM M. M. & AMBRE J. J. (1978) Pharmacokinetics of Etomidate, a new intravenous anaesthetic. *Anesthesiology* **49**, 274.

100. VAUGHAN D. P. & TUCKER G. T. (1975) General theory for rapidly establishing steady state drug concentrations using two consecutive constant rate I. V. infusions. *Eur. J. Clin. Pharmacol.* **9**, 235.

101. WAGNER J. G. (1974) A safe method for rapidly achieving plasma concentration plateaus. *Clin. Pharmacol. Ther.* **16**, 691.

102. WALTERS F. J. M., WILKINS D. G., WILLATTS S. M., NICKLESS G. & SEAR J. W. (1982) Etomidate infusion for neuroanaesthesia. *Anaesthesia*, Volume of Summaries, VIth European Congress of Anaesthesiology, London. Abstract 358, p. 199.

103. WATKINS J., CLARK A., APPLEYARD T. N. & PADFIELD A. (1976) Immune-mediated reactions to Althesin (Alphaxalone). *Br. J. Anaesth.* **48**, 881–6.

104. WEYL R., UNAL B. & ALPER Y. (1958) Clinical evaluation of a new ultrashort-acting oxygen barbiturate for intravenous anaesthesia. *Surg. Gynecol. Obstet.* **107**, 588.

105. HEBRON B. S., EDBROOKE D. L., MATHER S. J. & NEWBY D. M. (1983) Pharmacokinetics of etomidate associated with a prolonged intravenous infusion. *Br. J. Anaesth.* **55**,

106. LEDINGHAM I. McA. & WATT I. (1983) Influence of sedation on mortality in critically ill multiple trauma patients. *Lancet* **i**, 1270.

107. DOENICKE A. (1983) Etomidate. *Lancet* **ii**, 168.

108. FÉLLOWS I. W., BYRNE A. J. & ALLISON S. P. (1983) Adrenocortical suppression with Etomidate. *Lancet* **ii**, 54.

8 Benzodiazepines

J. G. REVES

The benzodiazepines are a highly versatile group of drugs enjoying widespread use in anaesthesia practice. Their versatility is based on the diversity of the compounds which allows the anaesthesiologist to pick the appropriate drug for a particular need. Among the many benzodiazepines (Fig. 8.1), seemingly minor variations in the chemical structures are associated with sometimes major differences in physicochemical properties, pharmacological activity and pharmacokinetics. The diversity of the benzodiazepines is especially apparent in regard to their pharmacokinetics, which are the subject of a number of reviews[18, 19, 23, 27, 30, 38, 39, 53, 54, 55, 60, 68, 69, 95, 100, 101, 132].

Biotransformation of the benzodiazpeines is particularly important for several reasons. Firstly, their biotransformation occurs in the liver and hepatic intrinsic clearance is the rate-limiting step in total body clearance of most benzodiazepines. Secondly, metabolism of the so-called 'prodrugs' accounts for their pharmacological activity; that is, the metabolic conversion of the inactive parent drug to an active metabolite. Thirdly, biotransformation of some of the active parent drugs to active metabolites contributes importantly to their effects. Finally, there are two fundamentally different pathways for the biotransformation of benzodiazepines: oxidation–reduction or Phase I reactions, and conjugation or Phase II reactions (Table 8.1). The significance of these two pathways will become obvious later.

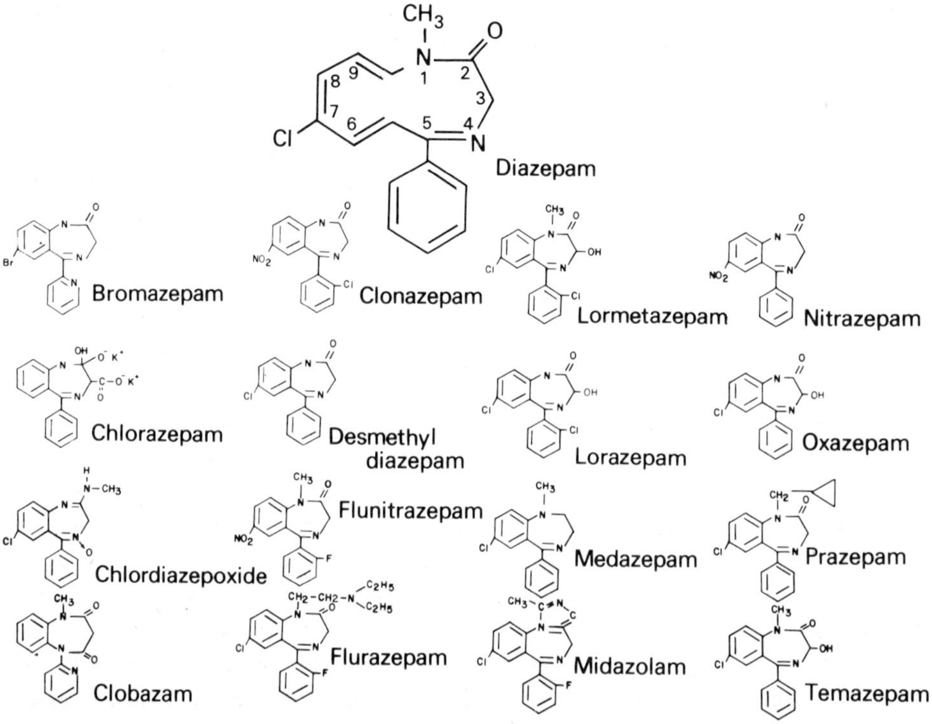

Chapter 8

Fig. 8.1 Structural differences among the major benzodiazepines. Diazepam with ring numbering is shown at the top. Note that all are 1–4-benzodiazepines except clobazam which is a 1,5-benzodiazepine. Lormetazepam, lorazepam, oxazepam and temazepam are 3 hydroxy-1,4-benzodiazepines.

Table 8.1 Metabolism of benzodiazepines.

Oxidation–reduction	Conjugation
Bromazepam	Lorazepam
Chlordiazepoxide	Lormetazepam
Clobazam	Oxazepam
Clonazepam	Temazepam
Clorazepate	
Diazepam	
Flunitrazepam	
Flurazepam	
Medazepam	
Midazolam	
Nitrazepam	
Prazepam	

Benzodiazepines share certain common pharmacodynamic properties. In general, particular drugs differ far more in potency than in the spectrum of their pharmacological effects, and the major difference between benzodiazepines administered in equipotent doses is their duration of action.

The purpose of this chapter is three-fold; to review the pharmacokinetics of benzodiazepines, to relate the pharmacokinetics to pharmacodynamics, and to summarise the clinical implications of this information for the anaesthesiologist.

PHARMACOKINETICS

Elimination kinetics

Despite the diversity noted above, the disappearance of all benzodiazepines from plasma exhibits first order kinetics, and can be described in almost all cases by a biexponential equation and a two-compartment model. The pharmacokinetics of benzodiazepines, in general, are not altered by route of administration, dose, or duration of therapy. But a consistent finding among the benzodiazepines is a large interindividual variability in their pharmacokinetics, and average values for pharmacokinetic variables sometimes represent misleading oversimplifications.

Greenblatt's classification of the benzodiazepines according to the range of elimination half-times is useful (Table 8.2)[60]. This classification is not entirely dependent on the half-life of the parent compound, but also takes into consideration the half-life of active metabolites. Therefore, a parent drug with a short elimination half-time and a major active metabolite with a long duration of action will be classified as long acting.

Table 8.2 A pharmacokinetic classification of benzodiazepine drugs on the basis of elimination half-life.

Long $(T_{\frac{1}{2}}^{\beta} > 24\,h)$	Intermediate $(T_{\frac{1}{2}}^{\beta}\,5–24\,h)$	Short $(T_{\frac{1}{2}}^{\beta} < 5\,h)$
Chlordiazepoxide	Alprazolam	Midazolam
Clobazam	Bromazepam	Triazolam
Clorazepate*	Clonazepam	
Desmethyldiazepam	Estazolam	
Diazepam	Flunitrazepam	
Flurazepam*	Lorazepam	
Medazepam*	Oxazepam	
Nitrazepam	Temazepam	
Prazepam*		

* Prodrugs for long lasting active metabolites. Classification after that of Greenblatt 1981[60].

Long-acting benzodiazepines

Chlordiazepoxide has a rapid distribution phase ($T_{\frac{1}{2}}^{\alpha}$ of approximately 10 minutes) in young healthy subjects[14, 56, 59, 62, 119]. The elimination half-time of chlordiazepoxide is 8–18 h in normal subjects[14, 15, 56, 58, 62, 99, 114, 115, 119, 120, 123]. It is categorised as a long acting benzodiazepine because one of its metabolites, desmethyldiazepam, is active and has a long $T_{\frac{1}{2}}^{\beta}$ (Table 8.3). The volume of distribution of chlordiazepoxide is relatively small (0.3–0.6 l kg^{-1}) compared to most benzodiazepines[14, 15, 56, 62, 114, 115, 119, 120, 123]. Total body clearance is slow, ranging from 0.21–0.56 ml kg^{-1} min^{-1}[14, 56, 62, 114, 119, 123]. Of the total chlordiazepoxide found in plasma, 94–97% is bound to protein[14, 99, 114, 115]. Clearance of the unbound drug has not been estimated by most investigators, but Roberts *et al* computed a free drug clearance of 15.6 ml kg^{-1} min^{-1} for 11 young healthy men and 8.7 ml kg^{-1} min^{-1} for 11 young healthy women; the difference was statistically significant[114].

Table 8.3 Pharmacokinetic characteristics of selected benzodiazepines in young healthy humans.

	$T_{\frac{1}{2}}^{\alpha}$ (min)	$T_{\frac{1}{2}}^{\beta}$ (h)	V_D (1 kg^{-1})	Total body clearance (ml min^{-1} kg^{-1})	Protein binding (%)
Chlordiazepoxide	1–15	8 – 18	0.3–0.6	0.21 –0.61	94 – 7
Desmethyldiazepam	36	41 –139	0.8–2.1	0.002–0.43	97
Diazepam	30–66	24 – 57	0.7–1.7	0.24 –0.53	96 – 9
Nitrazepam	?	24 – 31	2.4	?	88–97
Flunitrazepam	?	14 – 21	2.5–4.6	1.9– 5.6	80
Lorazepam	3–10	11 – 22	0.8–1.3	0.8– 1.8	85–93
Oxazepam	?	5 – 12	0.7–1.9	0.8– 2.8	87–97
Midazolam	6–15	1.7– 2.6	1.1–1.7	6.4–11.1	97

? = incomplete or inconclusive date. See text for elaboration and references.

Desmethyldiazepam per se has seldom been administered. It is an active metabolite of several benzodiazepines and its kinetics have mostly been investigated along with those of the parent drug (e.g. diazepam, chlordiazepoxide, clorazepate and prazepam). Different parent drugs presumably do not alter the elimination kinetics of desmethyldiazepam, but there are marked differences in the rate of appearance of desmethyldiazepam in plasma depending on the parent drug. Desmethyldiazepam has the lowest clearance and the longest half-time among the benzodiazepines included in this review. Its distribution half-time is 36 minutes[27]. The $T_{\frac{1}{2}}^{\beta}$ is 41–139 h[4, 11, 22, 67, 88, 113, 126]. The volume of distribution of desmethyldiazepam is 0.8–2.11 l kg^{-1} and there is some evidence that the V_D is greater in women than men[5, 11, 88, 113, 126].

Total body clearance varies widely (0.002–0.43 ml kg^{-1} min^{-1}) even in young healthy subjects[5, 88, 113, 126]. Protein binding of the drug in plasma averages 97 %[88, 126]. Free drug clearance averaged 12 ml kg^{-1} min^{-1} in 8 young males and 16 ml kg^{-1} min^{-1} in 7 young females[5].

Diazepam is the most extensively investigated benzodiazepine. Reported $T^{\alpha}_{\frac{1}{2}}$ values range from 30 to 66 minutes in normal healthy humans[36, 78, 83, 84, 86, 89, 107]. Most of the values for the $T^{\alpha}_{\frac{1}{2}}$ are in the 30–40 minute range, indicating a relatively slow distribution half-time compared to most other drugs used for the induction of anaesthesia. The $T^{\beta}_{\frac{1}{2}}$ is long, 24–57 hours in normal patients[2, 10, 17, 32, 36, 41, 66, 78, 80, 83, 84, 86, 89, 97, 98, 104, 106, 107]. A number of physiological and pharmacological factors alter these 'normal' values (*vide infra*). The volume of distribution of diazepam is large (0.7–1.7 l kg^{-1}), indicative of its widespread distribution to tissues[2, 17, 32, 36, 41, 78, 80, 83, 84, 86, 89, 97, 98, 106, 107]. The volume distribution is greater in patients with hepatic cirrhosis (1.74 l kg^{-1} vs. 1.13 l kg^{-1} for normal subjects) at least in part because of the significantly reduced plasma protein binding of diazepam in cirrhotic patients[86]. That is, measurements of plasma levels include both free and protein bound diazepam; reduced protein binding leaves more free drug to enter tissues and lowers the total (free and bound) diazepam in plasma; this results in a longer apparent distribution volume. In normal patients total body clearance of diazepam ranges from 0.24 to 0.53 ml kg^{-1} min^{-1}[2, 17, 32, 36, 41, 84, 86, 89, 98, 100, 104, 107] and 96–99 % of diazepam in plasma is bound to protein[1, 2, 36, 41, 74, 83, 84, 86, 89, 97, 104, 106, 116]. Free drug clearance ranges from 28 to 44 ml kg^{-1} min^{-1} and in young subjects it appears to be lower in males (29.9 ml kg^{-1} min^{-1}) than females (43.6 ml kg^{-1} min^{-1})[2, 41]. Two of the metabolites of diazepam, desmethyldiazepam and oxazepam, are pharmacologically active. The formation of the primary metabolite, desmethyldiazepam, is slow (Fig. 8.2) and its $T^{\beta}_{\frac{1}{2}}$ is much longer than that of diazepam.

Nitrazepam has a $T^{\beta}_{\frac{1}{2}}$ of 24–31 h, but no apparent long-acting metabolite[70, 72, 73, 75]. The volume of distribution is large (2.4–2.6 l kg^{-1}) and is significantly increased by age to 4.8 l kg^{-1}[70, 73]. Total clearance of nitrazepam in normal adults ranges from 0.9 to 1.0 ml kg^{-1} min^{-1} [57, 94]. Plasma protein binding is 88.97 %[72].

Flurazepam, like chlordiazepoxide, has a short $T^{\beta}_{\frac{1}{2}}$ of 2–3 h[79], but its active metabolite N-desalkylflurazepam is reported to have a $T^{\alpha}_{\frac{1}{2}}$ of 47–100 hours in one study[79], and 40–250 h in another[60]; this metabolite has the longest elimination half-time of any benzodiazepine.

Medazepam, prazepam and *chlorazepate* are the prodrugs for desmethyldiazepam. Medazepam is also biotransformed to diazepam.

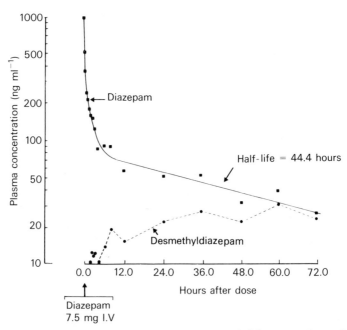

Fig. 8.2 Plasma concentrations of diazepam and desmethyldiazepam after a 7.5 mg intravenous dose of diazepam to a volunteer subject. Half-life = $T_{\frac{1}{2}}^{\beta}$. Redrawn from Greenblatt *et al.*[55]. Reprinted by permission from the *S. Med. J.* **71**, 2–9 (1978).

Intermediate-acting benzodiazepines

Flunitrazepam has a relatively rapid distribution phase such that two-thirds disappears from the plasma in 60 minutes[101]. The elimination half-time in healthy subjects is 14–19 h after single and steady-state oral administration studies, respectively. The volume of distribution is large, 2.5 l kg^{-1} after intravenous and 4.4–4.6 l kg^{-1} after oral administration. Total clearance ranges from 1.9 ml kg^{-1} min^{-1} after intravenous administration to 4.63–5.63 ml kg^{-1} min^{-1} after oral doses[16]. Protein binding (80%) of flunitrazepam is relatively low for a benzodiazepine[16]. Flunitrazepam is reduced in the liver and its metabolites are probably active; their elimination half-times are 23–31 h[19].

Lorazepam is very rapidly distributed from the plasma with a $T_{\frac{1}{2}}^{\alpha}$ of 3–10 minutes[42, 46, 48, 57]. The $T_{\frac{1}{2}}^{\beta}$ ranges from 11 to 22 hours[42, 44, 46, 48, 49, 50, 52, 57, 94, 128], and is significantly prolonged by liver disease[94], but unaffected by age[42], dose, or route of administration[57]. The volume of distribution varies from 0.8–1.3 l kg^{-1} in healthy man[42, 46, 48, 49, 57, 94], and is significantly increased by hepatic cirrhosis[94], but decreased by age[42]. Protein binding averages 85–93%[94, 95].

Oxazepam $T^\beta_{\frac{1}{2}}$ ranges from 5–12 hours with some suggestions that it is longer in females than in males (7.8 hours vs. 9.7 hours)[7, 8, 47, 88, 120, 124, 127]. Newborn infants have a markedly prolonged elimination half-time of 22 h[127]. The volume of distribution in healthy man ranges from 0.7 to 1.9 l kg^{-1}[7, 8, 47, 124, 127]. Plasma protein binding varies between 87 and 97%[47, 88, 124]. There are apparently no active metabolites of oxazepam.

Bromazepam, clonazepam, temazepam and *estazolam* have not been studied extensively in terms of pharmacokinetics, but their elimination half-times are in the intermediate range: estazolam—17 hours[3]; bromazepam—12 hours[81], temazepam—5–8 hours[12, 33, 118]. The $T^\gamma_{\frac{1}{2}}$ for temazepam is 30–49 minutes[12, 118]. Clonazepam has a $T^\beta_{\frac{1}{2}}$ of about 22 h, which is decreased to 15 h when clonazepam is combined with hepatic microsomal enzyme inducers like phenobarbital and diphenylhydantoin; the decrease in $T^\beta_{\frac{1}{2}}$ is due to an enhanced clearance[82, 90, 96]. Clonazepam has a large volume of distribution 3.1–3.3 l kg^{-1} in part due to its relatively low degree (i.e. 87%) binding to plasma proteins[82, 90].

Short-acting benzodiazepines

Midazolam has a 6–15 min $T^\gamma_{\frac{1}{2}}$, the shortest distribution half-time of all the benzodiazepines[6, 20, 51, 117, 130]. The elimination half-time ranges from 1.7 to 2.6 hours, again significantly shorter than other benzodiazepines[6, 20, 51, 108, 117, 125, 130]. Its distribution volume ranges from 1.1 to 1.7 l kg^{-1}[20, 51, 125], and plasma protein binding averages 97%[130].

Triazolam is a new short-lived benzodiazepine; a preliminary report shows that $T^\beta_{\frac{1}{2}}$ is 4.5 hours[102].

Factors altering elimination kinetics

There are a host of physiological, pharmacological, pathological, and probably environmental factors able to alter the pharmacokinetics of individual benzodiazepines. Some of these factors and the particular drugs demonstrated to be affected by them are listed in Table 8.4. It is important to understand that there are large gaps in our knowledge and that a substantial amount of research is in progress. Diazepam has been investigated most; other compounds have not been studied at all. Some consistent observations have been noted in regard to the biotransformation of benzodiazepines. The unsubstituted 3, 1–4-benzodiazepines (Table 8.1, Fig. 8.1) are biotransformed by oxidative or reductive pathways in the liver utilising P450 and other mixed function oxygenase enzymes whereas the 3-hydroxy benzodiazepines are biotransformed by glucuronide conjugation facilitated by a totally different set of hepatic enzymes. The

Table 8.4 Variables that alter the clearance and elimination half-life of selected benzo-diazepines.

	Age	Sex	History of smoking	Enzyme inhibition	Liver disease	Renal disease
Chlordiazepoxide	Yes	Yes	No	Yes	Yes	?
Diazepam	Yes	Yes	Yes	Yes	Yes	Yes
Desmethyldiazepam	Yes	Yes	?	Yes	Yes	?
Flunitrazepam	Yes	?	?	?	?	?
Lorazepam*	No	No	Yes	No	Yes/No	No
Midazolam	Yes	?	?	?	?	No
Oxazepam*	No	Yes	Yes	No	No	Yes/No

* = 3-hydroxy, 1-4 benzodiazepine; Yes = a significant effect; No = no significant effect; Yes/No = influence on $T_\frac{1}{2}^\beta$ not on clearance; and ? = incomplete or inconclusive data. See text for elaboration and references.

biotransformation reactions of the unsubstituted 3, 1–4-benzodiazepines are more sensitive to the factors that alter biotransformation than are conjugation reactions of the 3-hydroxy, 1–4-benzodiazepines.

Age affects both the $T_\frac{1}{2}^\beta$ and the clearance of chlordiazepoxide[58, 123], diazepam[32, 78, 86, 98], desmethyldiazepam[5, 87], flunitrazepam[101], nitrazepam[70, 73], and probably midazolam[Collier *et al.*, unpubl. data]. The data are quite clear for diazepam (Fig. 8.3) which is representative of most 1–4-benzodiazepines. An almost linear relationship between $T_\frac{1}{2}^\beta$ and age (r = 0.80–0.83) has been demonstrated and it has been noted that age and $T_\frac{1}{2}^\beta$ of diazepam have almost identical values ($T_\frac{1}{2}^\beta$ = 20 h at 20 years of age and 90 h at 80 years)[86, 97, 100]. Despite this close relationship, total drug

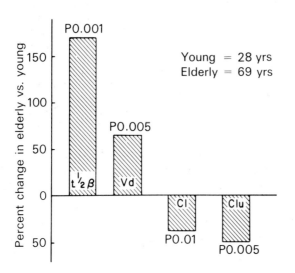

Fig. 8.3 The effects of age on diazepam pharmacokinetics are shown. Where $T_\frac{1}{2}^\beta$ = elimination half-time, V_D = volume of distribution, Cl = clearance of total drug, Cl_u = clearance of unbound drug, p = probability value, young group (n = 11) versus elderly (n = 11). Note that in elderly patients the $T_\frac{1}{2}$ and V_D are significantly greater and clearance smaller than in young patients. Drawn from Greenblatt *et al.*[41].

clearance does not consistently vary with age in the studies of Klotz[86]. On the other hand, unbound diazepam clearance is negatively correlated with age (r = −0.717) indicating that intrinsic clearance is indeed decreased by age. The distribution volume of diazepam also increases with age for reasons which are not clear[41, 78, 86, 97]. In contrast to these significant age-related alterations in the kinetics of diazepam and other 1-4-benzodiazepines, those of lorazepam and oxazepam are not so clearly affected by age[42, 47, 94, 124]. The association of age with lorazepam $T_{\frac{1}{2}}^{\beta}$, total clearance, intrinsic clearance and V_D are poor and insignificant[94]. Aging appears to have little or no effect on the conjugation of these compounds with glucuronic acid[94].

Gender has a pronounced effect on the pharmacokinetics of some benzodiazepines (Table 8.4). Chlordiazepoxide[114], diazepam[41, 98], desmethyldiazepam[4, 5], and oxazepam[47] have sex-related alterations in kinetics. The influence of gender has been clearly shown by MacLeod for diazepam (Fig. 8.4)[98]. In comparing young females to males, Greenblatt found a greater $T_{\frac{1}{2}}^{\beta}$ (18 %) reflecting a more rapid clearance of the unbound drug (46 %) as well as the offsetting factor of a larger distribution volume (36 %)[41]. Reasons for the different kinetic findings in males and females are not entirely clear.

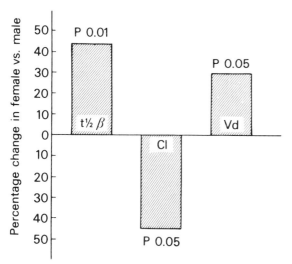

Fig. 8.4 The effects of gender on diazepam pharmacokinetics are shown. Where $T_{\frac{1}{2}}^{\beta}$ = elimination half-time, Cl = body clearance of total drug, V_D = volume of distribution, and P = probability value, women (n = 10) versus men (n = 9). Drawn from MacLeod *et al.*[98].

Race is a factor which affects pharmacokinetics of diazepam[36]; it has not been systematically studied in regard to the other benzodiazepines. Both the V_D and Cl of diazepam are greater in Caucasians than in Orientals, so that the $T_{\frac{1}{2}}^{\beta}$ is not different: V_D = 1.10 vs 0.88 l kg^{-1}, p = 0.07; Cl = 0.40 vs. 0.29 ml kg^{-1} min^{-1}, p = 0.01; $T_{\frac{1}{2}}^{\beta}$ = 29 vs. 39 hrs. Protein binding is the same (98 %) in both groups so that differences in V_D cannot be explained on this basis. Genetic differences in the biotransformation of diazepam are among the plausible explanations.

Hepatic enzyme induction/inhibition

Direct evidence of the influence of hepatic microsomal enzyme induction and inhibition on the kinetics of benzodiazepines is lacking. However, there are a number of observations which suggest that drugs or environmental factors inducing or inhibiting hepatic enzymes affect the pharmacokinetics of benzodiazepines. The effects of cigarette smoking are inconsistent. No change was found by some investigators for diazepam[84] or chlordiazepoxide[28]. Others have found that cigarette smoking is associated with increased total clearance and unbound clearance of diazepam[41], and total clearance of lorazepam[42] and oxazepam[47]. These latter findings may reflect hepatic microsomal enzyme induction. Antipyrine[107] and phenytoin[82] induce hepatic microsomal enzymes and significantly increase the clearance of diazepam (93 %) and clonazepam (46–58 %). The increased clearance is reflected in a significant reduction in the $T_{\frac{1}{2}}^{\beta}$ of both drugs (51 % for diazepam in the presence of antipyrine and a 31 % decrease for clorazepam in subjects receiving phenytoin).

Hepatic microsomal enzymes can be inhibited pharmacologically by drugs such as cimetidine and disulfiram. Cimetidine significantly (p = 0.012) prolonged the $T_{\frac{1}{2}}^{\beta}$ of diazepam from 34 to 51 hours (53 %) in healthy volunteers[89]. There was no effect on V_D, but total plasma clearance was significantly (p = 0.03) reduced from 19.9 ml/min to 11.4 ml/min (43 %). Cimetidine also impaired (p = 0.03) the elimination of desmethyldiazepam, prolonging its $T_{\frac{1}{2}}^{\beta}$ from 52 to 73 hrs (40 %) and decreasing plasma clearance from 12 to 8.6 ml min^{-1} (28 %) in healthy volunteers. In contrast, the disposition of oxazepam was not affected[88]. The significance of this study lies in its support of the hypothesis that fundamental differences in biotransformation of benzodiazepines account for differences in pharmacokinetics caused by concurrent drug administration. Enzyme inhibition of Phase I reactions alters pharmacokinetics of diazepam and desmethyldiazepam whereas neither the Phase II reactions nor the kinetics of oxazepam are influenced by the enzyme inhibition[88]. This hypothesis has also been supported by the observations that disulfiram did not affect the disposition of oxazepam, but significantly decreased the clearance of chlordiazepoxide, diazepam, and desmethyldiazepam[99, 121].

Studies of chronic administration of benzodiazepines raise the question of auto-enzyme induction/inhibition and associated changes in kinetics. Klotz has shown that the pharmacokinetics of an intravenous dose of diazepam are different in patients taking oral diazepam subchronically than in subjects given just a single injection[77, 83]. 'Sub-chronic' diazepam therapy was associated with a significant (p = 0.03) prolongation of $T_{\frac{1}{2}}^{\beta}$ from 36 hours to 53 hours, no change in protein binding or V_D, but a significant (p = 0.02) decrease in total clearance from 26 ml min^{-1} to 18.2 ml min^{-1}. It is possible that this prolongation in $T_{\frac{1}{2}}^{\beta}$ and decreased clearance was due to the inhibition of oxidation by the accumulation of the oxidative metabolite, desmethyldiazepam. However, others failed to demonstrate that the presence of desmethyldiazepam altered the kinetics of diazepam[2]. Lorazepam and nitrazepam administered on a chronic basis neither stimulate nor inhibit their own metabolism[50, 75]. Although there is no consensus, it appears that little auto-enzyme induction or inhibition occurs with the benzodiazepines.

Liver disease alters the pharmacokinetics of chlordiazepoxide[115, 120], diazepam[17, 85, 86], desmethyldiazepam[85], lorazepam[94], and oxazepam[124]. The effects of liver disease on diazepam pharmacokinetics are representative of the changes noted for the other benzodiazepines. Klotz, in an exhaustive study of the influence of liver diseases on diazepam pharmacokinetics, showed that patients with alcoholic cirrhosis (compared to age-matched control subjects) exhibited significant (p < .001) increases in $T^{\beta}_{\frac{1}{2}}$ from 47 to 106 hrs (126%) and had a larger V_D, 1.13 versus 1.74 (54%); the plasma clearance decreased from 45 to 25 ml min^{-1} (44%). Diazepam binding to plasma protein was slightly but significantly (p < .001) less (95.3 vs. 97.8%) in alcoholic cirrhosis. Viral hepatitis prolonged $T^{\beta}_{\frac{1}{2}}$ by 82% (33 vs. 60 h) reflecting a decreased plasma clearance, which returned to normal when the patients recovered from the active hepatitis[85, 86].

Similar kinetic changes were seen with chlordiazepoxide in patients with liver diseases (Fig. 8.5)[115, 120]. Cirrhosis prolonged the $T^{\beta}_{\frac{1}{2}}$ of lorazepam from 22 to 41 hours, but did not significantly change the total or unbound drug clearance. The increased $T^{\beta}_{\frac{1}{2}}$ appeared to be related to the increased V_D in cirrhosis, which was probably due to the decreased protein binding, from 93 to 89%[94]. Oxazepam disposition in cirrhotic patients was not altered significantly[120, 124]. Again, the fact that the pharmacokinetics of the 1, 3 hydroxy, 1,4 benzodiazepines, (oxazepam and lorazepam) are less altered by liver disease than those of the 1–4-benzodiazepines indicates that the glucuronide conjugation pathway is less vulnerable to the disease processes than is the microsomal oxidative–reductive drug metabolising system.

Renal disease does not markedly alter the pharmacokinetics of the few benzodiazepines for which it has been examined[7, 71, 74, 101, 128, 130]. There was a significant reduction in diazepam protein binding in renal failure patients and the clearance of total drug was significantly (p < 0.005) decreased from 0.9 to 0.3 ml kg^{-1} min^{-1}[74, 106]. The clearance of unbound diazepam was unaltered in renal disease. Midazolam pharmacokinetics were altered in the presence of severe renal disease; the clearance of unbound midazolam and the degree of binding to plasma protein were both reduced. The $T^{\beta}_{\frac{1}{2}}$ was prolonged and the patients slept longer than normal[130]. Oxazepam clearance was unaffected by renal disease though the $T^{\beta}_{\frac{1}{2}}$ was prolonged (from 24 to 91 h)[7]. Lorazepam kinetics were not altered by renal failure[128]. However, excretion of the inactive lorazepam-glucuronide metabolite was considerably slowed, with a corresponding increase in the $T^{\beta}_{\frac{1}{2}}$ of the glucuronide from the normal 20 hours up to the range of 72–136 h. In summary, renal disease does not predictably affect the

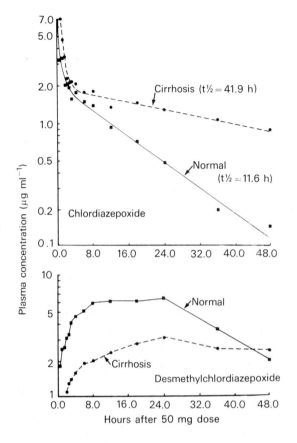

Fig. 8.5 Plasma concentrations of chlordiazepoxide and desmethylchlordiazepoxide for 48 hours after ten-minute intravenous infusion of 50 mg of chlordiazepoxide hydrochloride to two subjects. Also shown are pharmacokinetic functions for chlordiazepoxide. One subject was a healthy volunteer; the other was a patient with cirrhosis. Note the prolonged elimination half-life of chlordiazepoxide, and the delayed appearance of desmethylchlordiazepoxide in the patient with cirrhosis. Redrawn from Greenblatt *et al.*[55]. Reprinted by permission from the *S. Med. J.* **71**, 2–9 (1978).

pharmacokinetics of the unchanged benzodiazepines, but it will slow the excretion of water-soluble metabolites which are pharmacologically inactive.

Absorption kinetics

Benzodiazepines are commonly administered by routes other than intravenous injection, especially for preanaesthetic medication. The rate of absorption from the gastrointestinal tract or muscle obviously affects the rise and fall of blood levels and the onset, intensity, and duration of action. Terminology used to describe absorption kinetics includes: $T_{\frac{1}{2}}^{a}$, half-time for apparent first order absorption; T_{max}, time of the highest plasma concentration after administration; T_0, lag time or time elapsing prior to the start of first-order absorption; and bioavailability which is determined by comparing areas under the time vs. plasma concentration curves (AUC) after the same size dose is administered intravenously (i.v.) and by a non-intravenous route (e.g. $AUC_{oral}/AUC_{i.v.}$ = fraction of oral dose available systemically). Despite great interindividual variation in absorption kinetics, qualitative differences between drugs are

Table 8.5 Absorption kinetics of five benzodiazepines used for premedication in normal subjects.

	Oral				Intramuscular			
	T_0 (min)	$T^a_{\frac{1}{2}}$ (min)	T_{max} (min)	Bioavail-ability (%)	T_0 (min)	$T^a_{\frac{1}{2}}$ (min)	T_{max} (min)	Bioavail-ability (%)
Chlordiazepoxide	0–10	6–43	30–138	100	?	13–540*	456	86–100
Diazepam	12–17	19	30– 80	90–100	?	?	60 –90	80–100
Flunitrazepam	< 15	?	60– 90	80– 90	< 15	?	60	80– 90
Lorazepam*	9–17	14–22	60–150	90–100	0	12 –73	70–150	92–100
Midazolam	10–28	?	22– 44	high	NA	NA	NA	NA

* Boxenbaum has developed a model with two $T^a_{\frac{1}{2}}$, 13 min and 5 h (see text); NA = data not available; ? = incompleate or inconclusive data.

apparent. For the most part, absorption follows first-order kinetic patterns. Intramuscular absorption is less well studied than oral. In comparative investigations, some benzodiazepines absorbed rapidly when given orally are poorly absorbed after intramuscular administration, and vice versa. Table 8.5 contains absorption kinetic data of five benzodiazepines of interest to anaesthesiologists. The size of the dose does not seem to alter absorption kinetics, but other factors do (*vide infra*).

Chlordiazepoxide is more reliably absorbed after oral than after intramuscular administration[14, 15, 58, 61, 62, 63, 123]. Oral administration has a short lag time (0–10 min), and a relatively short absorption half-time of 6–43 minutes[14, 58, 63, 123]. Absorption was slower in elderly than in younger individuals, 20 minutes vs. 6 minutes[123]. The $T^a_{\frac{1}{2}}$ was prolonged by the concurrent administration of magnesium aluminum hydroxide (Maalox)[58]. Maalox decreased the peak concentration, but not the total absorption. Reasons for this are not entirely known, but two possibilities are a raised gastric pH increasing the concentration of the poorly soluble nonionised base, or more probably, a delay of gastric emptying[58]. Although chlordiazepoxide was completely absorbed by the oral route, the time to attain peak concentration (T_{max}) varied considerably, 30–138 min[14, 15, 63, 123].

The intramuscular administration of chlordiazepoxide is slow and erratic in comparison to oral administration[62]. The peak concentration following intramuscular administration of 50 mg of chlordiazepoxide resulted in the achievement of only 50% of the plasma level attained following oral administration of the same size dose[63]. The $T^a_{\frac{1}{2}}$ varied from 13 to 540 minutes[14, 63]. Boxenbaum used rather elegant pharmacokinetic modelling to describe both a rapid (13 min) and a slow absorption half-time (5 h)[14]. The smaller $T^a_{\frac{1}{2}}$ represents rapid absorption of the drug remaining in solution, whereas the larger $T^a_{\frac{1}{2}}$ reflects (theoretically) precipitation of the

Chapter 8

drug at the injection site in muscle and delay of absorption until it redissolves. Many benzodiazepines are relatively insoluble at physiological pH and may behave in a similar fashion, accounting for their varied and slow absorption after intramuscular injection. Maximum plasma concentrations occur approximately 8 hours after an i.m. injection, and though slow and variable, the intramuscular absorption of chlordiazepoxide is virtually complete 86–100%[14, 63].

Diazepam is also better absorbed after oral than after intramuscular administration. Peak drug levels occur 30–80 minutes after oral diazepam and are significantly greater than after the same dose injected intramuscularly[26, 43, 66, 80, 92]. Oral absorption is rapid with a lag time in normal subjects of 12–17 min, but the absorption half-time varies from 30 to 80 min[43, 64, 66, 80, 92]. The peak concentration is reduced and both T_0 and $T_{\frac{1}{2}}^a$ are prolonged by simultaneous administration of magnesium aluminum hydroxide (Maalox), aluminum hydroxide trisilicate (Gelusil), ethyl alcohol (as a commercial brand of 80 proof vodka), and a hearty breakfast[43, 64]. Bioavailability of oral diazepam is 100%, indicating no first pass removal by the liver[80].

Intramuscular absorption of diazepam is poor and irregular[100]. The peak plasma levels following similar doses of diazepam (10 mg) are 30–40% lower after IM than after PO administration[66, 92]. The reasons for the poor absorption of diazepam from intramuscular sites are not entirely understood, but one factor is the limited solubility of diazepam at physiological pH and the possibility of its precipitation at the injection site (as described above for chlordiazepoxide). The T_{max} is delayed, ranging from 60 to 90 minutes[66, 92]. Diazepam absorption from the deltoid muscle of the shoulder is more rapid than from the vastus lateralis of the thigh[92].

Flunitrazepam absorption kinetics have not been studied *per se*, but the existing data indicate that more than 80% of the dose is available after either oral or intramuscular administration[21]. Plasma concentrations after PO and IM administration are nearly identical[101], but more rapidly attained following IM injection in the vastus lateralis muscle than after oral injection[25].

Lorazepam absorption kinetics differ from those described above in that the oral and intramuscular routes are equally effective in achieving similar plasma concentrations in about the same time. The lag time following oral administration of lorazepam is 9–17 minutes and absorption is rapid ($T_{\frac{1}{2}}^a = 14$–22 min) and essentially complete (90–100% bioavailability). The T_{max} occurs between 1 and 2.5 hours[44, 48, 95]. Unlike most benzodiazepines, the peak blood levels are virtually identical after either intramuscular or oral administration[95]. There is little or no lag time following an IM injection; the T_{max} occurs in 1 to 2.5 hours and absorption is essentially complete, being 92–107%[44, 48, 95].

Midazolam absorption kinetics have been examined in only one study. It was rapidly absorbed following oral injection, the mean lag time ranging from 10 minutes with a 10 mg oral suspension to 28 minutes after a 10 mg tablet. The T_{max} occurred earlier (22 min) after the suspension compared to the tablet (44 min)[125]. Complete absorption of midazolam is suggested by the relatively high absorption constant values (Ka = 9.6), but comparisons based on AUC mg^{-1} of dose after IV and PO administration suggest that almost two-thirds of an oral dose is cleared by the liver during its first pass[125]. Midazolam has been injected IM, but kinetic data are not yet available[R. J. Fragen, pers. commun.].

Prodrugs, clorazepate and prazepam, are biotransformed to desmethyldiazepam, the active compound. The absorption of clorazepate and prazepam are very interesting examples of the impact of gastrointestinal absorption and hepatic metabolism on bioavailability. Fig. 8.6 illustrates the marked difference in the appearance of desmethyldiazepam in plasma after the administration of clorazepate (15 mg) and prazepam (20 mg). Both prodrugs ultimately produce similar concentrations of desmethyldiazepam, but the peak concentrations are higher and more rapidly achieved with clorazepate than prazepam. These differences are attributable to the facts that prazepam is metabolised in the liver and clorazepate is biotransformed in the gastrointestinal tract[54, 126]. T_{max} was 1.8 h with clordiazepate[122], whereas it was 2–4 hours for prazepam depending on whether a tablet or suspension were

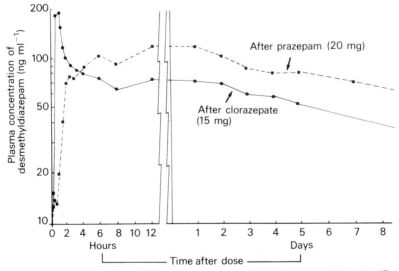

Fig. 8.6 Plasma concentration of desmethyldiazepam in a volunteer subject (a 67-year-old man) who ingested 20 mg of prazepam on one occasion and 15 mg of clorazepate on another occasion six months later. Redrawn from Greenblatt[38]. Reprinted by permission from *Psychosomatics* **21**, 9–14 (1980).

administered[126]. The $T_{\frac{1}{2}}^a$ was much smaller after oral injection of clorazepate (15 min) compared to 59–75 min for prazepam[4, 5, 113]. Intramuscular clorazepate has a $T_{\frac{1}{2}}^a$ of 11 min[113].

PHARMACODYNAMICS

Structure activity relationships

All benzodiazepines have hypnotic, sedative, anxiolytic, amnestic, anticonvulsant, and centrally produced muscle relaxant properties. But the drugs differ in their potency and efficacy in regard to each of the pharmacodynamic actions. The chemical structure of each drug dictates its particular physicochemical properties and pharmacokinetics, and in addition determines the tissue and receptor binding characteristics unique to each drug. From a structural standpoint, benzodiazepines are either 2-amino-4-oxides or 1,3-dihydro-2-ketones (Fig. 8.1); chlordiazepoxide is representative of the former class and diazepam of the latter. In both categories an electronegative group in position 7 is essential for psychopharmacological activity[53]. Likewise, structural changes cause differences in receptor binding: the rank order for synaptosomal binding is midazolam > clonazepam > lorazepam > flunitrazepam > diazepam > nitrazepam > flurazepam > bromazepam > oxazepam > clorazepate > and chlordiazepoxide > medazepam[103]. Marked physicochemical changes can result from minor structural alterations; for example, the pKa of diazepam is 3.5, that of midazolam is 6.0[26, 111]. The proportion of ionised and unionised forms of the drugs determines in large part the rate of their absorption from the GI tract and penetration of the blood–brain-barrier. The alkaline environment of the intestine enhances diazepam absorption and the pH of blood favours the entry of midazolam into the central nervous system.

Plasma concentrations and biological activity

The association between benzodiazepine concentrations in plasma and pharmaco-dynamics is controversial[9, 31, 62, 66, 67, 76, 91, 95, 100, 101, 105, 126]. The onset and initial intensity of the neuropharmacological actions of benzodiazepines tend to approximate the rate of rise and peak concentrations of the drugs in plasma after a single dose, but during the gradual decline of plasma levels in the elimination phase of a single dose and during chronic therapy the relationships between plasma levels and pharmacological effects are less evident. Also, there is marked interindividual variation, so that one patient may be wide awake and another barely arousable at the same drug level. For example, plasma levels of diazepam required for satisfactory sedation during cardioversion ranges from 0.16 to 2.68 μg/ml (a 15-fold difference) in patients of the same age and without liver or renal disease[112]. The multiplicity of neuropharmaco-logical effects of benzodiazepines further complicates the identification of relationships of drug concentrations to pharmacodynamics. Fig. 8.7 illustrates the change of plasma

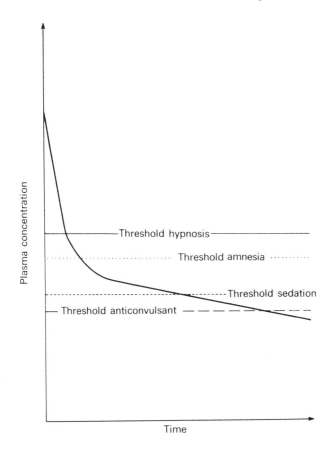

Plasma concentration

Threshold hypnosis

Threshold amnesia

Threshold sedation

Threshold anticonvulsant

Time

Fig. 8.7 A schematic semi-log plot of the drug concentration and therapeutic threshold effect relationship for benzodiazepines. Note each pharmacodynamic effect has a different plasma drug concentration threshold, and the hypnotic threshold occurs in the distribution phase of the drug, the sedation and anticonvulsant in the elimination phase, and the amnesia in the transition from elimination to distribution phase. Each benzodiazepine has unique plasma decay curves and therapeutic thresholds.

concentration over time in relation to hypothetical threshold concentrations for various neuropharmacological effects. Several points should be noted:

1   Each pharmacodynamic action has a different concentration threshold. The rank order probably is hypnosis > amnesia > sedation = anxiolysis > anticonvulsant.

2   Certain thresholds are crossed during the α or distribution phase of the plasma disappearance curve, while the drug concentration falls below the others during the elimination or β phase.

3   Each individual drug has its own unique plasma disappearance curve as well as pharmacodynamic threshold concentrations.

The importance of route of administration on the intensity and duration of effects is illustrated in Fig. 8.8. After the same size dose, marked effects can be expected with i.v., mild with oral, and minimal with i.m. administration. Few studies have demonstrated the plasma concentration threshold for specific effects of benzodiazepines, but Ghoneim has made a good start in associating certain tests of mental and psychomotor function with kinetic data for diazepam[36]. In Fig. 8.9, digit recall (a measure of

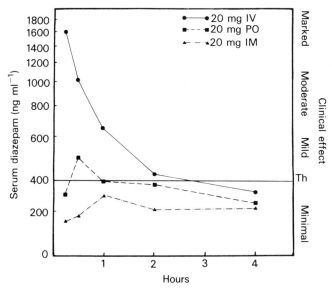

Fig. 8.8   The route of administration and clinical effects of diazepam are shown schematically in this illustration. Note highest serum drug levels are obtained most rapidly with intravenous diazepam. Oral administration produces higher and more rapid peaks in blood level than intramuscular. Clinical effects (sleepiness, impairment of mental arithmetic, amnesia, blurred vision and coordination) are all altered in a dose-related fashion. Minimal clinical effects are noted at blood levels less than $400\,mg\,ml^{-1}$ whereas more marked effects are encountered at blood levels of approximately $\geqslant 1000\,mg\,ml^{-1}$. This denotes therapeutic drug levels in these normal healthy volunteers. Drawn from data published by Hillestad *et al.*[66] 'Th' indicates the threshold concentration.

amnesic effects) and plasma drug levels after an intravenous injection of diazepam (0.2 mg/kg) in Caucasians are shown. Note that the peak effect on recall was found 30 min after administration and was still evident 2 hours after administration. The $T\frac{i}{2}$ for diazepam is 38 minutes, so it appears that the amnesic concentration threshold was crossed near the end of the distribution phase. Although not studied, awakening from the hypnotic effects of diazepam probably occurs earlier in the distribution phase, and for this reason, patients will awaken from a single intravenous dose of diazepam and still be amnesic for certain subsequent events.

Factors altering pharmacodynamics

A number of factors affect the pharmacodynamics of benzodiazepines. Although largely unexplored, certain factors appear to be important: acute versus chronic administration; dose; speed of IV injection; protein binding; age; and disease. Because of the pharmacokinetic characteristics of most benzodiazepines (i.e. a long $T\frac{\beta}{2}$, accumulation with chronic use), the results of acute versus chronic administration will

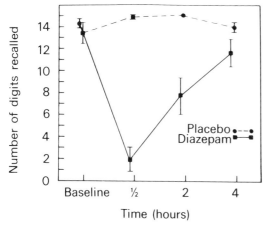

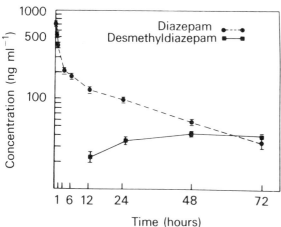

Fig. 8.9 Relationship of pharmacodynamics (number of digits recalled) and pharmacokinetics of diazepam (0.2 mg kg^{-1}) i.v. in 12 Caucasians. The time scales are different on each horizontal axis. Note diazepam reduces the mean ($\pm$SEM) number digits recalled, but by 4 hours the difference is not significantly different than baseline. The T$\frac{\alpha}{2}$ of diazepam levels mean ($\pm$SEM) is 0.63 hours. Note memory is impaired beyond the distribution phase of the drug (threshold approximately 200 ng ml^{-1}), but normal before significant accumulation of desmethyldiazepam. Redrawn from Ghoneim *et al.*[36] Reprinted by permission from *Clin. Pharmacol. Ther.* **29**, 749–56 (1981).

be different. If a significant drug level is present from the daily administration of a benzodiazepine, then an additional dose will produce higher drug levels and potentially greater effects than observed in a patient given the same size dose for the first time[15, 34, 62, 80, 83]. The effects of higher plasma concentrations will be reduced to the extent that tolerance develops during chronic therapy.

Pharmacodynamics of benzodiazepines are dose-related. The larger the dose, the more rapid the onset, the greater the intensity, and the longer the duration of action. Fig. 8.10 illustrates the relationship of increasing doses of midazolam on the probability of inducing sleep or anaesthesia and the rapidity of the induction[109, 110]. The relationships of dose to pharmacokinetics and pharmacodynamics are illustrated in Fig. 8.11. A 50% greater dose produces almost the same duration of sleep, but a more prolonged amnestic effect.

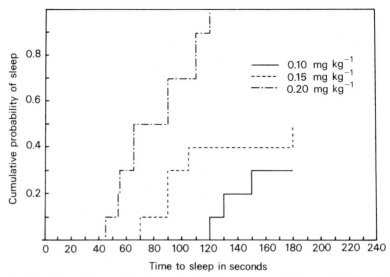

Fig. 8.10   The effects of increasing dose of midazolam on cumulative probability of inducing sleep (anesthesia induction) and on the time required for sleep (induction) to occur. Each group consists of healthy patients. Note the dose-related effects: with increasing dose the probability of induction increases and the time of induction decreases. Thus, with $0.20 \, \text{mg kg}^{-1}$ all patients were anesthetised within 110 seconds, whereas with $0.10 \, \text{mg kg}^{-1}$ only 30% were anesthetised between 120 and 180 seconds after the intravenous injection of midazolam.

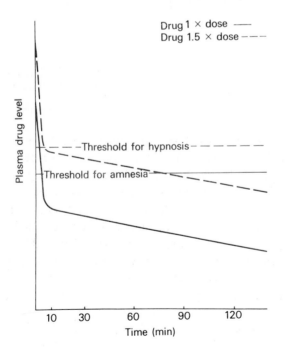

Fig. 8.11   A schematic semi-log plot of drug concentration and therapeutic threshold effect relationship for two dosages of the same drug. Note with a dose 50% higher the plasma disappearance curve is shifted upwards and to the right resulting in little change in time of hypnosis, but importantly longer time of amnesia.

Another pharmacodynamic consideration regarding benzodiazepines relates to their high degree of binding to protein. Only unbound drug crosses the blood–brain-barrier. The induction time of midazolam anaesthesia is approximately proportional ($r = 0.0524$, $p = 0.03$) to the concentrations of serum albumin in normal patients; that is, a lower level of serum albumin leaves a greater proportion of the drug free in plasma and able to enter the brain so that the induction time is also lower[110].

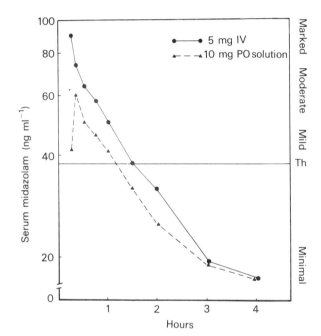

Fig. 8.12 Midazolam time effect relationship.

Although the effects of age, liver and renal diseases have been extensively evaluated on pharmacokinetics (*vide supra*), the impact of these factors on pharmacodynamics have not been investigated systemically. There are suggestions that elderly patients and patients with renal or liver disease may be more sensitive to a given plasma or tissue concentration of a benzodiazepine[13, 24, 37, 40, 42, 45, 68, 93, 129] (P. S. Collier *et al.* unpubl. data). Reasons for this are not clear, but changes in drug-receptor kinetics and interactions of benzodiazepines with metabolic byproducts accumulating in renal and liver failure are possibilities. There are intrinsic differences between drugs independent of their pharmacokinetics. Lorazepam has a shorter half-life and a greater clearance than diazepam, yet the amnestic actions of apparently equipotent doses of lorazepam last significantly longer than diazepam[31, 35]. This may be a reflection of lorazepam's greater affinity for and more prolonged occupation of benzodiazepine receptors.

CLINICAL IMPLICATIONS

The uses of benzodiazepines of interest to anaesthesiologists are listed in Table 8.6, and have changed little since they were reviewed a decade ago[30]. A number of clinical implications are apparent from a review of the pharmacokinetics and pharmaco-dynamics of benzodiazepines.

Table 8.6 Principle uses of selected benzodiazepines.

	Anesthesia induction agent	Anesthesia premedicant	Night hypnotic	In/outpatient anxiolytic	Anticonvulsant
Bromazepam				✓	
Clobazam					✓
Chlorazepate				✓	
Chlordiazepoxide		✓	✓	✓	
Clonzepam					✓
Diazepam	✓	✓	✓	✓	✓
Flunitrazepam	✓	✓	✓	✓	
Flurazepam			✓		
Lorazepam		✓	✓	✓	
Lormetazepam			✓		
Medazepam				✓	
Midazolam	✓	✓			
Nitrazepam			✓	✓	✓
Oxazepam		✓	✓	✓	
Prazepam				✓	
Temazepam			✓	✓	
Triazolam			✓	✓	

Drug selection is based primarily on elimination kinetics, for example, a short-lived drug (midazolam) for a short procedure or a longer lived compound (diazepam) for longer operations.

Route of administration is chosen on the basis of the absorption kinetics of each drug. For example, oral diazepam is rapid and dependable whereas intramuscular is not; lorazepam is dependable by both routes of administration.

Dose size is determined by route of administration and by factors that are known to alter pharmacokinetics and dynamics (i.e. tissue sensitivity to given drug concentration). Obviously, if similar plasma concentrations are desired to achieve similar therapeutic effects, the dosage must be adjusted according to the kinetics of absorption. It may be appropriate to lower the dosage of the benzodiazepine in patients taking benzodiazepines chronically, receiving cimetidine, or afflicted with renal or liver disease. Smokers and patients taking drugs which induce hepatic enzymes may require larger doses of benzodiazepines. Always it is important to remember that despite the general statements that can be made in regard to the pharmacokinetics and pharmacodynamics of benzodiazepines, individual patients vary greatly in their responses to the same size dose administered by the same route under similar circumstances. This variability does not reduce the value of the information reviewed in this chapter, but emphasises the need to expand that information so as to improve the efficiency with which the anaesthesiologist uses benzodiazepines in his patients, especially in view of the many variables encountered in the perioperative period that can affect both pharmacokinetics and dynamics.

ACKNOWLEDGEMENTS:

Rae Kerutis has laboured untiringly on the preparation of this manuscript with her usual level of excellence. Frank Hill's artistic talent is clear in the many illustrations that make the text more understandable. Drs Paul Samuelson and Ronald Vinik offered helpful constructive criticism in the preparation of the manuscript.

GLOSSARY

Generic	Trade
Bromazepam	Lectopam
Chlordiazepoxide	Librium
Clonazepam	Clonoptin, Rivotril
Clorazepate	Tranxene, Azene
Desmethyldiazepam	Nordiazepam
Diazepam	Valium-Roche, Diazemuls (Kabivitrum)
Flunitrazepam	Rohypnol
Flurazepam	Dalmane
Lorazepam	Ativan
Lormetazepam	Noctamid
Medazepam	Nobrium
Midazolam	Dobralam
Nitrazepam	Mogadon
Oxazepam	Serax, Serenid
Prazepam	Verstran
Temazepam	Restoril, Cerepax, Levanxol, Euhypnos, Normosin
Triazolam	Halcion

REFERENCES

1. ABEL J. G., SELLERS E. M. & NARANJO C. A. (1979) Inter- and intra-subject variation in diazepam free fraction. *Clin. Pharmacol. Ther.* **26**, 247–55.

2. ABERNETHY D. R. & GREENBLATT D. J. (1981) Effects of desmethyldiazepam on diazepam kinetics: a study of effects of a metabolite on parent drug disposition. *Clin. Pharmacol. Ther.* **29**, 757–61.

3. ALLEN M. D., GREENBLATT D. J. & ARNOLD J. D. (1979) Single- and multiple-dose kinetics of estazolam, a triazolo benzodiazepine. *Psychopharmacology* **66**, 267–74.

4. ALLEN M. D., GREENBLATT D. J. & HARMATZ J. S. (1979) Single-dose kinetics of prazepam, a precursor of desmethyldiazepam. *J. Clin. Pharmacol.* **19**, 445–50.

5. ALLEN M. D., GREENBLATT D. J. & HARMATZ B. A. (1980) Desmethyldiazepam kinetics in the elderly after oral prazepam. *Clin. Pharmacol. Ther.* **28**, 196–202.

6. ALLONEN H., ANTILLA V. & KLOTZ U. (1981) Effect kinetics of midazolam a new hypnotic benzodiazepine derivative. *Arch. Pharmacol.* **316**, R74.

7. ALVAN G. & ODAR-CEDERLOF I. (1978) The pharmacokinetic profile of oxazepam. *Acta Psychiatr. Scand.* **274**, 47–55.

8. ALVAN G., SIWERS B. & VESSMAN J. (1977) Pharmacokinetics of oxazepam in healthy volunteers. *Acta Pharmacol. Toxicol.* **40**, 40–51.

9. BAIRD E. S. & HAILEY D. M. (1972) Delayed recovery from a sedative: correlation of the plasma levels of diazepam with clinical effects after oral and intravenous administration. *Br. J. Anaesth.* **44**, 803–7.

10. BERLIN A., SIWERS B. & AGUREIL S. (1972) Determination of bioavailability of diazepam in various formulations from steady state plasma concentration data. *Clin. Pharmacol. Ther.* **13**, 733–44.

11. BERTLER A., LINDGREN S. & MALMGREN H. (1980) Pharmacokinetics of dipotassium chlorazepate in patients after repeated 50 mg oral doses. *Psychopharmacology* **71**, 165–7.

12. BITTENCOURT P., RICHENS A. & TOSELAND P. A. (1979) Pharmacokinetics of the hypnotic benzodiazepine, temazepam. *Br. J. Clin. Pharmacol.* **8**, 37s–38s.

13. Boston Collaborative Drug Surveillance Program, Boston University Medical Center (1973) Clinical depression of the central nervous system due to diazepam and chlordiazepoxide in relation to cigarette smoking and age. *New Engl. J. Med.* **288**, 277–80.

14. BOXENBAUM H. G., GEITNER K. A. & JACK M. L. (1977) Pharmacokinetic and biopharmaceutic profile of chlordiazepoxide HCl in healthy subjects: single-dose studies by the intravenous, intramuscular, and oral routes. *J. Pharmacokinet. Biopharm.* **5**, 3–23.

15. BOXENBAUM H. G., GEITNER K. A. & JACK M. L. (1977) Pharmacokinetic and biopharmaceutic profile of chlordiazepoxide HCl in healthy subjects: multiple-dose oral administration. *J. Pharmacokinet. Biopharm.* **5**, 25–39.

16. BOXENBAUM H. G., POSMANTER H. N. & MACASIEB T. (1978) Pharmacokinetics of flunitrazepam following single- and multiple-dose oral administration to healthy human subjects. *J. Pharmacokinet. Biopharm.* **6**, 283–93.

17. BRANCH R. A., MORGAN M. H. & JAMES J. (1976) Intravenous administration of diazepam in patients with chronic liver disease. *Gut* **17**, 975–83.

18. BREIMER D. D. (1977) Clinical pharmacokinetics of hypnotics. *Clin. Pharmacokin.* **2**, 93–109

19. BREIMER D. D. (1979) Pharmacokinetics and metabolism of various benzodiazepines used as hypnotics. *Br. J. Clin. Pharmacol.* **8**, 7S–13S

20. BROWN C. R., SARNQUIST F. H. & CANUP C. A. (1979) Clinical, electroencephalographic, and pharmacokinetic studies of a water-soluble benzodiazepine, midazolam maleate. *Anesthesiology* **50**, 467–70.

21. CANO J. P., SOLIVA M. & HARTMANN D. (1977) Bioavailability from various galenic formulations of flunitrazepam. *Arzneim-Forsch* **27**, 2383–8.

22. CARRIGAN P. J., CHAO G. C. & BARKER W. M. (1977) Steady-state bioavailability of two clorazepate dipotassium dosage forms. *J. Clin. Pharmacol.* **17**, 18–28

23. CARSTENSEN J. T., SU K. S. E. & MADDRELL P. (1971) Thermodynamic and kinetic aspects of parenteral benzodiazepines. *Bull. Parenteral Drug Assoc.* **25**, 193–202.

24. CASTLEDEN C. M., GEORGE C. F. & MARCER D. (1977) Increased sensitivity to nitrazepam in old age. *Br. Med. J.* **1**, 10–12

25. CLARKE R. S. J., DUNDEE J. W. & McGOWAN W. A. W. (1980) Comparison of the subjective effects and plasma concentrations following oral and I.M. administration flunitrazepam in volunteers. *Br. J. Anaesth.* **52**, 437–45.

26. CROOKS J., O'MALLEY K. & STEVENSON I. H. (1976) Pharmacokinetics in the elderly. *Clin. Pharmacokinet.* **1**, 280–96.

27. CURRY S. H. & WHELPTON R. (1979) Pharmacokinetics of closely related benzodiazepines. *Br. J. Clin. Pharmacol.* **8**, 15S–21S.

28. DESMOND P. V., ROBERTS R. K. & WILKINSON G. R. (1979) No effect of smoking on metabolism of chlordiazepoxide. *New Engl. J. Med.* **300**, 199–200.

29. DESILVA A. F. & PUGLISI C. V. (1970) Determination of medazepam (nobrium), diazepam (valium) and their major biotransformation products in blood and urine by electron capture gas-liquid chromatography. *Anal. Chem.* **42**, 1725–36.

30. DUNDEE J. W. & HASLETT W. H. K. (1970) The benzodiazepines. A review of their actions and uses relative to anesthetic practice. *Br. J. Anaesth.* **42**, 217–34.

31. DUNDEE J. W., McGOWAN W. A. W. & LILBURN J. K. (1979) Comparison of the actions of diazepam and lorazepam. *Br. J. Anaesth.* **51**, 439–46.

32. EATMAN F. B., COLBURN W. A. & BOXENBAUM H. G. (1977) Pharmacokinetics of diazepam following multiple-dose oral administration to healthy human subjects. *J. Pharmacokinet. Biopharm.* **5**, 481–94.

33. FUCCELLA L. M. (1979) Bioavailability of temazepam in soft gelatin capsules. *Br. J. Clin. Pharmacol.* **8**, 31S–35S.

34. GAMBLE J. A. S., DUNDEE J. W. & GRAY R. C. (1976) Plasma diazepam concentrations following prolonged administration. *Br. J. Anaesth.* **48**, 1087–90.

35. GEORGE K. A. & DUNDEE J. W. (1977) Relative amnesic actions of diazepam, flunitrazepam and lorazepam in man. *Br. J. Clin. Pharmacol.* **4**, 45–50.

36. GHONEIM M. M., KORTTILA K. & CHIANG C. K. (1981) Diazepam effects and kinetics in caucasians and orientals. *Clin. Pharmacol. Ther.* **29**, 749–56.

37. GREENBLATT D. J. (1979) Reduced serum albumin concentration in the elderly: a report from the Boston collaborative drug surveillance program. *J. Am. Geriatr. Soc.* **27**, 20–2.

38. GREENBLATT D. J. (1980) Pharmacokinetic comparisons. *Psychosomatics* **21**, 9–14.

39. GREENBLATT D. J. (1981) Clinical pharmacokinetics of oxazepam and lorazepam. *Clin. Pharmacokinet.* **6**, 89–105.

40. GREENBLATT D. J. & ALLEN M. D. (1978) Toxicity of nitrazepam in the elderly: a report from the Boston Collaborative Drug Surveillance Program. *Br. J. Clin. Pharmacol.* **5**, 407–13.

41. GREENBLATT D. J., ALLEN M. D. & HARMATZ J. S. (1980) Diazepam disposition determinants. *Clin. Pharmacol. Ther.* **27**, 301–12.

42. GREENBLATT D. J., ALLEN M. D. & LOCNISKAR A. (1979) Lorazepam kinetics in the elderly. *Clin. Pharmacol. Ther.* **26**, 103–13.

43. GREENBLATT D. J., ALLEN M. D. & MACLAUGHLIN D. S. (1978) Diazepam absorption: effect of antacids and food. *Clin. Pharmacol. Ther.* **24**, 600–609.

44. GREENBLATT D. J., ALLEN M. D. & MACLAUGHLIN D. S. (1979) Single- and multiple-dose kinetics of oral lorazepam in humans: the predictability of accumulation. *J. Pharmacokinet. Biopharm.* **7**, 159–79.

45. GREENBLATT D. J., ALLEN M. D. & SHADER R. I. (1977) Toxicity of high-dose flurazepam in the elderly. *Clin. Pharmacol. Ther.* **21**, 355–61.

46. GREENBLATT D. J., COMER W. H. & ELLIOTT H. W. (1977) Clinical pharmacokinetics of lorazepam. III. Intravenous injection. Preliminary results. *J. Clin. Pharmacol.* **17**, 490–94.

47. GREENBLATT D. J., DIVOLL M. & HARMATZ J. S. (1980) Oxazepam kinetics: effects of age and sex. *J. Pharmacol. Exp. Ther.* **215**, 86–91.

48. GREENBLATT D. J., FRANKE K. & SHADER R. I. (1978) Analysis of lorazepam and its glucuronide metabolite by electron-capture gas-liquid chromatography. *J. Chromatogr.* **146**, 311–20.

49. GREENBLATT D. J., JOYCE T. H. & COMER W. H. (1977) Clinical pharmacokinetics of lorazepam. II. Intramuscular injection. *Clin. Pharmacol. Ther.* **21**, 222–30.

50. GREENBLATT D. J., KNOWLES J. A. & COMER W. H. (1977) Clinical pharmacokinetics of lorazepam. IV. Long-term oral administration. *J. Clin. Pharmacol.* **17**, 495–500

51. GREENBLATT D. J., LOCKNISKAR A. & OCHS H. R. (1981) Automated gas chromatography for studies of midazolam pharmacokinetics. *Anesthesiology* **55**, 176–9.

52. GREENBLATT D. J., SCHILLINGS R. T. &

KYRIAKOPOULOS A. A. (1976) Clinical pharmacokinetics of lorazepam. I. Absorption and disposition of oral C-lorazepam. *Clin. Pharmacol. Ther.*, 329–41.

53. GREENBLATT D. J. & SHADER R. I. (1974) *Benzodiazepines in Clinical Practice.* Raven Press, New York City.

54. GREENBLATT D. J. & SHADER R. I. (1978) Prazepam and lorazepam, two new benzodiazepines. *New Engl. J. Med.* **299**, 1342–4.

55. GREENBLATT D. J. & SHADER R. I. (1978) Pharmacokinetic understanding of anti-anxiety drug therapy. *South Med. J.* **71**, 2–9.

56. GREENBLATT D. J., SHADER R. I. & FRANKE K. (1977) Kinetics of intravenous chlordiazepoxide: sex differences in drug distribution. *Clin. Pharmacol. Ther.* **22**, 893–903.

57. GREENBLATT D. J., SHADER R. I. & FRANKE K. (1979) Pharmacokinetics and bioavailability of intravenous, intramuscular, and oral lorazepam in humans. *J. Pharm. Sci.* **68**, 57–63.

58. GREENBLATT D. J., SHADER R. I. & HARMATZ J. S. (1976) Influence of magnesium and aluminum hydroxide mixture on chlordiazepoxide absorption. *Clin. Pharmacol. Ther.* **19**, 234–9.

59. GREENBLATT D. J., SHADER R. I. & HARMATZ J. S. (1977) Absorpton rate, blood concentrations, and early response to oral chlordiazepoxide. *Am. J. Psychiatry.* **13**, 559–62.

60. GREENBLATT D. J., SHADER R. I. & HARMATZ J. S. (1981) Benzodiazepines: a summary of pharmacokinetic properties. *Br. J. Clin. Pharmacol.* **11**, 11–16.

61. GREENBLATT D. J., SHADER R. I. & KOCH-WESER J. (1974) Slow absorption of intramuscular chlordiazepoxide. *New Engl. J. Med.* **291**, 1116–18.

62. GREENBLATT D. J., SHADER R. I. & MACLEOD S. M. (1978) Clinical pharmacokinetics of chlordiazepoxide. *Clin. Pharmacokin.* **3**, 381–94.

63. GREENBLATT D. J., SHADER R. I. &
    MACLEOD S. M. (1978) Absorption of
    oral and intramuscular chlordiazepoxide.
    Eur. J. Clin. Pharmacol. **13**, 267–74.

64. GREENBLATT D. J., SHADER R. I. &
    WEINBERGER D. R. (1978) Effect of a
    cocktail on diazepam absorption.
    Psychopharmacology **57**, 199–203.

65. HAILEY D. M. & BAIRD E. S. (1979)
    Plasma concentrations of medazepam
    and its metabolites after oral administra-
    tion. *Br. J. Anaesth.* **51**, 493–6.

66. HILLESTAD L., HANSEN T. & MELSOM H.
    (1974) Diazepam metabolism in normal
    man. I. Serum concentrations and clinical
    effects after intravenous, intramuscular,
    and oral administration. *Clin. Phar-
    macol. Ther.* **16**, 479–84.

67. HILLESTAD L., HANSEN T. & MELSOM H.
    (1974) Diazepam metabolism in normal
    man. II. Serum concentration and clinical
    effect after oral administration and cumu-
    lation. *Clin. Pharmacol. Ther.* **16**, 485–9.

68. HOYUMPA A. M. Jr. (1978) Disposition
    and elimination of minor tranquilizers in
    the aged and in patients with liver disease.
    South Med. J. **71**, 23–8.

69. HUMPEL M., NIEUWEBOER B. & MILIUM
    W. (1980) Kinetics and biotransform-
    ation of lormetazepam. *Clin. Pharmacol.
    Ther.* **28**, 673–9.

70. IISALO E., KANGAS L. & RUIKKA I. (1977)
    Pharmacokinetics of nitrazepam in
    young volunteers and aged patients. *Br.
    J. Clin. Pharmacol.* **4**, 646–7.

71. KAMPF D., HUEMPEL M. & LERCHE U.
    (1981) Effects of uremia and hemo-
    dialysis on lormetazepam disposition.
    Clin. Pharmacol. Ther. **30**, 77–85.

72. KANGAS   L.,   ALLONEN   H.   &
    LAMMINTAUSTA R. (1979) Pharmaco-
    kinetics of nitrazepam in saliva and
    serum after a single oral dose. *Acta
    Pharmacol. Toxicol.* **45**, 20–4.

73. KANGAS L., IISALO E. & KANTO J. (1979)
    Human pharmacokinetics of nitrazepam:
    effect of age and diseases. *Eur. J. Clin.
    Pharmacol.* **15**, 163–170.

74. KANGAS L., KANTO J. & FORSSTROM J.
    (1976) The protein binding of diazepam
    and N-demethyldiazepam in patients
    with poor renal function. *Clin. Nephrol.*
    5, 114–118.

75. KANGAS L., KANTO J. & LEHTINEN V.
    (1979) Long-term nitrazepam treatment
    in psychiatric out-patients with insomnia.
    Psychopharmacology **63**, 63–6.

76. KANTO J. (1981) Benzodiazepines as oral
    premedicants. *Br. J. Anaesth.* **53**, 1179–
    88.

77. KANTO J., IISALO E. & LEHTINEN V.
    (1971) The concentrations of diazepam
    and its metabolites in the plasma after an
    acute   and   chronic   administration.
    Psychopharmacologia **36**, 123–31.

78. KANTO J., MAENPAA M. & MANTYLA R.
    (1979) Effect of age on the pharmaco-
    kinetics of diazepam given in conjunction
    with spinal anesthesia. *Anesthesiology* **51**,
    154–9.

79. KAPLAN S. A., DESILVA J. A. F. & JACK
    M. L. (1973) Blood level profile in man
    following chronic oral administration of
    flurazepam hydrochloride. *J. Pharm. Sci.*
    62, 1932–5.

80. KAPLAN S. A., JACK M. L. & ALEXANDER
    K. (1973) Pharmacokinetic profile of
    diazepam in man following single intra-
    venous and oral and chronic oral ad-
    ministrations. *J. Pharm. Sci.* **62**, 1789–
    96.

81. KAPLAN S. A., JACK M. L. & WEINFELD
    R. E. (1976) Biopharmaceutical and clini-
    cal pharmacokinetic profile of brom-
    azepam. *J. Pharmacokinet. Biopharm.* **4**,
    1–16.

82. KHOO K. C., MENDELS J. & ROTHBART
    M. (1980) Influence of phenytoin and
    phenobarbital on the disposition of a
    single oral dose of clonazepam. *Clin.
    Pharmacol. Ther.* **28**, 368–75.

83. KLOTZ U., ANTONIN K. H. & BIECK P. R.
    (1976) Comparison of the pharmacokin-
    etics of diazepam after single and sub-
    chronic doses. *Eur. J. Clin. Pharmacol.*
    10, 121–6.

84. KLOTZ U., ANTONIN K. H. & BIECK P. R. (1976) Pharmacokinetics and plasma binding of diazepam in man, dog, rabbit, guinea pig and rat. *J. Pharmacol. Exp. Ther.* **199**, 67–73.

85. KLOTZ U., ANTONIN K. H. & BRUGEL H. (1977) Disposition of diazepam and its major metabolite desmethyldiazepam in patients with liver disease. *Clin. Pharmacol. Ther.* **21**, 430–6.

86. KLOTZ U., AVANT G. R. & HOYUMPA A. (1975) The effects of age and liver disease on the disposition and elimination of diazepam in adult man. *J. Clin. Invest.* **55**, 347–59.

87. KLOTZ U. & MULLER-SEYDLITZ P. (1979) Altered elimination of desmethyldiazepam in the elderly. *Br. J. Clin. Pharmacol.* **7**, 119–20.

88. KLOTZ U. & REIMANN I. (1980) Influence of cimetidine on the pharmacokinetics of desmethyldiazepam and oxazepam. *Eur. J. Clin. Pharmacol.* **18**, 517–20.

89. KLOTZ U. & REIMANN I. (1980) Delayed clearance of diazepam due to cimetidine. *New Engl. J. Med.* **302**, 1012–14.

90. KNOP H. J., VAN DER KLEIJN E. & EDMUNDS L. C. (1975) Pharmacokinetics of clonazepam in man and laboratory animals. In Schneider H. *et al.* (eds.) *Clinical Pharmacology of Anti-Epileptic Drugs*, pp. 247–59. Springer, Berlin.

91. KORTTILA K. & LINNOILA M. (1975) Recovery and skills related to driving after intravenous sedation: dose-response relationship with diazepam. *Br. J. Anaesth.* **47**, 457–63.

92. KORTTILA K. & LINNOILA M. (1975) Absorption and sedative effects of diazepam after oral administration and intramuscular administration into the vastus lateralis muscle and the deltoid muscle. *Br. J. Anaesth.* **47**, 857–62.

93. KORTTILA K., SAARNIVAARA L. & TARKKANEN J. (1978) Effect of age on amnesia and sedation induced by flunitrazepam during local anaesthesia for bronchoscopy. *Br. J. Anaesth.* **50**, 1211–18.

94. KRAUS J. W., DESMOND P. V. & MARSHALL J. P. (1978) Effects of aging and liver disease on disposition of lorazepam. *Clin. Pharmacol. Ther.* **24**, 411–19.

95. KYRIAKOPOULOS A. A., GREENBLATT D. J. & SHADER R. I. (1978) Clinical pharmacokinetics of lorazepam: a review. *J. Clin. Psychiatry.* **39**, 16–23

96. LAI A. A., LEVY R. H. & CUTLER R. E. (1978) Time-course of interaction between carbamazepine and clonazepam in normal man. *Clin. Pharmacol. Ther.* **24**, 316–23.

97. MACKLON A. K., BARTON M. & JAMES O. (1980) The effect of age on the pharmacokinetics of diazepam. *Clin. Sci.* **59**, 479–83.

98. MACLEOD S. M., GILES H. G. & BENGERT B. (1979) Age- and gender-related differences in diazepam pharmacokinetics. *J. Clin. Pharmacol.* **19**, 15–19.

99. MACLEOD S. M., SELLERS E. M. & GILES H. G. (1978) Interaction of disulfiram with benzodiazepines. *Clin. Pharmacol. Ther.* **24**, 583–9.

100. MANDELLI M., TOGNONI G. & GARATTINI S. (1978) Clinical pharmacokinetics of diazepam. *Clin. Pharmacokinet.* **3**, 72–91.

101. MATTILA M. A. K. & LARNI H. M. (1980) Flunitrazepam: A review of its pharmacological properties and therapeutic use. *Drugs* **20**, 353–74.

102. METZLER C. M., KO H. & ROYTER M. E. (1977) Bioavailability and pharmacokinetics of orally administered triazolam in normal subjects. *Clin. Pharmacol. Ther.* **21**, 111–12.

103. MOHLER H. & OKADA T. (1978) Biochemical identification of the site of action of benzodiazepines in human brain by ^{3}H-diazepam binding. *Life Sci.* **22**, 985–96.

104. MOORE R. G. & MCBRIDE W. G. (1978) The disposition kinetics of diazepam in pregnant women at parturition. *Eur. J. Clin. Pharmacol.* **13**, 275–84.

105. NICHOLSON A. N. (1979) Performance studies with diazepam and its hydroxylated metabolites. *Br. J. Clin. Pharmacol.* **8**, 39s–42s.

106. OCHS H. R., GREENBLATT D. J. & KASCHEL H. J. (1981) Diazepam kinetics in patients with renal insufficiency or hyperthyroidism. *Br. J. Clin. Pharmacol.* **12**, 829–32.

107. OHNHAUS E. E., PARK B. K. & COLOMBO J. P. (1979) The effect of enzyme induction on diazepam metabolism in man. *Br. J. Clin. Pharmacol.* **8**, 557–63.

108. PUGLISI C. V., MEYER J. C. & D'ARCONTE L. (1978) Determination of water soluble imidazo-1,4-benzodiazepines in blood by electro-capture gas-liquid chromatography and in urine by differential pulse polarography. *J. Chromatograph.* **145**, 81–96.

109. REVES J. G., CORSSEN G. & HOLCOMB C. (1978) Comparison of two benzodiazepines for anaesthesia induction: midazolam and diazepam. *Can. Anaesth. Soc. J.* **25**, 211–14.

110. REVES J. G., NEWFIELD P. & SMITH L. R. (1981) Influence of serum protein, serum albumin concentrations and dose on midazolam anaesthesia induction times. *Can. Anaesth. Soc. J.* **28**, 556–60.

111. REVES J. G., SAMUELSON P. N. & VINIK H. R. (in press) Midazolam. In Brown B. R. (ed.), *Contemporary Anesthesia Practice*. F. A. Davis, Philadelphia.

112. REIDENBERG M., LEVY M. & WARNER H. (1978) Relationship between diazepam dose, plasma level, age, and central nervous system depression. *Clin. Pharmacol. Ther.* **23**, 371–4.

113. REY E., D'ATHIS P. & GIRAUX P. (1979) Pharmacokinetics of clorazepate in pregnant and non-pregnant women. *Eur. J. Clin. Pharmacol.* **15**, 175–80.

114. ROBERTS R. K., DESMOND P. V. & WILKINSON G. R. (1979) Disposition of chlordiazepoxide: sex differences and effects of oral contraceptives. *Clin. Phar-*

macol. Ther. **25**, 826–31.

115. ROBERTS R. K., WILKINSON G. R. & BRANCH R. A. (1978) Effect of age and parenchymal liver disease on the disposition and elimination of chlordiazepoxide (librium). *Gastroenterology* **75**, 479–85.

116. ROUTLEDGE P. A., KITCHELL B. B. & BJORNSSON T. D. (1980) Diazepam and N-desmethyldiazepam redistribution after heparin. *Clin. Pharmacol. Ther.* **27**, 528–32.

117. SARNQUIST F. H., MATHERS W. D. & BLASCHKE T. F. (1979) Steady-state pharmacokinetics of midazolam maleate. *Anesthesiology* **51**, S41.

118. SCHWARZ H. J. (1979) Pharmacokinetics and metabolism of temazepam in man and several animal species. *Br. J. Clin. Pharmacol.* **8**, 23S–29S.

119. SCHWARTZ M. A., POSTMA E. & GAUT Z. (1971) Biological half-life of chlordiazepoxide and its metabolite, demoxepam, in man. *J. Pharm. Sci.* **60**, 1500–3.

120. SELLERS E. M., GREENBLATT D. J. & GILES H. G. (1979) Chlordiazepoxide and oxazepam disposition in cirrhosis. *Clin. Pharmacol. Ther.* **26**, 240–6.

121. SELLERS E. M., MACLEOD S. M. & GREENBLATT D. J. (1977) Influence of disulfiram and disease on benzodiazepine disposition. *Clin. Pharmacol. Ther.* **21**, 117.

122. SHADER R. I., GOERGOTAS A. & GREENBLATT D. J. (1978) Impaired absorption of desmethyldiazepam for clorazepate by magnesium aluminum hydroxide. *Clin. Pharmacol. Ther.* **24**, 308–15.

123. SHADER R. I., GREENBLATT D. J. & HARMATZ J. S. (1977) Absorption and disposition of chlordiazepoxide in young and elderly male volunteers. *J. Clin. Pharmacol.* **17**, 709–18.

124. SHULL H. J., WILKINSON G. R. & JOHNSON R. (1976) Normal disposition of oxazepam in acute viral hepatitis and cirrhosis. *Ann. Intern. Med.* **84**, 420–5.

125. SMITH M. T., EADIE M. J. & BROPHY T. O. (1981) The pharmacokinetics of midazolam in man. *Eur. J. Clin. Pharmacol.* **19**, 271–8.

126. SMITH M. T., EVANS L. E. J. & EADIE M. J. (1979) Pharmacokinetics of prazepam in man. *Eur. J. Clin. Pharmacol.* **16**, 141–7.

127. TOMSON G., LUNELL N. O. & SUNDWALL A. (1979) Placental passage of oxazepam and its metabolism in mother and newborn. *Clin. Pharmacol. Ther.* **25**, 74–81.

128. VERBEECK R., TJANDRAMAGA T. B. & VERBERCKMOES R. (1976) Biotransformation and excretion of lorazepam in patients with chronic renal failure. *Br. J. Clin. Pharmacol.* **3**, 1033–9.

129. VINIK R., REVES J. G. & NIXON D. (1981) Midazolam induction and emergence in renal failure patients. *Anesthesiology* **55**, A262.

130. VINIK H. R., REVES J. G. & GREENBLATT D. J. (1982) Pharmacokinetics of midazolam in renal failure patients. *Anesthesiology* **57**, A366.

131. VIUKARI M. & LINNOILA M. (1977) Serum medazepam, diazepam, and n-desmethyldiazepam levels after single and multiple oral doses of medazepam. *Ann. Clin. Res.* **9**, 284–6.

132. WILKINSON G. R. & SCHENKER S. (1975) Drug disposition and liver disease. *Drug. Metab. Rev.* **4**, 139–75.

9 Pharmacokinetics and Dynamics of Narcotic Analgesics

CARL C. HUG JR.

The anaesthesiologist uses narcotic analgesics for preanaesthetic medication; to supplement regional and general anaesthesia; as primary anaesthetic agents; and for relief of pain. Despite the long history of their use for these different purposes, the anaesthesiologist of today is still faced with the challenge of using the narcotic analgesics efficiently; that is, for maximum benefit of the patient with a minimum of acute and chronic toxicity. For example, concerns about ventilatory depression and the development of drug dependence lead many practitioners to prescribe fixed doses at fixed intervals. The result is poor control of pain, the predominant cause of complaints among post-surgical patients interviewed at the time of their discharge from the hospital[147].

The challenge of efficiency in the use of narcotic analgesics intraoperatively is even more difficult. The simultaneous use of fully paralysing doses of muscle relaxants obliterates the somatic signs of anaesthetic depth and there are recurring reports of awareness and recall of intraoperative events by the patient[90]. The use of autonomic sympathetic and cardiovascular responses as indicators of inadequate anaesthetic depth is less than completely reliable and in some instances may be dangerous (i.e. tachycardia and hypertension in the patient with coronary artery disease). Moreover, it is a common belief among anaesthesiologists that it is much easier to prevent cardiovascular stimulation than it is to control it once it occurs. Consequently, there is a strong tendency to use large, often excessive doses of a narcotic analgesic, with the result of prolonged postoperative ventilatory depression requiring mechanical ventilatory support or the use of narcotic antagonists, both choices having substantial drawbacks (monetary costs, risks of complications)[40, 65, 66, 119].

Beyond these imposing challenges, the anaesthesiologist is faced with variability in the patients' responses to the narcotic analgesics. To date there has been little progress made in distinguishing the two primary sources of variability: pharmacodynamic (i.e. the tissue responsiveness to a given drug concentration) and pharmacokinetic (i.e. the drug concentration resulting from a given dose).

Investigations of the kinetics of narcotic analgesic disposition offer the following
1   distinguishing pharmacodynamic and kinetic causes of variability;
2   recognising potential problems in the choice of a particular narcotic analgesic and its dose;
3   defining the drug concentrations associated with desired effects and undesirable toxicity;
4   designing an optimal dosage regimen for a given clinical situation;
5   monitoring narcotic analgesic therapy; and
6   predicting recovery from its effects.

The emphasis of this chapter will be on the three narcotic analgesics most widely used by anaesthesiologists and most thoroughly studied in terms of pharmacokinetics. Morphine, pethidine (meperidine, Demerol), and fentanyl (Sublimaze) have many similarities in their biological disposition and also some important differences. Not all of the details have been determined for any one of the three, but cautious speculation based on the general principles of pharmacokinetics is appropriate and useful to the anaesthesiologist.

Among new narcotic analgesics undergoing clinical trials, alfentanil (Alfenta, Rapifen) is particularly interesting to anaesthesiologists from a pharmacokinetic viewpoint; it will be discussed under the heading 'Clinical Applications' near the end of this chapter (p. 215).

SITES OF NARCOTIC ANALGESIC ACTION

With the exceptions of their actions on smooth muscle and mast cells (histamine release), the most important effects of the narcotic analgesics result from their actions within the central narvous system (CNS) (Table 9.1). It is clear that most of the effects result from their interactions with specific opioid receptors that are discretely located in certain areas of the CNS[58, 84]. In contrast to the general anaesthetics which potentially act on all cells, the actions of the narcotic analgesics are quite selective and limited. There is every reason to believe that the intensity of the effect is proportional to the concentration of narcotic analgesic at the site of action, because each effect can be characterised by a log-dose vs. response relationship, and because morphine and the other narcotic agonists interact competitively with the narcotic antagonists[78, 92, 145].

Table 9.1   Narcotic analgesic effects and sites of action.

CNS Actions
Analgesia (↓ autonomic, endocrine, and somatic responses to noxious stimulation)*
Sleep (unconsciousness in extremely high doses)*
Antitussive (↓ response to endotracheal tube and manipulation of the airway)*
Nausea, retching, vomiting
Ventilatory depression (cause of death)
Muscular rigidity (anaesthetic doses)
Dysphoria, euphoria
Psychological and physical dependence

Peripheral Actions
Histamine release
Vasodilation
Smooth muscle
   spasm (e.g. biliary colic)
   ↓ acetylcholine release from parasympathetic nerves (e.g. inhibition of contraction of guinea
      pig ileum)
Cardiac depression (certain analgesics in high doses)

No effects on
Cardiac or vascular responses to sympathomimetics
Autoregulation of cerebral and renal blood flow
Liver or renal function
Fetal development (providing normal hygiene and nutrition are maintained)
Malignant hyperthemia

---

* Useful to the anaesthiologist

It should be noted that the individual effects of a single narcotic analgesic do not always have the same dose-concentration–response relationships[78]. Moreover, the affinities of the individual narcotic analgesics for the opioid receptors differ to a considerable degree; differences in receptor affinity may be reflected not only in terms of concentration vs. response relationships (pharmacodynamics), but also in pharmaco-kinetic terms (e.g. duration of action).

It is also clear that narcotic analgesic binding to specific opioid receptors represents a very minute fraction of the total amount of drug entering the CNS. There is considerable non-specific binding of the narcotic analgesics to tissues[51, 75]. In fact, the administration of a narcotic antagonist in doses sufficient to completely antagonise narcotic analgesic effects results in inconsistent and small changes in the CNS concentrations of the agonist[106].

When considering the relationships between plasma concentrations of a narcotic analgesic and the intensity of its actions within the CNS, several important points must be kept in mind.

1 The only certain way to define a plasma concentration vs. response relationship precisely is to establish steady-state conditions with complete equilibrium of drug concentrations between plasma and the drug receptor sites. Such conditions can be achieved by continuous administration of drug (e.g. by infusion) under constant physiological conditions[109].

2 The relationship can be estimated somewhat less precisely by correlating drug effects and plasma concentrations after the distribution phases of a single dose are completed and a pseudoequilibrium exists between plasma and tissue concentrations of the drug. At least in the case of lipid-soluble drugs able to equilibrate rapidly across membranes, the drug concentrations in tissues will decline in parallel with its concentrations in plasma during the elimination phase (especially if the rate constant for elimination is slow relative to the rate constants for dissociation of the drug-receptor complex and for movement of the drug out of tissue into plasma). In fact, useful correlations have been made between log-concentrations and the analgesic and ventilatory depressant effects of meperidine and fentanyl, two very lipid soluble narcotic analgesics[4, 98]. On the other hand, no direct correlations between plasma levels of morphine and either its CNS concentrations or the intensity of effects have been demonstrated after a single dose; morphine leaves the CNS slowly as a result of its limited lipid solubility[33, 42, 73, 115, 156].

3 Little or no direct relationship between log concentration and effect is likely to be apparent when there is a rapid rate of change in the plasma concentration of a drug such as that occurring immediately after its injection. The relationship will be even more remote (indirect) in the case of a drug penetrating membranes slowly (e.g. morphine), for a drug dissociating from its receptors at a slower rate than that at which it is eliminated from plasma (e.g. lofentanil[J. Leysen, unpubl. obs.]), and under circumstances of poor tissue perfusion resulting in slow delivery of the drug to and removal from its sites of action (e.g. in shock[10]).

4 Finally, it is important to understand exactly what the narcotic analgesic assay measures in plasma or blood[55]. Most assays measure the total drug in plasma, including free and protein-bound, ionised and unionised. These variables must be taken into account when interpreting pharmacokinetic data and attempting to relate it to the pharmacodynamic actions of the drug. Of course, it is absolutely essential that the assay measures only the unchanged, pharmacologically active narcotic analgesic and not its metabolites. These and other caveats that should be borne in mind are discussed in more detail in a recent review[55].

INDIVIDUAL FACTORS IN THE DISPOSITION OF NARCOTIC ANALGESICS

Absorption

Oral

The narcotic analgesics are rarely administered orally because their systemic availability is low and erratic. It is erratic because the narcotic analgesics have prominent effects on gastrointestinal function that add to numerous other factors affecting the absorption of orally administered drugs[9]. It is low because all of the narcotic analgesics ionise as organic bases in the acidic medium of the stomach and the ionised forms do not readily penetrate the gastric mucosa. The narcotic analgesics are less ionised in the alkaline milieu of the small intestine and probably penetrate the intestinal mucosa readily. However, once they enter the portal venous circulation they are carried to the liver, which removes them efficiently from the blood and biotransforms them into inactive metabolites* [20, 95, 143]. There is also the possibility that morphine is taken up and metabolised by the intestinal mucosa or by intestinal bacteria[32, 76].

Pethidine is used orally in some circumstances and its systemic availability has been determined to average approximately 52% (range 47–61%) of the ingested dose in volunteers[95]. Given the facts that morphine and fentanyl have characteristics similar to pethidine (i.e. a clearance approximating hepatic blood flow, minimal elimination by extra-hepatic routes, blood to plasma concentration ratio approximating unity), it is predictable that their bioavailability after oral administration would be similarly low[155]. Indeed, the plasma concentrations of morphine after an oral dose were approximately one-half those found after the same size dose was injected parenterally in volunteers[20] (Fig. 9.1). An estimate of bioavailability of orally ingested morphine in these volunteers (0.30) agrees closely with the oral bioavailability of morphine (0.38) measured in patients with advanced malignancy[126].

---

* Codeine may represent an exception since it has a methyl group at the phenolic position which otherwise is readily conjugated to glucuronic acid. The removal of the methyl group in the liver releases morphine, some of which escapes conjugation and enters the systemic circulation; low concentrations of morphine account for the weak analgesic effects of orally administered codeine[43].

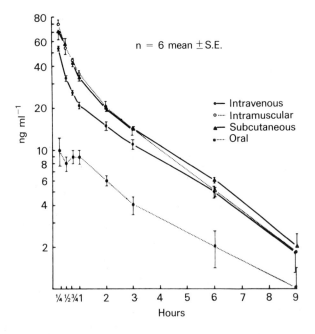

Fig. 9.1 Plasma concentrations of unchanged morphine in volunteers given a 5.75 mg/m² dose (approximately 10 mg) by one of the routes of administration indicated. Reproduced with permission from Brunk S. F. and Delle M. (1974) *Clin. Pharmacol. Ther.* **16**, 51–57, [20].

Alfentanil is a new narcotic analgesic with a relatively high lipid solubility and relatively low hepatic clearance (*vide infra*). Theoretically, its absorption from the intestine should be complete and its presystemic clearance low. If so, most of a dose ingested orally or administered rectally should reach the systemic circulation. The potential applications of this drug are considered near the end of this chapter.

Intramuscular and subcutaneous

Subcutaneous injections are seldom used these days, and there are no studies of blood levels of the narcotic analgesics in man given to them subcutaneously, except for morphine. Brunk and Delle found nearly identical plasma concentrations of morphine in volunteers receiving the same dose of the drug either subcutaneously or intramuscularly (Fig. 9.1)[20].

The uptake of morphine and of pethidine from intramuscular injection sites was relatively efficient in volunteers and maximum plasma concentrations of the drugs were found between 15 and 60 minutes after injection[20, 94, 139, 141]. The kinetics of fentanyl absorption from parenteral injection sites have not been reported, but the intensity of analgesia and other CNS effects were maximal within 20 minutes after an intramuscular injection in adult surgical patients[41]. This observation and the similarity of its physicochemical properties to those of pethidine, are strongly suggestive of efficient absorption of fentanyl after parenteral administration to normal adults.

Detailed studies of the absorption of pethidine from intramuscular injection sites revealed that more than 80% of an analgesic dose was absorbed within 6 hours and that the absorption processes exhibited biphasic kinetics. Initially, the absorption of approximately two-thirds of the dose was rapid ($T_{\frac{1}{2}}$ = 28 min) but then it continued at a slower rate ($T_{\frac{1}{2}}$ = 5.3 h)[94].

These data from normal volunteers given a single injection into gluteal muscle may not always apply to patients, especially under circumstances of abnormal perfusion of the injection site. Peripheral vasoconstriction due to pain, hypvolaemia, hypotension, hypothermia, infusion of vasoconstrictors, or any other cause will almost certainly slow the absorption of the narcotic analgesics. Correction of these abnormalities may lead to an unexpected increase in the rate of absorption and to excessive drug effects, especially after multiple injections have been given to compensate for the inadequate effects of the initial dose[52]. Autonomic and haemodynamic factors probably contribute to the erratic absorption of pethidine and morphine reported in surgical patients[94, 95, 124]. The erratic relief of postoperative pain has been attributed to the variability of plasma levels of pethidine after its intramuscular injection[4].

Given the likelihood of variable perfusion of parenteral injection sites in patients following surgery, it is unreasonable to administer the narcotic analgesics by other than intravenous injection when an intravenous cannula is present. Moreover, the intravenous route offers the additional advantages of (1) avoiding the discomfort of the injection needle; (2) rapid onset of analgesia; (3) ease of titration of the dose according to response; (4) progressive decline of plasma levels with a correspondingly progressive reduction in the risks of toxicity; and (5) the likelihood that the signs of overdosage will be manifest early when the physician or nurse administering the drug are still observing the patient closely.

Although it is true that the peak concentrations of drug in plasma will be higher and the decline of drug concentrations more rapid after intravenous than after intramuscular injection, the differences are relatively small (Fig. 9.1) and not likely to be consistent under the variable conditions encountered clinically. The use of intravenous infusions (see below) can extend the duration of drug action and smooth out the peaks and valleys of drug concentrations associated with intermittent injections by either the intravenous or intramuscular routes.

Epidural and intrathecal

The administration of narcotic analgesics by these routes is intended to focus their actions on the pain transmission pathways in the spinal cord[18, 123]. Nevertheless, it is clear that some, if not all, of the dose eventually reaches the systemic circulation. In the case of small doses administered intrathecally, the systemic concentrations are likely to be small because the drug is distributed among body tissues and eliminated, as after any other route of administration. Larger doses administered epidurally can be expected to result in plasma levels of narcotic analgesics similar in magnitude to those produced by an intramuscular or subcutaneous injection of the same size dose.

In fact, plasma levels of pethidine rose more slowly after epidural injection than after intramuscular administration, but they eventually reached the lower range of plasma concentrations associated with systemic side-effects and analgesia[50]. The latter may contribute to the overall effects of epidural analgesia, but the relatively rapid onset and especially the long duration of regional analgesia indicate that the local action of pethidine on the spinal cord is the predominant one.

In the case of morphine, the rise and decline of plasma concentrations measured after an epidural injection were quantitatively similar to those found after an intramuscular injection[18, 20, 123, 154]. Because of the lack of a clear-cut, direct relationship between plasma levels of morphine and its analgesic effect (see p. 190), it is difficult to estimate the contribution of systemically absorbed morphine to its effects after epidural administration. At least during the first hour after an epidural dose of 10 mg, morphine concentrations remained above the minimum plasma level ($19 \ \mathrm{ng \ ml^{-1}}$) associated with satisfactory relief of postoperative pain by intravenously administered morphine[18, 146]. Subsequently, the plasma levels declined and it is improbable that systemically absorbed morphine contributed to the sustained regional analgesia. It may be that the systemic uptake of morphine from the epidural space contributes to the onset of analgesia and to side-effects observed soon after an epidural injection. Delayed and sustained effects more likely result from its persistent action on the spinal cord and to its rostral diffusion in cerebrospinal fluid to the brain stem and other higher centres containing opioid receptors[18].

Many studies of the pharmacokinetics of epidurally administered narcotic analgesics are in progress; the results will contribute greatly to our understanding of the role of systemic absorption in the production of analgesia and side-effects. In the meantime, the obvious potential for systemic absorption of narcotic analgesics from the epidural space strongly supports the recommendation to limit the dose if the local actions are to predominate. This recommendation is also supported by observations of the limited benefits and increased side-effects resulting from morphine doses exceeding 10 mg in adults [7, 18, 19, 120, 123, 125].

Distribution

Factors affecting the rate and extent of narcotic analgesic uptake by tissues include lipid solubility, ionisation, binding to plasma proteins and to tissue components (Table 9.2).

Lipid solubility is the most important factor determining the rate of narcotic analgesic entry and exit from the CNS. Highly lipid soluble drugs such as fentanyl equilibrate rapidly across the membranes separating plasma, brain tissue and cerebrospinal fluid,

Table 9.2 Physicochemical factors affecting the disposition of narcotic analgesics[100].

Factor	Morphine	Pethidine	Fentanyl	Alfentanil
pKa	7.9	8.5	8.4	6.5
Percent unionised at pH 7.4	23	7	9	89
Octanol: water partition coefficients				
Unionised base	6	525	11 220	145
Ionised form	—	—	0.5	0.07
Apparent at pH 7.4	1.4	39	955	126
Ratio to morphine	1	28	676	89
Free fraction in human plasma (%)	70	30	16	8
'Relative potential' for entering CNS*	1	12	156	10

* Apparent partition coefficient at pH 7.4 multiplied by the free fraction of drug in plasma and divided by the value for morphine.

and they have a rapid onset of action after either intravenous administration or injection into the cerebral ventricles[84, 149]. The short duration of action of lipid soluble narcotic analgesics correlates with their prompt egress from the CNS as their plasma levels fall rapidly during the distribution phase following a single intravenous dose of moderate size[70, 71].

Morphine and other less lipophilic analgesics enter the CNS somewhat more slowly and have a modest delay in reaching their peak effect after an intravenous injection[73, 149, 156]. The onset of some of their CNS effects, e.g. ventilatory depression, is evident almost immediately after an intravenous bolus dose[C. C. Hug Jr, pers. obs.]. The surprising observation is the delayed occurrence of morphine's peak action after its injection into the lateral cerebral ventricle[149]. The basis for the presumably slow entry of morphine into brain from CSF is unknown, but it may reflect the long diffusion paths from the ependymal cells lining the ventricle to sites of action deep within the brain. The rate of onset after intraventricular injection clearly correlates with lipid solubility among the narcotic analgesics[153]. Lipid solubility also correlates with the relatively long duration of action and slow egress of the less lipid soluble narcotic analgesics from the CNS[42, 58, 73, 105, 115, 149].

Lipid solubility is obviously important in the accumulation of narcotic analgesics in adipose tissue. The fat : plasma partition coefficient for fentanyl is 35:1, compared to 0.8:1 for morphine[71, 72]. Accumulation of fentanyl in fat and its slow re-entry into the circulation (analogous to halothane) has been cited as one factor in its relatively long elimination half-time ($T^{\beta}_{\frac{1}{2}}$; see p. 200).

Ionisation of the narcotic analgesics as weak organic bases is a significant factor in that it

1   reduces their lipid solubility,

2   decreases their binding to plasma proteins, and

3   affects their partitioning between plasma and fluids differing from plasma in pH.

pH-dependent partitioning is an important factor in the overall disposition of drugs with pKa values (Table 9.2) close to the pH of plasma[127]. The phenomenon is particularly evident in the accumulation of the narcotic analgesics in the acidic medium of the stomach and in the clearance of the unchanged (i.e. not metabolised) drugs by the kidney[2, 28, 29, 37, 48, 143].

The significance of gastric accumulation of pethidine and fentanyl in the overall disposition of these drugs in the body is still being debated. Given an average gastric volume of 100 ml with a pH of 4.5 in the fasting patient, as much as 16% of a dose of fentanyl (pKa = 8.43) may be present in the stomach near the end of the distribution phases one hour after an intravenous bolus injection*. This calculation indicates the potential for a substantial accumulation of *unchanged* fentanyl in the stomach. Similar degress of accumulation of pethidine and morphine are likely. The points of debate concern the fate of narcotic analgesics entering the stomach.

Although 9% of a fentanyl dose was recovered in faeces, very little of it was present as the unchanged drug[98]. One possibility is that the drug was metabolised within the intestinal tract by mucosal cells or by bacteria, as has been claimed for morphine[76]. Another and more likely possibility is that the drug was reabsorbed from the alkaline milieu of the small intestine and cleared from the portal blood by the liver, which biotransformed fentanyl and excreted the metabolites into bile. No quantitative data are yet available concerning these or any other possibilities.

The other point of debate concerns the role of 'gastric fentanyl' in the recurrence of ventilatory depression after the patient appears to have recovered[7]. Transient small elevations of fentanyl concentrations in plasma have been observed during the elimination phase[98, 143]. One proposed mechanism is the intestinal reabsorption of 'gastric fentanyl' following periodic gastric emptying. (The other proposed mechanism is the reuptake of fentanyl from skeletal muscle; see p. 200.) The high first-pass hepatic clearance of fentanyl from the portal circulation reduces the impact of this reabsorption, but the possibility that 30–50% of the intestinal drug may be able to enter the systemic circulation (see Oral Absorption above), makes this mechanism a plausible explanation for the fluctuations in plasma levels of fentanyl. On the other hand, these fluctuations are so small that they are an unlikely explanation for the recurrence of ventilatory depression (see Clinical Applications, p. 215).

Ionisation of the narcotic analgesics in the glomerular filtrate reduces their reabsorption by the renal tubules[24]. Theoretically, excretion of the unchanged drug in urine could be enhanced by acidification of the urine and reduced by its alkalinisation. This has been shown to be true for pethidine and its active metabolite, norpethidine[2, 28, 29, 136, 137]. This possible therapeutic approach to the treatment

---

* To the extent that gastric blood flow limits the delivery of fentanyl to the stomach, lesser amounts of fentanyl will accumulate.

of overdosage has not attracted much interest in the face of current management techniques involving the use of the narcotic antagonist, naloxone, and mechanical support of ventilation.

Plasma protein binding of the narcotic analgesics varies in degree and in relation to their lipid solubility (Table 9.2). The unbound drug is able to penetrate capillary and cellular membranes much more rapidly than the bound drug. So it is to be expected that alterations of protein binding will alter the disposition of the narcotic analgesics, especially those that are more extensively bound. The importance of this expectation in terms of free drug concentration is dampened to a considerable degree by the fact that the volumes of distribution of morphine, pethidine and fentanyl are very large. Hence, any decrease in their binding to plasma protein is likely to produce an insignificant increase in the plasma concentrations of the unbound drug, because the increment of free drug will be diluted by its widespread distribution to extravascular tissues. Similarly, any decrease in free drug concentration as a result of its increased binding to plasma proteins will be blunted by the movement of relatively small amounts of drug into plasma from the large tissue stores. More than 90% of the unchanged narcotic analgesic in the body is located extravascularly after completion of the distribution phases. In fact, no correlation has been found between the free fraction of pethidine and its volume of distribution[95, 97].

The impact of plasma protein binding on the hepatic elimination of the narcotic analgesics may be significant under certain conditions. As the liver is able to clear the plasma of both free and protein-bound forms of most narcotic analgesics (i.e. non-restrictive clearance), a decrease in protein binding may reduce the amount of drug delivered to the liver per unit time and thereby decrease the rate of drug elimination (clearance) from the body[155]. As yet, however, no correlation has been demonstrated between the free fraction and the clearance of the narcotic analgesics; it has been looked for specifically in the case of pethidine[97].

Despite its apparently limited significance, the following observations about the plasma protein binding of narcotic analgesics are worthy of note. With the possible exception of pethidine in some subjects, the proportion of narcotic analgesic in plasma bound to protein is independent of the drug concentration, at least in the ranges encountered in the clinical use of these drugs for analgesia and anaesthesia. The degree of binding is proportional to protein concentration, is increased with increasing pH and vice versa. The binding is readily reversible (i.e. by decreasing the drug concentration) and is relatively non-specific (i.e. naloxone and the other narcotic analgesics and antagonists do not compete for opioid binding sites on albumin, alpha-1-acid glycoprotein, or the other proteins in plasma) [60, 73, 97, 98, 100, 112, 117, 118].

It should be noted that all currently described analytical methods for the narcotic analgesics measure both the free and bound drug in plasma (and probably in all other types of specimens as well). Thus, changes in the degree of binding may be reflected in the total concentration measured, and yet for the reasons given above, there may be little or no change in the concentration of the unbound, pharmacologically active drug.

Tissue Uptake.   The narcotic analgesics are distributed by the circulating plasma to all tissues and organs of the body. The rate and extent of their uptake varies considerably for the different drugs and for the different tissues in the case of any one narcotic analgesic.

The *rate* at which an individual tissue takes up a drug depends upon the tissue blood flow, the permeability coefficient of the drug for membranes in that tissue, and the concentration gradient of free drug between plasma and the tissue. Immediately after an initial intravenous injection, the concentration gradient from plasma to tissue is infinitely large. But as the drug accumulates in the tissue, and as the drug concentration in plasma declines (due to distribution and elimination processes), the plasma-to-tissue concentration gradient falls and the rate of uptake slows. Eventually the gradient will be zero (equilibrium); then it will be reversed due to the continuing decline of drug concentrations in plasma. With a concentration gradient from the tissue to plasma there will be a net movement of drug molecules out of the tissue into the plasma. This last phase is often described as a *pseudoequilibrium* when the *rates of decline* of drug concentrations in the tissue and plasma are the *same*, as is usually the case for drugs with high permeability coefficients (highly lipid soluble drugs) able to equilibrate rapidly between tissues and plasma[62].

The *extent* of drug uptake by a particular tissue depends on the length of time that a plasma-to-tissue concentration gradient is maintained relative to the time required for that tissue to equilibrate with plasma, and on the plasma/tissue partition coefficient for the drug. The latter reflects all the factors that influence the equilibration of the free, unionised drug across the capillary membrane. A drug will tend to distribute more to a tissue in which it is bound, ionised, actively transported, or otherwise sequestered by cells[62]. Three important points should be kept in mind when considering the tissue/plasma partition coefficient of drugs:

1   Currently used analytical methods measure the total drug content in tissues and plasma, that is, both ionised and unionised as well as protein-bound and unbound forms of the drug.

2   The degree of drug ionisation and binding can change independently on either side of the membrane, and thus, the partition coefficient may vary depending on physiological conditions.

3   In most cases, the intensity of response by a tissue or organ is proportional to the number of drug-receptor complexes formed, and the formation of complexes is proportional to the concentration of the free drug at the receptor site. Fortunately, the non-specific (i.e. non-receptor) binding of the drug is also proportional to the free drug

concentration, so that the intensity of response is also proportional to the total tissue concentration of the drug at steady state in most cases. The latter may not be true under conditions of changing drug concentrations when the rates of drug association and dissociation from its specific receptors differ from the rates at which it is bound and released from non-specific sites.

With these principles in mind, let us consider similarities and differences in the tissue uptake of morphine and fentanyl, representing the extremes of lipid solubility among the commonly used narcotic analgesics.

In terms of the CNS, there is a considerable blood–brain-barrier to morphine. So that its rates of entry and exit are relatively slow[42, 58, 73, 83, 100, 115, 116, 149].

In contrast, fentanyl appears to equilibrate rapidly across the cerebral capillary membranes. The brain/plasma partition coefficient for fentanyl is approximately 3[71]. The cerebrospinal fluid/plasma concentration ratio is less than 1, reflecting the binding of fentanyl to plasma proteins and equilibration of the free drug between plasma and CSF* (CSF contains little protein).

The affinity of morphine and brain is somewhat difficult to characterise. In the rat, the brain/plasma partition coefficient averages 0.57 in the pseudoequilibrium phase[72]. In the dog, studies of morphine distribution under equilibrium conditions have not been reported, and a partition coefficient cannot be estimated. It is evident however, that brain and CSF levels of morphine are considerably higher than those in plasma two or more hours after a single injection[42, 73, 105, 115]. The explanation for this apparent species difference is not clear. In the dog, the higher levels in the CNS relative to plasma may reflect the restricted exit of morphine from the CNS and CSF [149]. The *in vitro* uptake of morphine by rat and dog brain (cerebrocortical) slices is similar and the low tissue/plasma concentration ratios (1.5) are not suggestive of a high affinity between morphine and the overall brain[131]. On the other hand, morphine appears to have a high affinity for specific opioid receptors; these receptors represent such a small portion of the overall mass of brain that their uptake of morphine (and other narcotic analgesics) is not obviously reflected in studies of whole brain or even grossly dissected areas of the CNS[84, 87, 90, 105, J. Leysen. unpubl. obs.]. To some extent, the uptake of narcotic analgesics by opioid receptors may be reflected in the subcellular distribution of the drugs[75, 91].

Another striking and important contrast in the tissue uptake of morphine and fentanyl is evident in fat. Under pseudo-equilibrium conditions (i.e. after completion of the distribution phases), the fat/plasma partition coefficients for morphine and fentanyl were 0.8 and 35, respectively[71, 72]. There are several potential (unproven) pharmacokinetic implications of this difference.

---

* Approximately 50% of fentanyl in plasma was bound to protein under the conditions of the experiments in which the CSF/plasma concentration ratio for fentanyl was 0.5[70]. A somewhat lower CSF/plasma ratio would be anticipated with the higher percentage of fentanyl binding to plasma proteins under normal conditions (Table 9.2).

1   The large capacity of fat increases the volume of distribution for fentanyl and prolongs its elimination half-time relative to that of morphine. Given the similarly high perfusion-limited clearance of both drugs by the liver, the longer half-time of fentanyl reflects its relatively slow return from fat (high affinity, low perfusion) to the circulation from which it can be eliminated.

2   Given the low blood flow to fat, a relatively small portion of a single intravenous dose will be distributed there because the plasma to fat concentration gradient declines rapidly. With repeated injections or a continous infusion over a long period, fentanyl will accumulate in fat to a substantial degree and when administration of the drug is discontinued, the persistent slow release of fentanyl from fat will maintain plasma (and CNS) levels for a prolonged period and a slow recovery will be evident. Such accumulation and prolongation of recovery will not occur with morphine.

3   Should the dosage of either fentanyl or morphine be based on lean or total body weight? Based on the limited potential of fat to take up morphine, its dosage is more appropriately based on lean (or ideal) body weight. In the case of fentanyl, a definite recommendation cannot yet be made. Although the potential for its uptake by fat is great, the uptake occurs relatively slowly (low perfusion of fat), and has a limited impact on the overall distribution of a single dose (rapid decline of plasma levels). Thus, when plasma levels are not maintained by continuous or repeated administration of fentanyl, the use of lean body weight seems appropriate. The issue is further clouded for fentanyl because some investigators have been unable to find a correlation between total body weight and the volume of distribution of fentanyl[16]. The same lack of a correlation between distribution volume and total body weight is noted for pethidine, a relatively lipid-soluble narcotic analgesic for which tissue distribution data are lacking[95]. However, the plasma concentration of pethidine at steady-state during continuous infusion of the drug was inversely proportional to body weight[5]. This suggests that clearance of pethidine is proportional to total body weight.

Except for the CNS and fat, the patterns of morphine and fentanyl distribution among body tissues are similar. The so-called vessel-rich group of tissues, including lung, heart, kidney and liver, appear to equilibrate so rapidly with plasma that they cannot be distinguished kinetically from plasma or from one another and therefore can be grouped together in the central compartment of a pharmacokinetic model. Skeletal muscle equilibrates a little more slowly with plasma. Its affinity for fentanyl and morphine is modest (T/P ratios of 4 and 2, respectively), but its large mass makes it a significant depository of these drugs, perhaps the predominant member of a group of tissues that are represented by a peripheral compartment in a pharmacokinetic model[71, 72].

Given the large proportion of the dose that is distributed to skeletal muscle, it is conceivable that changes in muscle perfusion could affect the overall pharmacokinetics of the narcotic analgesics. For example, transient elevations of fentanyl concentrations in plasma were noted in volunteers during fentanyl's elimination phase and in association with their ambulation following a 2–3 hour period at bedrest[98]. The increased perfusion of muscle related to its increased activity may have mobilised fentanyl that had been deposited there during the distribution phase. This same phenomenon may occur in patients once they begin to move spontaneously following general anaesthesia. However, the clinical significance of this phenomenon remains to be demonstrated, especially since the actual increases in fentanyl concentrations were much too small to be responsible for any significant change in ventilation.

Elimination

Biotransformation, primarily in the liver, is by far the most important mechanism for the elimination of all of the narcotic analgesics from man and animals[102]. The metabolites are for the most part inactive, or at least much less potent that the parent drug (Tables 9.3–9.5). There are a few notable exceptions.

Norpethidine, the N-demethylated derivative of pethidine, in a CNS stimulant, and its accumulation (likely after repeated oral doses or in the presence renal failure) has been associated with a variety of manifestations, including convulsions[101, 144]. In

Table 9.3 Biotransformation of pethidine (meperidine) [95].

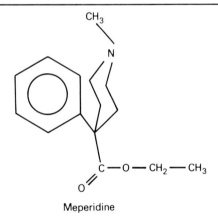

Meperidine

Ester hydrolysis (pethidinic acid*) }
N-Demethylation (norpethidine* †) } ⟶ Norpethidinic acid*
N-Oxidation (of pethidine and the above metabolites)
Para-hydroxylation (on aromatic ring)
Conjugation reactions with
   pethidinic acid*
   norpethidinic acid*
   para-hydroxyl group

* Major metabolites in man
† Only metabolite detected in blood of man

Table 9.4   Biotransformation of morphine[102].

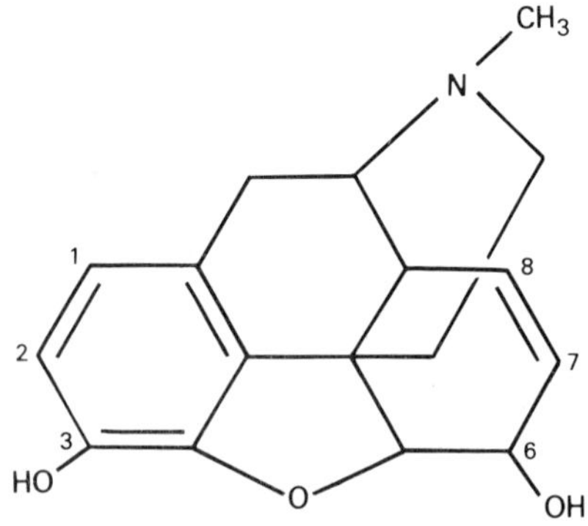

Morphine

Phenolic-(3)-hydroxyl group
    glucuronic acid conjugation (morphine-3-glucuronide)*
    sulphate conjugation (morphine ethereal sulphate)
    O-methylation (codeine)
Alcoholic-(6)-hydroxyl group
    glucuronic acid conjugation (morphine-6-glucuronide)
Piperidine nitrogen
    N-demethylation (normorphine)
    N-oxidation (morphine-N-oxide)
Phenolic ring (No. 2 carbon)
    hydroxylation (2,3-dihydrodiol, catechol or quinone-type metabolites)
Double bond (No. 7–8 carbons)
    oxidation (dihydromorphinone)

* Major metabolite in man

the presence of chlorpromazine, volunteers excreted greater amounts of norpethidine and norpethidinic acid than in its absence, indicating enhanced N-demethylation of the drug[138]. The authors suggested that the metabolites were responsible for the increased signs and symptoms of cardiac and CNS side-effects in these volunteers. The overall kinetics of unchanged pethidine were the same in the presence and absence of chlorpramazine[138].

Conjugation of morphine with glucuronic acid is the principal route of its biotransformation (Table 9.4). Morphine-3-glucuronide is pharmacologically inactive probably because it penetrates the blood–brain-barrier very slowly and is readily excreted by the kidney[73]. But in patients with renal failure, prolonged narcotic effects of morphine have been noted and it has been suggested that the accumulation of morphine glucuronide may be responsible[36, 73]. With the maintenance of high blood levels for long periods, even the most polar compounds can penetrate membranous barriers such as those of the CNS. Both morphine-3-glucuronide and morphine-6-glucuronide have been shown to have narcotic analgesic effects when injected directly

Table 9.5 Biotransformation of fentanyl[53, 134].

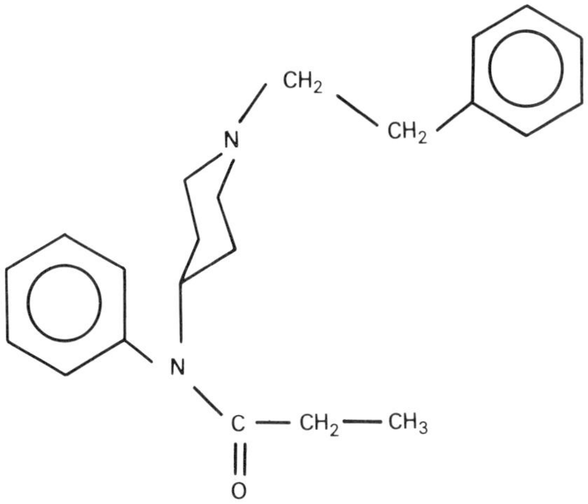

Fentanyl

Amide hydrolysis (despropionyl fentanyl) ⎱
N-dealkylation (nor-fentanyl)* ⎰ ————————————→ Despropionyl nor-fentanyl
Oxidation of propionyl side-chain
Hydroxylation (of fentanyl and above metabolites)
   propionyl chain*
   piperidine ring*
   aromatic rings
Conjugation of hydroxylated metabolites

* Major metabolites in man

into the CNS[129].† Morphine-6-glucuronide is a minor metabolite in man under normal circumstances, but it is claimed to have prolonged analgesic effects even after systemic administration to animals[102, 157]. In addition to their slow entry and accumulation within the CNS, it is also conceivable that the glucuronide conjugates are hydrolysed in plasma to release morphine which can enter the CNS[150].

None of the metabolites of fentanyl have significant pharmacological activity, and the drug has been used without incident in patients with renal failure (Table 9.5)[30].

† Morphine-3-glucuronide is inactive on the guinea pig ileum[129]. This strongly suggests that it will be inactive as an analgesic. The 3-phenolic hydroxyl is a key radical in the analgesic potency of morphine analogues; potency is reduced when this hydroxyl group is blocked. For example, codeine is much less potent than morphine due to the presence of a methoxy group in 3-position. The activity of morphine-6-glucuronide on the guinea pig ileum has not been tested, but the 6-alcoholic group is not essential for analgesic activity, and there is evidence that morphine-6-glucuronide is a potent analgesic[102, 157].

Excretion of the narcotic analgesics and their metabolites occurs primarily by way of the kidney although small amounts have been detected in saliva and other exocrine fluids including the milk of lactating subjects[102]. Variable and relatively small amounts of parenteral doses have been recovered in faeces, predominantly as metabolites[37, 98, 152].

Very little of the unchanged drug appears in urine under normal conditions. However, as noted above, acidification of urine may enhance the excretion of the unchanged drug by reducing its reabsorption from the glomerular filtrate in the renal tubules (see p. 196).

PHARMACOKINETICS

For obvious reasons, the study of drug disposition in humans is usually limited to the measurement of drug concentrations in blood and excreta. Determinations of the rates of change in drug levels in blood or plasma over time enables one to summarise the overall impact of the individual factors discussed above on the disposition of the drug and to make inferences about the relationship between drug dosage and plasma concentration, and under certain conditions, between drug concentration and the intensity of effect. Pharmacokinetic studies are usually based on intraveneous drug administration, which avoids the variability associated with absorption processes and also simplifies the interpretation of the data. This is the case with the currently available information for the narcotic analgesics in man.

Because of the great potency of the narcotic analgesics, studies of their pharmaco-kinetics have been limited until recently by the lack of sufficiently sensitive analytical methods that specifically measure only the unchanged drug and not its metabolites. The first breakthrough in pharmacokinetic investigations of analgesic doses of morphine and fentanyl in man resulted from the development of radioimmunoassays (RIA), some of which are not specific for the unchanged drug[27, 56, 135]. The data from studies based on unspecific RIA's are not useful for pharmacokinetic purposes and for the most part have not been included in this review. It should be noted that since the concentrations of morphine and fentanyl metabolites may exceed those of the unchanged drugs in plasma by more than ten times, the assay specificity must be very high indeed. For example, if the assay is only ten times more sensitive to the unchanged drug than it is to a metabolite, the presence of the latter in a ten-fold higher concentration will lead to a two-fold error in the estimate of the concentration of the unchanged drug in the sample.

Most of the investigations of pethidine utilised a specific gas chromatographic method[95, 96].

Normal volunteers

The pharmacokinetic parameters for morphine, fentanyl, and pethidine are summarised in Tables 9.6–9.8. The decline in plasma levels in all cases could be described by a two or three exponential equation. All three narcotic analgesics underwent rapid distribution to body tissues (distribution half-times ranged from 1.7 to 17 min), and all three drugs have a large distribution volume (range $3–6\,l\,kg^{-1}$) indicative of their extensive uptake by body tissues. Uptake by lipid components is probably a major factor in the case of the lipophilic drugs, fentanyl and pethidine. The relatively low affinity of morphine for fat makes it likely that its extensive uptake results from binding to other tissue components.

In most cases, the clearance of all three drugs approached the blood flow of liver ($18–21$ ml $kg^{-1}\,min^{-1}$)[155]. Several implications of this coincidence should be noted.
1   In view of their very limited elimination at non-hepatic sites, it is likely that their clearance is dependent on liver blood flow.
2   Their clearance by the liver is non-restrictive; that is, the drug bound to plasma protein and transported in blood cells is removed along with the free drug during the passage of blood through the liver.
3   The rate of their elimination by the liver is also dependent on their total concentration in blood. Their very large distribution volume means that their blood concentration is low relative to the total amount of drug in the body. Their reuptake from body tissues, especially fat with its low perfusion, is a rate-limiting factor in their elimination. Reductions of their protein binding and uptake by blood cells may also reduce their clearance, because the total drug content of blood traversing the liver will be less.

The small differences in the elimination half-times for the three narcotic analgesics reflect the small differences in their distribution volumes (V_D) and in their clearances (Cl):

$$T_{\frac{1}{2}}^{\beta} = \frac{0.69\ V_D}{Cl}$$

Incidentally, I have chosen to express the pharmacokinetic variables in terms of body weight despite the apparent lack of correlation that has been noted for fentanyl and meperidine. This is justified by the recognition of dose-response relationships and dose-concentration relationships with the dose being measured in terms of body weight in both cases. Furthermore, species and age comparisons are facilitated by this means. Finally, as noted above, the relationship to body weight may become more apparent when it is expressed as lean body mass (see p. 200).

Surgical patients

Consistent differences in pharmacokinetic variables are not evident for surgical patients compared to volunteers (Tables 9.6–9.8). Those differences that are evident

Table 9.6 Morphine pharmacokinetics.

Investigator	n	Age (y)	Intravenous dose	Half-times Distribution $T_{\frac{1}{2}}^{\pi}$ (min)	$T_{\frac{1}{2}}^{\alpha}$ (min)	Elimination $T_{\frac{1}{2}}^{\beta}$ (h)	Distribution volumes Initial (l kg^{-1})	Total (l kg^{-1})	Clearance (ml kg^{-1} min^{-1})
Volunteers									
Brunk et al.[20–23]	42	20–60	10 mg	—	—	1.9–2.6	—	—	—
Stanski et al.[141]	6	26–32	10 mg	—	1.7	2.9	0.33	3.2	15
Surgical patients with various anesthetics									
Stanski et al.[141]	4	61–80	1 mg kg^{-1}	1.3	20	4.5	0.10	4.7	12
Dahlstrom et al.[31]	16	1–15	0.15 mg kg^{-1}	2.4	13	2.2	0.04	1.2	6.4
Murphy & Hug[108]	10	18–39	0.05–0.2 mg kg^{-1}	1.2	9	1.7	0.13	3.4	23
Tamsen[34, 146]	10	22–58		1.3	13	2.8	—	6.2	21
Post-surgical patients									
Tamsen[34, 146]	10	22–58	1–4 mg h^{-1} × 18 ± 6 h	0.9	9.8	1.9	—	3.7	21
Cancer patients									
Sawe et al.[126]	7	49–76	4 mg kg^{-1}	—	2.4	3.1	0.39	2.1	10

Table 9.7 Fentanyl pharmacokinetics.

Investigator	n	Age (y)	Intravenous dose	Half-times			Distribution volumes		Clearance (ml kg⁻¹ min⁻¹)
				Distribution		Elimination	Initial (1 kg⁻¹)	Total (1 kg⁻¹)	
				$T_{\frac{1}{2}}^{\pi}$ (min)	$T_{\frac{1}{2}}^{\alpha}$ (min)	$T_{\frac{1}{2}}^{\beta}$ (h)			
Volunteers									
McClain & Hug[98]	5	22–29	6.4 µg kg⁻¹	1.7	13	3.7	0.36	4.0	13
Bower & Hull[16]	7	24–60	2.4 µg kg⁻¹	—	4.1	3.1	0.88	4.7	22
Bower et al.[15]	8	—	200 µg	—	—	—	~0.85	~4.6	~10
							(~ estimated for 70 kg subject)		
Surgical patients with various anesthetics									
Schleimer et al.[128]*†	14	28–69	3–30 µg kg⁻¹	0.7–1.6	5.1–21	1.7–5.8	0.04–0.13	0.7–2.0	3.6–5.2
Fung & Eisele[47]*‡	14	20–30	2–4 µg kg⁻¹	3.1	26	1.7–14	0.12–1.27	1.0–2.6	1.9–6.3
Fung & Moore*‡	8	34±17	4 µg kg⁻¹	1.4	6.0	2.0	0.15	0.77	5.1
Hengstmann et al.[57]*‡	5	23–38	500 µg	—	1.4	2.4	0.07	1.2	6.9
Lauven et al.[85]	8	32–56	500 µg	—	1.2	2.4	—	—	—
Koska et al.[81]	6	45–60	7.2 µg kg⁻¹	—	—	3.3	—	3.2	11
Cardiac surgical patients subjected to extracorporeal circulation									
Bovill & Sebel[13]	5	45–65	60 µg kg⁻¹	—	—	7.1	—	—	—
Koska et al.[81]	6	45–60	7.2 µg kg⁻¹	—	—	5.2	—	—	—
Hug & Moldenhauer[69]	18	—	75–107 µg kg⁻¹§	—	—	11	—	7.9	7.6

* Specificity of RIA has been called into question
† Sampled for only 2 hours after injection
‡ Sampled for only 4–5 hours after injection
§ Priming infusion 54 µg kg⁻¹ in 20 min followed by maintenance infusion of 0.15 or 0.3 µg kg⁻¹ min⁻¹ for 3–4 h.

Table 9.8 Pethidine pharmacokinetics.

Investigator	n	Age (y)	Intravenous dose	Half-times Distribution (min)	Elimination (h)	Distribution volumes Initial (1 kg⁻¹)	Total (1 kg⁻¹)	Clearance (ml kg⁻¹ min⁻¹)
Volunteers								
Klotz et al.[79]	8	25–55	$0.8\,mg\,kg^{-1}$	11	3.2	1.5	4.2	16
McHorse et al.[99]	10	18–34	$0.8\,mg\,kg^{-1}$	—	3.4	—	5.9	~18
Mather et al.[97]	4	24–49	50 mg	7.1	3.7	1.2	3.7	14
Dunkerley et al.[37]	6	20–32	50 mg	—	3.8	—	—	~17
Stambaugh et al.[139]	6	21–30	50 mg	4.2	3.9	—	~2.8	~10
Fung et al.[46]	3	21±0.5	100 mg	17	4.1	1.8	3.4	10
Pond et al.[121]	6	40±10	$0.8\,mg\,kg^{-1}$	—	5.2	—	4.7	12
Verbeeck et al.[148]	6	23–31	25 mg	—	6.7	0.7	4.2	7.5
Neal et al.[113]	4	—	$0.8\,mg\,kg^{-1}$	—	3.6	—	~3.3	~13
Surgical patients with various anaesthetics								
Mather et al.[97]	29	18–73	50 mg	3.3	3.1	0.6	2.6	12
Koska et al.[80]	6	—	$5\,mg\,kg^{-1}$	—	4.4	—	3.7	10
Tamsen[146]	12	20–53	100–200 mg	6.0	4.7	—	4.3	8.8
Post-surgical patients								
Tamsen[146]	12	20–53	$12–50\,mg\,hr^{-1}$	5.2	2.9	—	3.1	12
Austin et al.[5]	10	29–67	$24\,mg\,hr^{-1}$	30	5.5	2.2	3.8	8.7
Pregnant patients at term								
Kuhnert et al.[82]	10	15–28	50 mg	4.7	2.4	—	~3.2	~15
Morgan et al.[104]	7	16–30	50 mg	—	3.7	—	2.7	11
Patients with liver disease								
CIRRHOSIS								
Klotz et al.[79]	10	37–55	$0.8\,mg\,kg^{-1}$	16	7.0	2.5	5.8	10
Neal et al.[113]	8	39–57	$0.8\,mg\,kg^{-1}$	—	6.0	—	~3.8	~8.2
Pond et al.[121]	5	50±11	$0.8\,mg\,kg^{-1}$	—	11.4	—	5.2	5.6
HEPATITIS								
McHorse et al.[99]	14	18–48	$0.8\,mg\,kg^{-1}$	—	7.0	—	5.6	~9.3
RECOVERED FROM HEPATITIS								
McHorse et al.[99]	5	18–23	$0.8\,mg\,kg^{-1}$	—	3.2	—	—	~17

(~ estimated for 70 kg subject)

probably reflect the impact of variables in experimental and clinical conditions and some of these variables are discussed individually below. Most importantly, changes in tissue perfusion associated with anaesthetic and surgical procedures can be expected to alter the distribution and elimination of narcotic analgesics. None of the studies summarised in the tables included any attempt to control haemodynamic variables, and in the case of cardiac surgical patients there were direct interventions on cardiovascular function.

Variables potentially affecting the pharmacokinetics of narcotic analgesics in man

Dose-size may alter pharmacokinetics in two general ways: (a) conversion of rate-limiting steps from first-order (drug-concentration-dependent) kinetics to zero-order (concentration-independent) kinetics; (b) dose-dependent pharmacological actions of the drug which affect its disposition. The relationship of dose and kinetics is particularly important for the narcotic analgesics that may be used in very low doses for analgesia and in extremely high doses for anaesthesia (e.g. fentanyl in doses ranging from 1.5 μg kg^{-1} for analgesia up to 150 μg kg^{-1} for anaesthesia). To date, none of the important drug dispositional factors has been described by other than first-order kinetics. There is no evidence of their saturation within the range of concentrations encountered clinically after either analgesic or anaesthetic doses. In fact, intravenous doses of fentanyl in the range 2.5–640 μg kg^{-1} exhibited virtually the same pharmacokinetics in the dog[111]. Factors other than dose (e.g. altered perfusion of tissues) are probably responsible for the differences described in the kinetics of analgesic and anaesthetic doses of fentanyl in volunteers and patients.

The dose-dependent hypotension produced by morphine is the most likely cause of the small, but definite differences noted in the kinetics of its disposition in dogs given 0.3 or 2 mg kg^{-1} doses intravenously[73]. Unfortunately, most authors to date have failed to describe the haemodynamic and other effects of drugs during pharmacokinetic studies. Certainly the cardiovascular system plays the central role in the absorption, distribution, biotransformation and excretion of drugs.

The kinetics of pethidine disposition appear to be independent of dose in the range 50–375 mg in adults[80].

Age-related differences in the pharmacokinetics of narcotic analgesics are of con-siderable interest in the light of clinical impressions that the very young and the elderly and 'sensitive' to the actions of these drugs. Although the newborn rat does not have a fully developed blood–brain-barrier to morphine[83], only small differences have been found in the sensitivity of newborn humans to the analgesic and ventilatory depressant effects of morphine and pethidine compared to adults[31, 153]. Moreover, only minor and insignificant differences in the pharmacokinetics of intravenous morphine were noted among children ranging in age from 1 month to 15 years, and the average data closely resembled that reported for normal adults[31]. (In this study, five of the paediatric patients exhibited unusual differences in the disposition of morphine, but the differences were spread among all age groups.) It is interesting to note that there appears to be a correlation between the upper limits of age and elimination half-time of morphine among the patient groups summarised in Table 9.6. The apparently greater $T_{\frac{1}{2}}^{\beta}$ for older patients was not evident within the individual studies, and it was not consistently related to changes in distribution volume and clearance. Also, this trend is not evident in the data for either fentanyl or pethidine (Tables 9.7 and 9.8).

Among the elderly, two pharmacokinetic observations may be significant in explaining their relatively greater responses to a given dose of either pethidine or morphine. In the case of pethidine the unbound fraction of the drug in plasma is likely to be greater than 0.4 in patients over 45 years, whereas it is less than 0.4 in younger subjects[97]. At least in the first 5 minutes after an intravenous injection of morphine, the serum levels of the unchanged drug were as much as 1.5 times greater in patients over 50 years in age than in younger patients given the same 10 mg/70 kg dose*[11]. Amongst other possibilities, the cardiovascular changes associated with aging may slow the early distribution of morphine to peripheral tissues so that the decline of morphine levels in plasma is slower (and the CNS levels may be higher) in the older patient.

Gender. The elimination half-time of a preanaesthetic dose of morphine (0.15 mg, intramuscularly) was reported to be shorter in female ($T_{\frac{1}{2}}^{\beta} = 110$ min) than in male surgical patients ($T_{\frac{1}{2}}^{\beta} = 173$ min)[124]. The RIA used in the study undoubtedly measured some of the morphine glucuronide in plasma as morphine, especially at later times after injection when the conjugate levels are more than ten times greater than those of the unchanged drug[108]. The rate of glucuronide conjugation of morphine in rats is strongly influenced by testosterone and oestradiol, but these hormones are not thought to important factors in the biotransformation of morphine in humans[102].

Surgical operations introduce many factors that may be expected to affect the disposition of drugs. Several differences have been noted in the disposition of narcotic analgesics in surgical patients compared to volunteers (Tables 9.6–9.8)[95, 97]. Preoperative anxiety leading to vasoconstriction has been offered as an explanation for the slower absorption of pethidine from intramuscular injection sites and for its reduced volume of distribution in surgical patients compared to volunteers[94].

A shorter distribution half-time, a reduced initial volume of distribution, and the tendency for the clearance and the steady-state distribution volume to be lower have

---

* Although the RIA used in this study was not completely specific for unchanged morphine, the observations in the first minutes after injection are probably valid because the levels of conjugated morphine should be low relative to the unchanged drug and interfere minimally with the RIA of samples taken within the first few minutes after a single intravenous dose.

also been attributed to a reduction in tissue perfusion and hepatic blood flow in surgical patients given pethidine[95, 97]. The causes of these changes have not been identified, but it is interesting to note that plasma concentrations of pethidine increased rather suddenly upon the induction of anaesthesia with any one of several anaesthetics[97]. For the most part, the above differences between volunteers and surgical patients were small and clinically insignificant. Similarly small and insignificant differences have been evident in comparisons of pharmacokinetic studies of morphine and fentanyl in volunteers and general surgical patients.

Cardiopulmonary bypass. More substantial differences in fentanyl pharmacokinetics have been noted in patients undergoing cardiac surgery including extracorporeal circulation (Table 9.7). It appears that the three-fold increase in the elimination half-time of fentanyl was associated with a doubling of the distribution volume and a halving of the clearance rate[69]. Our preliminary data with alfentanil, a low clearance narcotic analgesic (see p. 223), indicate that a three-fold increase in elimination half-time was related exclusively to an increase in distribution volume with no change in alfentanil clearance[68].

   In regard to extracorporeal circulation there are several points to be kept in mind in the use of the narcotic analgesics.

1 Their plasma concentrations are not likely to be affected substantially by the haemodilution because most of the drug is in peripheral tissues (large V_D) and only a relatively small amount of the dose remains in the circulating blood. Hence, any alterations of the blood volume, pH, protein content, or haematocrit will likely be minimised by movement of relatively small proportions of the narcotic analgesic between peripheral tissues and blood. Dilution of plasma proteins will reduce the protein-binding and the total (i.e. free and bound) concentration of narcotic analgesic in plasma, but will probably have minimal effects on the concentration of the free (pharmacologically active) drug. Of course, a lower concentration of the total drug in plasma will be reflected in an inversely proportional increase in the volume of distribution.

2 Alterations in tissue perfusion may lead to changes in the rate of decline of plasma levels of the narcotic analgesics as their entry into or removal from storage and elimination sites are correspondingly altered. Of particular interest may be the effect of excluding the lungs from the circulation because they appear to have a very large capacity to take up (and to release) a large variety of organic bases, including probably all of the narcotic analgesics[26, 71, 72].

3 Hypothermia is known to reduce the rate of drug biotransformation reactions, and it is likely that this is true for the narcotic analgesics.

4 To the extent that the circulatory system is altered after cardiopulmonary bypass (including the use of inotropic and vasoactive drugs), the disposition of all drugs, including the narcotic analgesics, can be expected to be affected.

Anaesthesia. The pharmacokinetic impact of anaesthetic drugs in distinction to all the other variables attending surgical operations cannot be estimated from the human studies available to date. General and regional anaesthesia would be expected to affect the pharmacokinetics of narcotic analgesics insofar as anaesthesia is associated with changes in ventilation and pH, cardiac output and tissue perfusion, hepatic and renal function, and other factors known to influence the distribution and elimination of drugs. As yet there have been no systematic studies of the effects of anaesthesia on the pharmacokinetics of narcotic analgesics. Independent pharmacokinetic studies in animals in the awake and anaesthetised states have produced quantitatively different results, but it is difficult, if not impossible, to relate the differences to anaesthesia *per se* because of the many other potential and often obscure differences in experimental procedures[12, 111, 112].

Ventilation and acid–base balance can affect a number of important variables in the disposition of drugs, and may be especially important in the case of narcotic analgesics with pKa values close to the pH of plasma. The role of pH differences between plasma and the gastric lumen, and between plasma and renal tubular fluid have been considered above (see p. 196).

From the point of view of the central nervous system and the overall kinetics of drug disposition, the consequences of changes in ventilation and acid–base balance can be expected to be complex. For example, in the case of fentanyl, respiratory acidosis would
1   increase the proportion of drug that is ionised in plasma ($\downarrow$CNS penetration);
2   increase the ionisation of drug in brain ($\uparrow$accumulation and retention within the CNS),
3   decrease the binding of drug to plasma protein ($\uparrow$CNS penetration); and
4   increase cerebral blood flow ($\uparrow$delivery during the onset or distribution phase and removal during the recovery or elimination phase).

In the face of such complexities, it is not surprising that the available data fail to present a clear picture of the effects of ventilatory changes on the distribution of fentanyl between plasma and the brain[1]. It is reported that hypocapnia had no effect on the elimination of fentanyl in surgical patients[49].

The effects of respiratory acidosis and alkalosis on the disposition of morphine have also been examined in the dog[42, 115]. Hypocapnic, alkalotic dogs exhibited plasma levels of morphine 10–30 % higher than those observed in animals with a normal Pa_{CO_2} and pH (normal ventilation as well as increased ventilation with CO_2 added to this inspired gas). The higher plasma levels were reflected in a correspondingly smaller distribution volume and a slightly lower clearance of morphine from plasma (perhaps to some degree due to greater renal tabular reabsorption of morphine from an alkaline glomerular filtrate). The elimination half-time was unchanged. It should be noted, however, that an increase in pH would increase the binding of morphine to plasma proteins and raise the plasma concentration of *total* morphine measured by the RIA. Thus, the pharmacokinetic interpretation of the results is still uncertain.

The cerebral cortical levels of morphine were 30–70% higher in the hypocapnic than in the normocapnic animals throughout the 4-hour experimental period. The higher CNS to plasma concentration ratio may reflect the fact that a greater proportion of the morphine in plasma would be unionised in the alkalotic animals and able to enter the CNS more readily in spite of the other changes that can be presumed to have occurred (i.e. reduced cerebral blood flow, increased binding of morphine to plasma proteins, corresponding changes in the $Paco_2$ and pH of brain extracellular fluid)[115].

Hypercapnia ($Paco_2$ 69 mmHg, pHa 7.15) produced in the dog by the addition of CO_2 to inspired gas also resulted in slightly (20%) higher CNS levels of morphine in the first few minutes after its intravenous injection, possibly the result of 80% higher plasma levels of morphine, its lesser binding to plasma proteins, and the presumably greater cerebral blood flow. A more impressive consequence of the respiratory acidosis was the slower rate of decline of CNS morphine levels in hypercapnic compared to normocapnic dogs ($T_{\frac{1}{2}}$CNS 6.9 vs. 4.1 h, respectively). This slower egress of morphine was attributed to greater ionisation of the drug within the CNS where the pH would also be reduced by the hypercapnia. It could not be explained by changes in the overall pharmacokinetics of morphine because the plasma levels were essentially the same as were the rates of their decline ($T_{\frac{1}{2}}^{\beta} = 1.1$ hour) beyond the first hour after the intravenous injection[42].

Liver function. Because the primary site of biotransformation of all of the narcotic analgesics is the liver, it is predictable that alterations of liver perfusion and function will affect the elimination of these drugs from the body. As expected, the total absence of liver function resulted in a marked prolongation of the actions and sojourn of narcotic analgesics in the body[67, 74]. Lesser degrees of hepatic impairment have not been investigated for their effects on narcotic analgesic pharmacokinetics except in the case of pethidine (Table 9.8). Such information is obviously important to the anaesthesiologist who frequently chooses a narcotic analgesic over a potent inhalational anaesthetic for the management of patients with hepatic disease.

In the case of meperidine, both cirrhosis and acute viral hepatitis resulted in similar reductions of plasma clearance and corresponding prolongations of the elimination half-times in patients. Distribution volumes were essentially unchanged. Pharmacokinetic variables reverted to normal after the patients recovered from viral hepatitis (Table 9.8).

The clinical implications of these observations are:

1 The initial dose required to achieve a given plasma and CNS concentration will be the same in patients with and without liver disease. Of course, to the extent that the liver disease impairs CNS functions (e.g. ammonia toxicity, hepatic encephalopathy), both

the dose and concentration required to produced a given degree of CNS depression will be less.

2   The duration of action of a given dose will be prolonged and the maintenance of drug effects will require smaller repeat doses or a longer dosage interval.

3   The ability to measure drug levels in plasma of patients with liver disease would be useful in guiding the administration of narcotic analgesics and in predicting the rate of recovery from their effects. It should be noted that the common clinical tests of liver function have not proven to be useful predictors of the rate of pethidine elimination in patients with either cirrhosis or acute viral hepatitis[95, 99].

4   Should the physician consider the oral administration of pethidine to patients with impaired hepatic function, he will have to allow for the increased bioavailability resulting from reduced pre-systemic clearance of pethidine from the portal circulation.

Renal disease. As noted above (p. 204), the kidneys provide the primary route of elimination of metabolites produced by hepatic biotransformation of the narcotic analgesics. Thus, accumulation of these metabolites can be anticipated in the face of impaired renal function, and to the extent that the metabolites are pharmacologically active, their effects will become significant. The accumulation of norphethidine and morphine-glucuronide have been implicated in the prolonged or toxic effects of morphine and pethidine in patients with renal disease (see pp. 201–2). Fentanyl metabolites have little or no pharmacological activity and the drug has been used without incident in anephric patients[30].

Drug interactions. Although there are numerous important interactions between the narcotic analgesics and a variety of drugs from other classes, few of these have been shown to be on a pharmacokinetic basis[88, 95, 138]. Specifically, Brunk *et al.* have shown that the parmacokinetics of morphine are not altered by the simultaneous administration of aspirin, guanethidine, or propranolol[21, 22, 23]. The increased N-demethylation of pethidine in the presence of chlorpromazine has been noted above (p. 202).

Certainly there is the possibility that other drugs can alter the disposition of narcotic analgesics (e.g. anaesthetic-induced alterations of hepatic blood flow) and vice versa (e.g. narcotic analgesic-induced changes in gastrointestinal function, respiratory acidosis)[95, 97]. There is no consistent evidence that drugs known to induce enzymatic activity in the hepatic microsomal system have an effect on the elimination of morphine or pethidine in man[95, 102]. The effect of hepatic enzyme induction on fentanyl elimination has not been examined in man or animals.

As noted above (p. 190), the specific narcotic antagonists do not consistently or markedly affect the distribution or elimination of the narcotic agonists.

Shock. The central role played by the cardiovascular system in the absorption, distribution and elimination of drugs makes it all but certain that haemodynamic alterations, especially those of an extreme nature, will alter the pharmacokinetics of the narcotic analgesics. Although formal and systematic experiments have not yet been reported, there are seemingly obvious consequences of shock on the disposition of narcotic analgesics. Absorption from parenteral injection sites will be impaired and the intensity of the effects unpredictable. Should multiple injections be given to compensate for slow absorption, the restoration of circulatory function may lead to an unexpected increase in morphine effects[52]. Although intravenous administration would eliminate the variability associated with erratic absorption, the smaller circulating blood volume and reduced tissue perfusion should lead to a smaller volume of distribution and a reduced rate of decline of plasma levels. Hence, more intense and longer lasting effects may be expected from a given dose of any of the narcotic analgesics administered to a patient in shock.

CLINICAL APPLICATIONS

As suggested above, the practical benefits of knowledge about the pharmacokinetics of narcotic analgesics are to be realised in more efficient use of these drugs for anaesthesia and analgesia. That is, rapidly providing the dose and drug concentration sufficient for the desired intensity of effect without causing toxicity or prolonged recovery due to an excessive dose or concentration. Of course, the very nature of a particular narcotic analgesic may limit the ability of the anaesthetist to manipulate the rate of onset and the duration of its actions. In such cases, knowledge of the kinetics of drug disposition enables the anaesthetist to recognise limits of a particular drug and to choose the most appropriate drug available for his purposes.

In this section, the potential usefulness of narcotic analgesic pharmacokinetics will be considered in regard to

1   Understanding their duration of action;
2   developing more efficient methods of their administration; and
3   recognising the potential for new drug developments.

The keys to realising these practical objectives are (a) definition of the relationships among dose, concentration, and intensity of effects and (b) recognition of factors contributing to variability in the responses of different patients, or even the same patient under different conditions, to a given dose of a narcotic analgesic. Pharmacokinetic variability has already been considered.

Pharmacodynamic variability

It is not our purpose to review the pharmacodynamic factors affecting the responsiveness of an individual to a given dose or concentration of a narcotic analgesic (Table 9.9). Rather it is to emphasise that such factors exist and that, in fact, the ultimate quantitation of their impact awaits the design of studies taking pharmacokinetic

Table 9.9   Factors affecting responses to narcotic analgesics.

Dose, CNS concentration of narcotic analgesic
Age and physical status of patient
Intensity of pain or noxious stimulation
Psychological and environmental conditions
Sleep
Other drugs
Tolerance

factors into account. For example, how does one evaluate the effect of a preanaesthetic medication on the requirements for fentanyl in anaesthesia unless the timing of the measurements is kept constant among experimental subjects in relation to the pharmacokinetics of both the premedicant and fentanyl. Ideally, the measurement of such drug interactions would be made under steady-state conditions, or at least at a time when the concentrations of the two drugs are known and changing slowly.

The anaesthesiologist can recognise the importance of such considerations and possibly identify some of the most important factors from his knowledge of their impact on the dosage or partial pressure requirements for general anaesthetics. The concept of MAC (minimum alveolar concentration) for inhalational anaesthetics has contributed immensely to our understanding and efficient use of them[122]. Similar concepts[121a] need to be utilised for intravenous drugs, including the narcotic analgesics (see Chapter 7).

Concentration vs. effect relationships

Morphine.   Because of the slow equilibration of morphine between plasma and its sites of action within the CNS, almost all studies to date have failed to find a meaningful correlation between morphine concentrations in plasma and the intensity of its effects. One possible exception is the study by Tamsen and his colleagues who measured plasma morphine levels during patient-controlled analgesic therapy in the postoperative (abdominal laparotomy) period[34, 146]. They found a reasonably constant rate of morphine consumption (2.6 ± 1.2 SD mg h^{-1}) that resulted in a relatively narrow range of fluctuation in morphine concentrations during self-administered therapy that provided satisfactory relief of pain in each patient (21 ± 12 SD ng ml^{-1} of plasma). There was a four-fold variation among patients in the MEC (minimum effective concentration $= 16 \pm 9$ SD ng ml^{-1}) of morphine, that is, the concentration at which patients self-administered another intravenous dose (2 or 3 mg i.v. bolus) to control pain. Although this variability may seem to be too great to be useful in the practical management of pain, it must be remembered that current analgesic dosage regimens for morphine (and the other narcotic analgesics) produce plasma levels that often fluctuate by more than 50-fold and exceed the MEC by 10 to 20 times during the course of therapy. Given the narrow range between analgesic and ventilatory-depressant doses, the efficiency of morphine therapy can certainly stand some improvement, and the observations of Tamsen *et al.* indicate that it is feasible for a drug like morphine.

The minimum plasma levels of morphine required to maintain a stable 'anaesthetic' state have not been defined. Dahlstrom *et al.* have suggested that a minimum plasma level of morphine is approximately 65 ng ml^{-1} (95 % confidence limits of 43 to 83 ng ml^{-1}) for adequate supplementation of 70 % nitrous oxide anaesthesia for general surgery in children less than 15 years of age[31]. Intravenous doses of 1–2 mg kg^{-1} result in plasma concentrations that fall from a peak of 500–1000 ng ml^{-1} soon after injection to 100–200 ng ml^{-1} within the first 60 minutes after injection (distribution phase). Subsequently they decline with $T^{\beta}_{\frac{1}{2}}$ of 4.5 h (elimination phase)[63, 141].

It is not surprising that 1–2 mg kg^{-1} doses of morphine alone are inadequate to maintain general anaesthesia in the absence of nitrous oxide or other CNS depressants[66, 89]. In fact, morphine alone is able to produce a maximal reduction of 65 % in enflurane MAC only at doses exceeding 5 mg kg^{-1} in the dog[110]. Assuming dose-independent pharmacokinetics, an intravenous dose of 5 mg kg^{-1} would produce plasma levels greater than 400 ng ml^{-1} during the first hour after its injection[73]. Thus, 1–2 mg kg^{-1} doses of morphine that produce less than one-half this '65 % anaesthetic-sparing' concentration beyond 1 hour after their administration cannot be expected to provide anaesthesia.

Pethidine. Because of its depressant effects on the cardiovascular system, the use of pethidine in anaesthesia has been confined to a relatively low and narrow range of doses (0.3–1.5 mg kg^{-1}) that are useful in producing analgesia and in supplementing nitrous oxide and other inhalational anaesthetics. Studies of the analgesic and ventilatory depressant effects of these doses and their resultant plasma concentrations have been reported by several groups of investigators. The results are summarised in Table 9.10.

Fentanyl. Studies of the relationship of fentanyl concentrations to the intensity of its effects are just beginning to be reported. Such information is badly needed because this narcotic analgesic is being used in doses of 1–150 μg kg^{-1} or more by anaesthesiologists. Moreover, the pharmacokinetic characteristics of fentanyl administered by intermittent intravenous doses make the interpretation of dose-response relationships extremely difficult because of

1   the marked fluctuation of plasma and brain levels;
2   the accumulation of fentanyl after repeated doses; and
3   the progressive lengthening of its duration of action after larger or repeated doses[70, 98].

Fortunately, there is a close relationship between plasma and brain levels of this

Table 9.10 Pethidine effects vs. its concentrations in plasma[95].

Pethidine concentration in plasma (ng ml^{-1})	Effects
100–200	Mild analgesia and sedation Impaired psychomotor performance Dry mouth, light-headedness Detectable, mild ventilatory depression
200–500	Moderate analgesia and euphoria Nausea, visual disturbances Increased intrabiliary pressure Moderate ventilatory depression
> 500	Strong analgesia Marked ventilatory depression in the absence of pain

lipophilic drug, and there also are close relationships between its plasma concentrations and the intensity of its analgesic, anaesthetic and ventilatory depressant effects under steady or pseudosteady state conditions that exist after the distribution phase is completed[49, 69, 70, 98, 109, 149]. These relationships are summarised in Table 9.11.

Table 9.11 Fentanyl effects vs. its concentrations in plasma[1a, 1b, 49, 98, 103, 109].

Fentanyl concentration in plasma (ng ml^{-1})	Effect
> 1	Slight analgesia and ventilatory depression
> 3	Analgesia and 50% decrease in ventilatory response to carbon dioxide
8–10	50% decrease in MAC
> 20	Unconsciousness and 65% decrease in MAC

With the relationships of concentration vs. effect in mind, it is possible to use pharmacokinetic data and concepts

1 to explain differences in the duration of action of the various narcotic analgesics and also differences for the same narcotic analgesic under different conditions; and

2 to devise dosage regimens consonant with more efficient use of the narcotic analgesics in anaesthesia and analgesia.

Duration of action

Why does the duration of fentanyl action vary with the dose administered? In the case of small intravenous doses, the concentrations of fentanyl fall below threshold levels during the relatively rapid distribution phases (Fig. 9.2). After large intravenous doses, the distribution phases are completed before the fentanyl concentrations decline to threshold levels, and recovery depends on the relatively slow elimination of fentanyl from the body. The same concepts apply to its progressively increasing duration of action after repeated small doses, which lead to its accumulation in tissues and a reduction of the effectiveness of distribution mechanisms in lowering fentanyl concentrations to threshold (Fig. 9.3)[70].

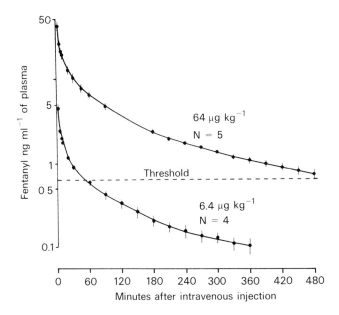

Fig. 9.2 Concentrations of fentanyl in plasma of dogs given either a 6.4 or a 64 μg kg^{-1} dose of fentanyl intravenously at time zero[70, 112].

Why does ventilatory depression recur after a period of time during which the patient appears to have recovered from its effects?[7]. As noted above, the re-entry of fentanyl into plasma from the gastrointestinal tract (see p. 196) and skeletal muscle (see p. 200) may result in transient, small increases in its plasma levels[98, 143]. However, a more likely explanation for recurrent ventilatory depression is an increase in the sensitivity of the brain stem respiratory centres as the patient is left undisturbed and falls asleep. Sleep alone decreases the ventilatory response to carbon dioxide and appears to interact synergistically with the depression produced by a narcotic analgesic[8, 44]. The low levels of fentanyl persisting during the slow elimination phase may then become effective in depressing ventilation. Still other factors such as anaesthesia with nitrous oxide[1a] may alter the patient's sensitivity to the ventilatory depressant effects of the residual concentrations of fentanyl (Table 9.9).

Why is morphine a long-acting narcotic analgesic when its elimination half-time is shorter than that of either fentanyl or pethidine? As noted above (pp. 190, 195), the

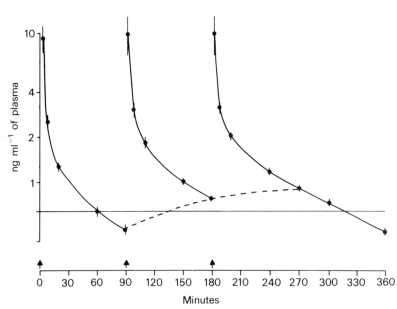

Fig. 9.3 Plasma concentrations of fentanyl in dogs given three intravenous bolus doses of fentanyl $(6.4\,\mu g\,kg^{-1})$ at 90 minute intervals (arrows). Accumulation of fentanyl is evident as higher concentrations at any time interval after each injection, and also as a progressive lengthening of the time required for the concentration to decline to the threshold level after each injection (i.e. 60, 90, 120 min). The dashed line connects the points at 90 minutes after each dose[70, 112].

decline of morphine concentrations in brain is much slower than the elimination of morphine from plasma. It appears that its slow exit from the CNS is related to its low lipoidal solubility[149]. Other narcotic analgesics that are lipid-soluble are long-acting because of their slow dissociation from opiate receptors (e.g. lofentanil)[J. Leysen, unpubl. obs.] or because of their slow elimination from plasma (e.g. methadone $T_{\frac{1}{2}}^{\beta} = 35\,h$)[54].

Why does ventilatory depression recur after a dose of naloxone sufficient to fully antagonise the effects of morphine? Although naloxone is a competitive antagonist of morphine and presumably displaces morphine from specific opiate receptors, it probably does not markedly reduce the total amount of morphine in the brain[77, 91, 106]. Although very limited pharmacokinetic data are available for naloxone, it appears that this lipophilic antagonist is eliminated rapidly from brain due primarily to its redistribution to other tissues[114]. As naloxone concentrations in brain decline, the residual morphine in brain can once again occupy opioid receptors and produce its effects, including ventilatory depression.

Does tolerance to the actions of narcotic analgesics result from alterations in their pharmacokinetics? No, all the available evidence points to a reduced sensitivity of the CNS to the actions of narcotic analgesics. There is no evidence that alterations in the absorption, distribution, biotransformation or excretion of narcotic analgesics are responsible for the development of tolerance to their actions[61, 102].

Studies involving measurements of drug concentrations in plasma would be useful in defining the degree of tolerance development. Although acute tolerance has been demonstrated under certain experimental conditions in animals after continuous infusion of a narcotic analgesic for 4–6 hours, it has not been observed when these drugs have been administered continuously to maintain presumably stable plasma concentrations for anaesthetic (hours) or analgesic (1–2 days) purposes[3, 39, 70, 93, 103, 109, 146].

Toward more efficient use of narcotic analgesics

The basic conflict in the ultisation of narcotic analgesics is the production of both analgesia and ventilatory depression by similar doses and concentrations. Several points must be borne in mind when considering these relationships.

1   Pain and noxious stimulation antagonise the ventilatory depressant effects[38].

2   Sleep and nitrous oxide anaesthesia augment the ventilatory depressant effects[1a, 8, 44].

3   It is often necessary to accept moderate degrees of ventilatory depression and hypercapnia providing there is no contraindication to it (e.g. pathological elevation of intracranial pressure) in order to achieve satisfactory control of pain.

4   The higher the dose (and concentration) of a narcotic analgesic needed intraoperatively, the longer the postoperative period required for recovery of satisfactory spontaneous ventilation[103, T. H. Stanley pers. commun.].

Despite these circumstances, it appears to be feasible to use the narcotic analgesics both to achieve satisfactory anaesthetic conditions while permitting a predictable recovery of spontaneous ventilation, and to relieve postoperative pain while the patient maintains satisfactory spontaneous ventilation[1a]. The keys to these achievements are the recognition of the concentration-response relationships and knowledge of the pharmacokinetics of the particular narcotic analgesic to be used.

A combination of priming and maintenance infusion of fentanyl have been used to produce and maintain anaesthesia for cardiac surgery[69, 103]. The benefits of this approach compared to repeated intravenous bolus doses are

1   the maintenance of a stable level of anaesthesia until the end of surgery without excessive accumulation of fentanyl;

2   a more predictable rate of recovery, albeit quite prolonged because of the long elimination half-time of fentanyl; and

3   a means of assessing the factors affecting the concentrations required for a given depth of anaesthesia.

In the postoperative period, it is feasible to maintain continuously satisfactory relief of pain while avoiding excessive CNS and ventilatory depression. One method involves the use of priming and sustaining infusions of pethidine[64, 140], fentanyl or alfentanil[1a, 1b]. Another method employs a device by which the patient can regulate his own degree of pain relief and timing of narcotic analgesic administration[34, 146]. Ventilatory depression has not been encountered in the initial trials of either of these methods of administering pethidine. Of course, larger numbers of patients will have to be studied in order to define the appropriate limits of dosage and to identify the factors that may suddenly alter the patient's responsiveness to a given concentration or dose. The on demand intravenous self-administration of a narcotic analgesic (i.e. titration of dose and concentrations vs. effect) offers a means of obtaining these data.

Development of new drugs

It is worthwhile considering the possibilities for developing a narcotic analgesic with the shortest possible elimination half-time. Such a drug would be ideal for short-term use when there is likely to be intense noxious stimulation for only a brief period. A short elimination half-time facilitates a rapid achievement of stable plasma levels by continuous intravenous infusion as well as a rapid recovery when the infusion is discontinued. An example of such a drug is succinylcholine ($T_{\frac{1}{2}}^{\beta}$ = 4.5 min). What are the possibilities for a very short acting narcotic analgesic?

The pharmacokinetic possibilities can be considered from the perspective of following relationships:

$$T_{\frac{1}{2}}^{\beta} = \frac{0.69\ V_d}{Cl}$$

where $T_{\frac{1}{2}}^{\beta}$ = terminal elimination half-time,
V_d = total volume of distribution,
Cl = clearance of the drug from the body,
and 0.69 is the natural logarithm of 2 used to relate the elimination rate constant (k) to the half-time:

$$T_{\frac{1}{2}}^{\beta} = \frac{0.693}{k}$$

Thus, either a decrease in distribution volume or an increase in clearance will result in a shorter elimination half-time. Since most of the narcotic analgesics including morphine, pethidine and fentanyl, are cleared at a nearly maximal rate by the liver (flow-dependent, high extraction compounds), it is not possible to shorten the elimination half-time substantially by developing a compound with a higher intrinsic rate of clearance by the liver[155]. A compound with a smaller distribution volume remains a possibility for a shorter-acting narcotic analgesic. One such compound, alfentanil, is now undergoing clinical trials.

The pharmacokinetic features of alfentanil are summarised in Tables 9.2 and 9.12.

Table 9.12 Alfentanil pharmacokinetics.

| Investigator | n | Age (y) | Intravenous dose (μg kg⁻¹) | Half-times | | | Distribution volumes | | Clearance (ml kg⁻¹ min⁻¹) |
				Distribution $T_{\frac{1}{2}}^{\pi}$ (min)	Distribution $T_{\frac{1}{2}}^{\alpha}$ (min)	Elimination $T_{\frac{1}{2}}^{\beta}$ (h)	Initial (l kg⁻¹)	Total (l kg⁻¹)	
Volunteers									
Bower & Hull[16]	7	24–60	2.4	—	—	1.6	0.16	0.39	3.4
	7	24–60	14	—	—	1.6	0.18	0.53	3.2
Surgical patients with various anaesthetics									
Schüttler & Stoeckel[130]	7	36±7	~80	3.4	19	1.4	0.11	0.56	4.9
Bovill et al.[14]	6	22–64	50	1.4	9.5	1.5	0.12	1.0	7.7
	5	19–63	125	1.0	13	1.4	0.08	0.59	5.1
Camu et al.[25]	5	33–55	120	3.5	17	1.6	0.22	1.0	8.3
Fragen et al.[45]	5	29–48	260	—	5.1	1.5	—	0.42	3.3
Cardiac surgical patients subjected to extracorporeal circulation (CPB)									
Hug et al.[68]	5	40–58	125 before CPB	—	5.4	1.3	0.10	0.32	3.0
	5	40–58	125 after CPB	—	22	3.3	0.26	0.89	3.3

Although its clearance is one-half that of fentanyl (see Table 9.7), its distribution volume is only one-fifth of fentanyl; hence, its elimination half-time is less than one-half that of fentanyl (1.5 vs. 3.7 hrs). The basis of the lower distribution volume of alfentanil compared to fentanyl appears to be a much lower lipoidal solubility, that limits its entry into cells (e.g. RBC) and tissues, especially fat. Despite its lesser lipoidal solubility, more of the alfentanil present in plasma at pH 7.4 is in the unionised form (89 % compared to 9 % for fentanyl) and so its onset of action is comparably rapid (see Table 9.2). It would appear that alfentanil would be a better drug than fentanyl for use by continuous intravenous infusion for anaesthetic purposes of short duration (Fig. 9.4) [1a, 142]. In fact, the clinical trials demonstrate a rapid recovery from its effects whether it is administered by a continuous infusion[1a, 1b, 3] or by repeated intravenous injections of bolus doses[3, 14, 35].

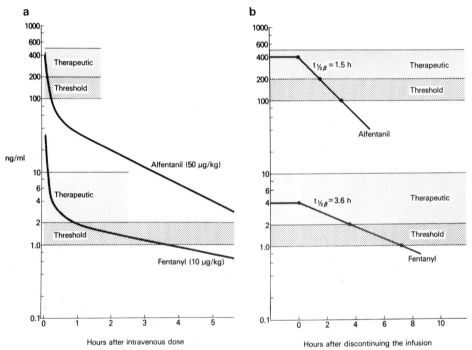

Fig. 9.4(a)   A comparison of the plasma decay curves of a single i.v. bolus dose of fentanyl and alfentanil. The solid line is the predicted plasma concentration in a single patient with representative pharmacokinetics. While the equivalent alfentanil dose is 5 times that of fentanyl, during the first 2 h after injection the alfentanil plasma concentrations are 14 to 25 times higher. This is in part due to the smaller volume of distribution of alfentanil. (b) Assuming that a steady-state plasma level of the narcotic analgesic has been maintained in the effective range, the rate of decline of drug concentrations will be determined by the elimination half-life. In this example, concentrations compatible with satisfactory spontaneous ventilation will be reached in two half-times: 3 h for alfentanil and 7.2 h for fentanyl.[142] (From Stanski & Hug, *Anesthesiology*, with permission.).

What is still needed?

The two essential elements to practical applications of pharmacokinetics on a broad scale are a reliable measure of the intensity of drug action and a means of rapidly measuring (i.e. monitoring) drug concentrations in plasma and other biological specimens. Both of these have been more or less lacking for the narcotic analgesics in the setting of surgical anaesthesia.

What is a reliable 'end-point' of anaesthesia produced by a narcotic analgesics alone or in combination with a hypnotic or nitrous oxide? Somatic signs (e.g. movement, vocalisation, airway reflex activity) have traditionally been used to judge depth of anaesthesia. These signs are obtunded or eliminated by muscle relaxants which are frequently used in combination with the narcotic analgesics. Moreover, the light levels of anaesthesia produced by the narcotic analgesics are associated with maintenance of, or even an increase in skeletal muscle tone (i.e. rigidity), thus further indicating the administration of muscle relaxants. Awareness has been reported after very large doses of the narcotic analgesics, is usually undetectable in the paralysed subject, and probably occurs more often than we believe because of the frequent use of premedicant drugs that induce amnesia[69, 90, 103, 107]. Although they may not be recalled, episodes of awareness during an operation may be very frightening and uncomfortable to the patient even though he may not experience pain[68, 89, 90].

We have recently observed that it is possible to maintain satisfactory levels of anaesthesia (i.e. unconsciousness and suppression of sympathetic and haemodynamic responses to noxious stimulation) with fentanyl or alfentanil alone or in combination with nitrous oxide in the presence of normal muscular responses to peripheral nerve stimulation (train-of-4)[3, 69, 103]. During the induction of anaesthesia with alfentanil or fentanyl, almost all of the patients became rigid and had a marked decrease in their ventilatory compliance that required the administration of a muscle relaxant (either succinylcholine or pancuronium) to facilitate positive pressure ventilation in the presence of apnoea, also induced by the narcotic analgesic. However, most of the patients did not exhibit abnormally high muscle tone nor any significant decline of ventilatory compliance once they had recovered from the muscle relaxant (i.e. normal train-of-4). Under such circumstances it was possible to observe somatic signs of inadequate anaesthetic depth. Obviously, more or less complete muscular relaxation may be required for the surgical operation, but the benefits of being able to judge anaesthetic depth by somatic signs strongly justify the admonition to use minimally required degrees of paralysis and only for that portion of the operation in which relaxation is essential.

Anaesthetic depth in the paralysed patient may be estimated electroencephalographically, but the currently high costs and substantial inconvenience of EEG monitoring make this approach impractical in the everyday practice of anaesthesia[132, 133, 151].

The ability or inability of narcotic analgesics to suppress sympathetic and haemodynamic responses to noxious stimulation has been emphasised in most studies evaluating their usefulness as anaesthetics. However, suppression of these signs of stress is not a consistent indication of adequate anaesthetic depth, since it is not uncommon to observe purposeful movement in the absence of sympathetic and haemodynamic responses to noxious surgical stimulation[3]. And contrariwise, somatic signs of light anaesthesia are not always present in the unparalysed patient in whom hypertension and tachycardia occur in association with noxious stimulation.

Thus, a reliable end-point and graded response to anaesthetic doses of the narcotic analgesics remains to be identified, especially for use in the presence of muscular paralysis.

A means of estimating plasma concentrations of a narcotic analgesic in matter of minutes would be very useful in evaluating the adequacy of a dosage regimen to produce the desired plasma levels (pharmacokinetic variability); in recognising patients who are unusually sensitive or resistant to the drug's actions; in making a differential diagnosis of dose-related side effects or toxicity (e.g. prolonged ventilatory depression after anaesthesia); and in predicting the time required for recovery from narcotic analgesic effects. Experience in relating intravenous drug concentrations to methods of administration and to clinical effects should also improve the efficiency of narcotic analgesic use (as it has in the case of potent inhalational anaesthetics) and minimise the need for narcotic antagonists, which add their own risks to the recovery period (e.g. unmasking pain, inducing nausea and retching, producing hypertension and tachycardia) [40, 65, 66, 119].

GLOSSARY

Generic	Trade
Alfentanil	Rapifen
Fentanyl	Sublimaze
Morphine	—
Pethidine	
(USA Meperidine)	Demerol
Naloxone	Narcan

REFERENCES

1. AINSLIE S. G., EISELE J. H. JR. & CORKILL G. (1979) Fentanyl concentrations in brain and serum during respiratory acid–base changes in the dog. *Anesthesiology* **51**, 293–7.

1a. ANDREWS C. J. H., SINCLAIR M., DYE A., DYE J., HARVEY J. & PRYS-ROBERTS C. (1982) The additive effect of nitrous oxide on respiratory depression in patients having fentanyl or alfentanil infusions. *Br. J. Anaesth.* **54**, 1129.

1b. ANDREWS C. J. H., SINCLAIR M., PRYS-

ROBERTS C. & DYE A. (1983) The ventilatory effects during and after continuous infusion of fentanyl or alfentanil. *Br. J. Anaesth.* **55**, (in press).

2. ASATOOR A. M., LONDON D. R., MILNE M. D. & SIMENHOFF M. L. (1963) The excretion of pethidine and its derivatives. *Br. J. Pharmacol.* **20**, 285–98.

3. AUSEMS M. E., HUG C. C. JR. & DE LANGE S. (1983) Variable rate infusion of alfentanil as a supplement to nitrous oxide anesthesia for general surgery. *Anesth. Analg.* **62** (in press).

4. AUSTIN K. L., STAPLETON J. V. & MATHER L. E. (1980) Relationship between blood meperidine concentrations and analgesic response. *Anesthesiology* **53**, 460–6.

5. AUSTIN K. L., STAPLETON J. V. & MATHER L. E. (1980) Multiple intramuscular injection: a major source of variability in analgesic response to meperidine. *Pain* **8**, 47–62.

6. AUSTIN K. L., STAPLETON J. V. & MATHER L. E. (1981) Pethidine clearance during continuous intravenous infusions in postoperative patients. *Br. J. Pharmacol.* **1**, 25–30.

7. BECKER L. D., PAULSON B. A., MILLER R. D. SEVERINGHAUS J. W. & EGER E. I. II (1976) Biphasic respiratory depression after fentanyl-droperidol or fentanyl alone used to supplement nitrous oxide anesthesia. *Anesthesiology* **44**, 291–6.

8. BELLVILLE J. W., HOWLAND W. S., SEED J. C. & HOUDE R. W. (1959) The effect of sleep on the respiratory response to carbon dioxide. *Anesthesiology* **20**, 628–34.

9. BENET L. Z., GREITHER A. & MEISTER W. (1976) Gastrointestinal absorption of drugs in patients with cardiac failure. In Benet L. Z. (ed.), *The Effect of Disease States on Drug Pharmacokinetics*, pp. 33–50. American Pharmaceutical Association, Washington D.C.

10. BENOWITZ N., FORSYTH R. P., MELMON K. L. & ROWLAND M. (1974) Lidocaine disposition kinetics in monkey and man. II. Effects of hemorrhage and sympathomimetic drug administration. *Clin. Pharmacol. Ther.* **16**, 99–109.

11. BERKOWITZ B. A., NGAI S. H., YANG J. C., HEMPSTEAD J. & SPEATOR S. (1975) The disposition of morphine in surgical patients. *Clin. Pharmacol. Ther.* **17**, 629–35.

12. BOREL J. D., BENTLEY J. B. & GILLESPIE T. J. (1981) Pharmacokinetics of intravenous sufentanil. *Anesthesiology* **55**, A251.

13. BOVILL J. G. & SEBEL P. S. (1980) Pharmacokinetics of high-dose fentanyl. A study in patients undergoing cardiac surgery. *Br. J. Anaesth.* **52**, 795–802.

14. BOVILL J. G., SEBEL P. S., BLACKBURN C. L. & HEYKANTS J. (1982) The pharmacokinetics of alfentanil (R 39209): A new opioid analgesic. *Anesthesiology* **57**, 439–43.

15. BOWER S., HOLLAND D. E. & HULL C. J. (1976) The pharmacokinetics of fentanyl in man. *Br. J. Anaesth.* **48**, 1121.

16. BOWER S. & HULL C. J. (1982) The comparative pharmacokinetics of fentanyl and alfentanil. *Br. J. Anaesth.* **54**, 871–7.

17. BROMAGE P. R., CAMPORESI E. & CHESTNUT D. (1980) Epidural narcotics for postoperative analgesia. *Anesth. Analg.* **59**, 473–80.

18. BROMAGE P. R., CAMPORESI E. M., DURANT P. A. C. & NIELSON C. H. (1982) Rostral spread of epidural morphine. *Anesthesiology* **56**, 431–6.

19. BROMAGE P. R., CAMPORESI E. & LESLIE J. (1980) Epidural narcotics in volunteers: Sensitivity to pain and to carbon dioxide. *Pain* **9**, 145–60.

20. BRUNK S. F. & DELLE M. (1974) Morphine metabolism in man. *Clin. Pharmacol. Ther.* **16**, 51–7.

21. BRUNK S. F., DELLE M. & WILSON W. R. (1974) Morphine metabolism in man: Effect of aspirin. *Clin. Pharmacol. Ther.* **15**, 283–90.

22. BRUNK S. F., DELLE M. & WILSON W. R. (1974) Effect of propranolol on morphine metabolism. *Clin. Pharmacol. Ther.* **16**, 1039–44.

23. BRUNK S. F., DELLE M. & WILSON W. R. (1974) Morphine metabolism in man: Effect of guanethidine. *J. Clin. Pharmacol.* **14**, 581–7.

24. CAFRUNY E. J. (1971) Renal excretion of drugs. In La Du B. N., Mandel H. G., Way E. L. (eds.), *Fundamentals of Drug Metabolism and Drug Disposition*, pp. 119–30. Williams and Wilkins, Baltimore.

25. CAMU F., GEPTS E., RUCQUOI M. & HEYKANTS J. (1982) Pharmacokinetics of alfentanil in man. *Anesth. Analg.* **61**, 657–61.

26. CARTWRIGHT D. P., CHAPMAN J. C., DAVIES J. R. & SCOGGINS A. M. (1981) Pharmacokinetics of high-dose fentanyl. *Br. J. Anaesth.* **53**, 780.

27. CATLIN D. H. (1977) Pharmacokinetics of morphine by radioimmunoassay: The influence of immunochemical factors. *J. Pharmacol. Exp. Ther.* **200**, 224–35.

28. CHAN K., KENDALL M. J., MITCHARD M. & WELLS W. D. E. (1975) The effect of ageing on plasma pethidine concentration. *Br. J. Clin. Pharmacol* **2**, 297–302.

29. CHAN K., KENDALL M. J., WELLS W. D. E. & MITCHARD M. (1975) Factors influencing the excretion and relative physiological availability of pethidine in man. *J. Pharm. Pharmacol.* **27**, 235–41.

30. CORAL I. M., MOORE A. R. & STRUNIN L. (1980) Plasma concentrations of fentanyl in normal surgical patients and those with severe renal and hepatic disease. *Br. J. Anaesth.* **52**, 101P.

31. DAHLSTROM B., BOLME P., FEYCHTING H., NOACK G. & PAALZOW L. (1979) Morphine kinetics in children. *Clin. Pharmacol. Ther.* **26**, 354–65.

32. DAHLSTROM B. E. & PAALZOW L. K. (1978) Pharmacokinetic interpretation of the enterohepatic recirculation and first-pass elimination of morphine in the rat. *J. Pharmacokin. Biopharm.* **6**, 505–19.

33. DAHLSTROM B. E., PAALZOW L. K., SEGRE G. & AGREN A. J. (1978) Relation between morphine pharmacokinetics and analgesia. *Pharmacokin. Biopharm.* **6**, 41–53.

34. DAHLSTROM B., TAMSEN A., PAALZOW L. & HARTVIG P. (1983) Patient-controlled analgesic therapy IV: Pharmacokinetics and analgesic plasma concentrations of morphine. *Clin. Pharmacokin.* (in press).

35. DE LANGE S., DE BRUIJN N., STANLEY T. H. & BOSCOE M. J. (1981) Alfentanil-oxygen anesthesia: Comparison of continuous infusion and frequent bolus techniques for coronary artery surgery. *Anesthesiology* **55**, A42.

36. DON H. F., DIEPPA R. A. & TAYLOR P. (1975) Narcotic analgesics in anuric patients. *Anesthesiology* **42**, 745–7.

37. DUNKERLEY R., JOHNSON R., SCHENKER S. & WILKINSON G. R. (1976) Gastric and biliary excretion of meperidine in man. *Clin. Pharmacol. Ther.* **20**, 546–51.

38. ECKENHOFF J. E. & OECH S. R. (1960) The effects of narcotics and antagonists upon respiration and circulation in man. *Clin. Pharmacol. Ther.* **1**, 483–524.

39. ELLIOTT H. W., PARKER K. D., CRIM M., WRIGHT J. A. & NOMOF N. (1971) Actions and metabolism of heroin administered by continuous intravenous infusion to man. *Clin. Pharmacol. Ther.* **12**, 806–14.

40. ESTILO A. E. & COTTRELL J. E. (1982) Hemodynamic and catecholamine changes after administration of naloxone. *Anesth. Analg.* **61**, 349–53.

41. FINCH J. S. & DeKORNFELD T. J. (1967) Clinical investigation of the analgesic potency and respiratory depressant activity of fentanyl, a new narcotic analgesic. *J. Clin. Pharmacol.* **7**, 46–51.

42. FINCK A. D., BERKOWITZ B. A., HEMPSTEAD J. & NGAI S. H. (1977) Pharmacokinetics of morphine: Effects of

hypercarbia on serum and brain concentrations in the dog. *Anesthesiology* **47**, 407–10.

43. FINDLAY J. W. A., JONES E. C., BUTZ R. F. & WELCH R. M. (1978) Plasma codeine and morphine concentrations after therapeutic oral doses of codeine-containing analgesics. *Clin. Pharmacol. Ther.* **24**, 60–68.

44. FORREST W. H. JR. & BELLVILLE J. W. (1964) The effect of sleep plus morphine on the respiratory response to carbon dioxide. *Anesthesiology* **25**, 137–41.

45. FRAGEN R. J., BOOIJ L. H. D. J., BRAAK G. J. J., VREE T. B., HEYKANTS J. & CRUL J. F. (1983) Pharmacokinetics of alfentanil infusion in man. *Br. J. Anaesth.* (in press).

46. FUNG D. L., ASLING J. H., EISELE J. H. & MARTUCCI R. (1980) A comparison of alphaprodine and meperidine pharmacokinetics. *J. Clin. Pharmacol.* **20**, 37–41.

47. FUNG D. L. & EISELE J. H. (1980) Fentanyl pharmacokinetics in awake volunteers. *J. Clin. Pharmacol.* **20**, 652–8.

48. GESSNER T., TRUDNOWSKI R., RICO R. *et al.* (1976) Passage of intravenously administered pethidine into gastric juice in humans. *J. Pharm. Pharmacol.* **28**, 78–81.

49. GILL K. J., CARTWRIGHT D. P., SCOGGINS A., GRAY A. J. & PRYS-ROBERTS C. (1980) Ventilatory depression related to plasma fentanyl concentrations during and after anaesthesia. *Br. J. Anaesth.* **52**, 632P.

50. GLYNN C. J., MATHER L. E., COUSINS M. J., GRAHAM J. R. & WILSON P. R. (1981) Peridural meperidine in man: Analgesic response, pharmacokinetics and transmission into CSF. *Anesthesiology* **55**, 520–6.

51. GOLDSTEIN A. (1976) Opioid peptides (endorphins) in pituitary and brain. *Science* **193**, 1081–6.

52. GOODMAN L. S. & GILMAN A. (1956) *The Pharmacological Basis of Therapeutics*, 2nd edition., pp. 8–9. Macmillan, New York.

53. GOROMARU T., FURUTA T., BABA S., YOSHIMURA N., MIYAWAKI T., SAMESHIMA T., & MIYAO J. (1981) Metabolism of fentanyl in rats and man. *Anesthesiology* **55**, A173.

54. GOURLAY G. K., WILSON P. R. & GLYNN C. J. (1982) Pharmacodynamics and pharmacokinetics of methadone during the peri-operative period. *Anesthesiology* **57**, 458–67.

55. GREENE N. M. & HUG C. C. JR. (1982) Pharmacokinetics. In Kitahata L. M. & Collins J. G. (eds.), *Narcotic Analgesics in Anesthesiology*, pp. 1–42. Williams and Wilkins, Baltimore.

56. HENDERSON G. L., FRINCKE J., LEUNG C. Y., TORTEN M. & BENJAMINI E. (1975) Antibodies to fentanyl. *J. Pharmacol. Exp. Ther.* **192**, 489–96.

57. HENGSTMANN J. H., STOECKEL H. & SCHUTTLER J. (1980) Infusion model for fentanyl based on pharmacokinetic analysis. *Br. J. Anaesth.* **52**, 1021–5.

58. HERZ A. & TESCHEMACHER H. J. (1971) Activities and sites of antinociceptive action of morphine-like analgesics. In Harper N. J. and Simmonds A. B. (eds.), *Advances in Drug Research*, vol. 6, pp. 79–119. Academic Press, New York.

59. HESS R., HERZ A. & FRIEDEL K. (1971) Pharmacokinetics of fentanyl in rabbits in view of the importance for limiting its effect. *J. Pharmacol. Exp. Ther.* **179**, 474–84.

60. HOLLT V. & TESCHEMACHER H. J. (1975) Hydrophobic interactions responsible for unspecific bindings of morphine-like drugs. *Naunyn-Schmiedeberg's Arch. Pharmacol.* **288**, 163–77.

61. HUG C. C. JR. (1972) Characteristics and theories related to acute and chronic tolerance development. In Mule S. J. & Brill H. (eds.), *Chemical and Biological Aspects of Drug Dependence*, pp. 307–58. CRC Press, Cleveland, Ohio.

62. HUG C. C. JR. (1978) Pharmacokinetics of drugs administered intravenously. *Anesth. Analg.* **57**, 704–23.

63. Hug C. C. Jr. (1978) Pharmacokinetics of morphine during cardiac surgery. Abstracts of Scientific Papers, *American Society of Anesthesiologists*, Annual Meeting, Chicago, pp. 305–306.

64. Hug C. C. Jr. (1980) Improving analgesic therapy. *Anesthesiology* **53**, 441–3.

65. Hug C. C. Jr. (1981) What are the roles of narcotic analgesics in anesthesia? *Refresher Courses in Anesthesiology* **9**, 71–83.

66. Hug C. C. Jr. (1982) Anesthetic agents and the patient with cardiovascular disease. In Ream A. K. & Fogdall R. P. (eds.), *Acute Cardiovascular Management: Anesthesia and Intensive Care*, pp. 247–91. J. P. Lippincott, Philadelphia.

67. Hug C. C. Jr., Aldrete J. A., Sampson J. F. & Murphy M. R. (1979) Morphine anesthesia in patients with liver failure. *Anesthesiology* **51**, s30.

68. Hug C. C. Jr., de Lange S. & Burm A. G. L. (1983) Alfentanil pharmacokinetics in cardiac surgical patients before and after cardiopulmonary bypass (CPB). *Anesth. Analg.* **62**, 266.

69. Hug C. C. Jr. & Moldenhauer C. C. (1982) Pharmacokinetics and dynamics of fentanyl infusions in cardiac surgical patients. *Anesthesiology* **57 A**, 45.

70. Hug C. C. Jr. & Murphy M. R. (1979) Fentanyl disposition in cerebrospinal fluid and plasma and its relationship to ventilatory depression in the dog. *Anesthesiology* **50**, 342–9.

71. Hug C. C. Jr. & Murphy M. R. (1981) Tissue redistribution of fentanyl and termination of its effects in rats. *Anesthesiology* **55**, 369–75.

72. Hug C. C. Jr. & Murphy M. R. Tissue distribution of morphine in rats. (in preparation).

73. Hug C. C. Jr., Murphy M. R., Rigel E. P. & Olson W. A. (1981) Pharmacokinetics of morphine injected intravenously into the anesthetized dog. *Anesthesiology* **54**, 38–47.

74. Hug C. C. Jr., Murphy M. R., Sampson J. F., Terblanche J. & Aldrete J. A. (1981) Biotransformation of morphine and fentanyl in anhepatic dogs. *Anesthesiology* **55**, A 261.

75. Hug C. C. Jr. & Oka T. (1971) Uptake of dihydromorphine-^{3}H by synaptosomes. *Life Sci.* **10**, 201–13.

76. Iwamoto K. & Klaassen C. D. (1977) First-pass effect of morphine in rats. *J. Pharmacol. Exp. Ther.* **200**, 236–44.

77. Jaffe J. H. & Martin W. R. (1980) Opioid analgesics and antagonists. In Gilman A. G., Goodman L. S. & Gilman A. (eds.), *The Pharmacological Basis of Therapeutics*, 6th edition, pp. 494–534. Macmillan, New York.

78. Jasinski D. R. & Mansky P. A. (1972) Evaluation of nalbuphine for abuse potential. *Clin. Pharmacol. Ther.* **13**, 78–90.

79. Klotz U., McHorse T. S., Wilkinson G. R. & Schenker S. (1974) The effect of cirrhosis on the disposition and elimination of meperidine in man. *Clin. Pharmacol. Ther.* **16**, 667–75.

80. Koska A. J., Kramer W. C., Romagnoli A., Keats A. S. & Sabawala P. B. (1981) Pharmacokinetics of high-dose meperidine in surgical patients. *Anesth. Analg.* **60**, 8–11.

81. Koska A. J., Romagnoli A. & Kramer W. G. (1981) Effect of cardiopulmonary bypass on fentanyl distribution and elimination. *Clin. Pharmacol. Ther.* **29**, 100–5.

82. Kuhnert B. R., Kuhnert P. M., Tu A. S. L., Lin D. C. K. & Foltz R. L. (1979) Meperidine and normeperidine levels following meperidine administration during labor. I. Mother. *Am. J. Obstet. Gynec.* **133**, 904–8.

83. Kupferberg H. J. & Way E. L. (1963) Pharmacologic basis for the sensitivity of the newborn rat to morphine. *J. Pharmacol. Exp. Ther.* **141**, 105–112.

84. La Motte C. C., Collins J. G. & Robinson C. J. (1982) Endogenous opiate systems and opiate receptors. In Kitahata L. M. & Collins J. G. (eds.),

Narcotic Analgesics in Anesthesiology, pp. 43–56. Williams and Wilkins, Baltimore.

85. LAUVEN P. M., STOECKEL H., SCHUTTLER J. & SCHWILDEN H. (1981) Verhinderung des Fentanyl-rebound-Phanomens durch Cimetidin-Medikation. *Anaesthetist* **30**, 467–71.

86. LEVY W. J., SHAPIRO H. M., MARUCHAK G. & MEATHE M. S. (1980) Automated EEG processing for intraoperative monitoring: A comparison of techniques. *Anesthesiology* **53**, 223–36.

87. LOH H. H. & ROSS D. H. (eds.) (197) *Neurochemical Mecanisms of Opiates and Endorphins, Advances in Biochemical Psychopharmacology,* vol. 20, pp. 31–68. Raven Press, New York.

88. LONGNECKER D. E. (1981) Narcotics and narcotic antagonists. In Smith N. T., Miller R. D. & Corbascio A. N. (eds.), *Drug Interactions in Anesthesia,* pp. 221–9. Lea and Febiger, Philadelphia.

89. LOWENSTEIN E. (1971) Morphine 'anesthesia': A perspective. *Anesthesiology* **35**, 563–5.

90. MAINZER J. JR. (1979) Awareness, muscle relaxants and balanced anaesthesia. *Can. Anaesth. Soc. J.* **26**, 386–93.

91. MANARA L., ALDINIO C., CERLETTI C., COCCIA P., LUINI A. & SERRA G. (1978) *In vivo* tissue levels and subcellular distribution of opiates with reference to pharmacological action. In Adler M. W., Manara L. & Samanin R. (eds.), *Factors Affecting the Action of Narcotics,* pp. 271–96. Raven Press, New York.

92. MARTIN W. R. (1979) History and development of mixed opioid antagonists, partial antagonists and antagonists. *Br. J. Clin. Pharmacol.* **7**, 273s–9s.

93. MARTIN W. R., EADES C. G., THOMPSON J. A., HUPPLER & GILBERT P. E. (1976) The effects of morphine- and nalorphine-like drugs in the nondependent and morphine-dependent chronic spinal dog. *J. Pharmacol. Exp. Ther.* **197**, 517–32.

94. MATHER L. E., LINDOP M. J., TUCKER G. T. & PFLUG A. E. (1975) Pethidine revisited: plasma concentrations and effects after intramuscular injection. *Br. J. Anaesth.* **47**, 1269–75.

95. MATHER L. E. & MEFFIN P. J. (1978) Clinical pharmacokinetics of pethidine. *Clin. Pharmacokin.* **3**, 352–68.

96. MATHER L. E. & TUCKER G. T. (1974) Meperidine and other basic drugs: A general method for their determination in plasma. *J. Pharm. Sci.* **63**, 306–7.

97. MATHER L. E., TUCKER G. T., PFLUG A. E., LINDOP M. J. & WILKERSON C. (1975) Meperidine kinetics in man. *Clin. Pharmacol. Ther.* **17**, 21–30.

98. MCCLAIN D. A. & HUG C. C. JR. (1980) Intravenous fentanyl kinetics. *Clin. Pharmacol. Ther.* **28**, 106–14.

99. MCHORSE T. S., WILKINSON G. R., JOHNSON R. F. & SCHENKER S. (1975) Effect of acute viral hepatitis in man on the disposition and elimintion of meperidine. *Gastroenterology* **68**, 775–80.

100. MEULDERMANS W. E. G., HURKMANS R. M. A. & HEYKANTS J. J. P. (1982) Plasma protein binding and distribution of fentanyl, sufentanil, alfentanil and lofentanil in blood. *Arch. Int. Pharmacodyn. Ther.* **257**, 4–19.

101. MILLER J. W. & ANDERSON H. H. (1954) The effect of N-demethylation on certain pharmacological actions of morphine, codeine and meperidine in the mouse. *J. Pharmacol. Exp. Ther.* **112**, 191–6.

102. MISRA A. L. (1978) Metabolism of opiates. In Adler M. W., Manara L. & Samanin R. (eds.), *Factors Affecting the Action of Narcotics,* pp. 297–343. Raven Press, New York.

103. MOLDENHAUER C. C. & HUG C. C. JR. (1982) Continuous infusion of fentanyl for cardiac surgery. *Anesth. Analg.* **61**, 206.

104. MORGAN D., MOORE G., THOMAS J. & TRIGGS E. (1978) Disposition of meperidine in pregnancy. *Clin. Pharmacol. Ther.* **23**, 288–95.

105. MULE S. J. & WOODS L. A. (1962) Distribution of N-^{14}C-methyl labeled morphine. I. In central nervous system of nontolerant and tolerant dogs. *J. Pharmacol. Exp. Ther.* **136**, 232–41.

106. MULE S. J., WOODS L. A. & MELLETT L. B. (1962) Distribution of N-^{14}C-methyl labeled morphine. II. Effect of nalorphine in the central nervous system of nontolerant dogs and observations on metabolism. *J. Pharmacol. Exp. Ther.* **136**, 242–9.

107. MUMMANENI N., RAO T. L. K. & MONTOYA A. (1980) Awareness and recall with high-dose fentanyl-oxygen anesthesia. *Anesth. Analg.* **59**, 948–9.

108. MURPHY M. R. & HUG C. C. JR. (1981) Pharmacokinetics of intravenous morphine in patients anesthetized with enflurane-nitrous oxide. *Anesthesiology* **54**, 187–92.

109. MURPHY M. R. & HUG C. C. JR. (1982) The anesthetic potency of fentanyl in terms of its reduction of enflurane MAC. *Anesthesiology* **57**, 485–8.

110. MURPHY M. R. & HUG C. C. JR. (1982) The enflurane sparing effect of morphine, butorphanol, and nalbuphine. *Anesthesiology* **57**, 489–92.

111. MURPHY M. R. & HUG C. C. JR. (1982) Dose-independent pharmacokinetics of fentanyl. *Anesthesiology* **57** A, 347.

112. MURPHY M. R., OLSON W. A. & HUG C. C. JR. (1979) Pharmacokinetics of ^{3}H-fentanyl in the dog anesthetized with enflurane. *Anesthesiology* **50**, 13–19.

113. NEAL E. A., MEFFIN P. J., GREGORY P. B. & BLASCHKE T. F. (1979) Enhanced bioavailability and deceased clearance of analgesics in patients with cirrhosis. *Gastroenterology* **77**, 96–102.

114. NGAI S. H., BERKOWITZ B. A., YAN J. C., HEMPSTEAD J. & SPECTOR S. (1976) Pharmacokinetics of naloxone in rat and in man. *Anesthesiology* **44**, 398–401.

115. NISHITATENO K., NGAI S. H., FINCK A. D. & BERKOWITZ B. A. (1979) Pharmacokinetics of morphine: Concentrations in the serum and brain of the dog during hyperventilation. *Anesthesiology* **50**, 520–23.

116. OLDENDORF W. H., HYMAN S., BRAUN L. & OLDENDORF S. Z. (1972) Blood-brain barrier: Penetration of morphine, codeine, heroin and methadone after carotid injection. *Science* **178**, 984–6.

117. OLSEN G. D. (1975) Morphine binding to human plasma proteins. *Clin. Pharmacol. Ther.* **17**, 31–35.

118. OLSEN G. D., BENNETT W. M. & PORTER G. A. (1975) Morphine and phenytoin binding to plasma proteins in renal and hepatic failure. *Clin. Pharmacol. Ther.* **17**, 677–84.

119. PATSCHKE D., EBERLEIN H. J. & HESS W. (1977) Antagonism of morphine with naloxone in dogs: Cardiovascular effects with special reference to the coronary circulation. *Br. J. Anaesth.* **49**, 525–33.

120. PAULUS D. A., PAUL W. L. & MUNSON E. S. (1981) Neurological depression after intrathecal morphine. *Anesthesiology* **54**, 517–18.

121. POND S. M., TONG T., BENOWITZ N. L., JACOB P. & RIGOD J. (1981) Presystemic metabolism of meperidine to normeperidine in normal and cirrhotic subjects. *Clin. Pharmacol. Ther.* **30**, 183–8.

121a. PRYS-ROBERTS C. (1982) Cardiovascular effects of continuous intravenous anaesthesia compared with those of inhalational anaesthesia. *Acta Anaesth. Scand.* S**75**, 10–17.

122. QUASHA A. L. & EGER E. I. II (1981) MAC. In Miller R. D. (ed.), *Anesthesia*, vol 1, pp. 257–81. Churchill Livingstone, Edinburgh.

123. RAWAL N., SJOSTRAND U. & DAHLSTROM B. (1981) Postoperative pain relief by epidural morphine. *Anesth. Analg.* **60**, 726–31.

124. RIGG J. R. A., BROWNE R. A., DAVIS C., KHANDELWAL J. K. & GOLDSMITH C. H. (1978) Variation in the disposition of morphine after IM administration in surgical patients. *Br. J. Anaesth.* **50**, 1125–30.

125. SAMII K., CHAUVIN M. & VIARS P. (1981) Postoperative spinal analgesia with morphine. *Br. J. Anaesth.* **53**, 817–20.

126. SAWE J., DAHLSTROM B., PAALZOW L. & RANE A. (1981) Morphine kinetics in cancer patients. *Clin. Pharmacol. Ther.* **30**, 629–35.

127. SCHANKER L. S. (1971) Drug absorption. In La Du B. N., Mandel H. G. & Way E. L. (eds.), *Fundamentals of Drug Metabolism and Drug Disposition*, pp. 22–43. Williams and Wilkins, Baltimore.

128. SCHLEIMER R., BENJAMINI E., EISELE J. & HENDERSON G. (1978) Pharmacokinetics of fentanyl as determined by radioimmunoassay. *Clin. Pharmacol. Ther.* **23**, 188–94.

129. SCHULZ R. & GOLDSTEIN A. (1972) Inactivity of narcotic glucuronides as analgesics and on guinea-pig ileum. *J. Pharmacol. Exp. Ther.* **183**, 404–10.

130. SCHÜTTLER J. & STOECKE H. (1982) Alfentanil (R 39209) ein neues kurzwirkendes Opiod. *Anaesthesist* **31**, 10–14.

131. SCRAFANI J. T. & HUG C. C. JR. (1968) Active uptake of dihydromorphine and other narcotic analgesics by cerebral cortical slices. *Biochem. Pharmacol.* **17**, 1557–66.

132. SEBEL P. S., BOVILL J. G., WACQUIER A. & ROG P. (1981) Effects of high-dose fentanyl anesthesia on the electroencephalogram. *Anesthesiology* **55**, 203–11.

133. SMITH N. T. & DEMETRESCU M. (1980) The EEG during high-dose fentanyl anesthesia. *Anesthesiology* **53**, s7.

134. SOUDIJN W., VAN WIJNGAARDEN I. & JANSSEN P. A. J. (1974) Biotransformation of neuroleptanalgesics. *Int. Anesth. Clin.* **12**, 145–55.

135. SPECTOR S. (1971) Quantitative determination of morphine in serum by radioimmunoassay. *J. Pharmacol. Exp. Ther.* **178**, 253–8.

136. STAMBAUGH J. E. & WAINER I. W. (1975) Drug interactions I: meperidine and combination oral contraceptives. *J. Clin. Pharmacol.* **15**, 46–51.

137. STAMBAUGH J. E. & WAINER I. W. (1976) Metabolic studies of hydroxyzine and meperidine in human subjects. In J. J. Bonica & D. G. Albe-Fessard (eds.), *Advances in Pain Research and Therapy*, vol 1, pp. 559–65. Raven Press, New York.

138. STAMBAUGH J. E. JR. & WAINER I. W. (1981) Drug interaction: Meperidine and chloropromazine, a toxic combination. *J. Clin. Pharmacol.* **21**, 140–6.

139. STAMBAUGH J. E., WAINER I. W., SANSTEAD J. K. & HEMPHILL D. M. (1976) The clinical pharmacology of meperidine—comparison of routes of administration. *J. Clin. Pharmacol.* **16**, 245–56.

140. STAPLETON J. V., AUSTIN K. L. & MATHER L. E. (1979) A pharmacokinetic approach to postoperative pain: Continuous infusion of pethidine. *Anaesth. Intens. Care* **7**, 25–32.

141. STANSKI D. R., GREENBLATT D. J. & LOWENSTEIN E. (1978) Kinetics of intravenous and intramuscular morphine. *Clin. Pharmacol. Ther.* **24**, 52–9.

142. STANSKI D. R. & HUG C. C. JR. (1982) Alfentanil—A kinetically predictable narcotic analgesic. *Anesthesiology* **57**, 435–8.

143. STOECKEL H., HENGSTMANN J. H. & SCHUTTLER J. (1979) Pharmacokinetics of fentanyl as a possible explanation for recurrence of respiratory depression. *Br. J. Anaesth.* **51**, 741–5.

144. SZETO H. H., INTURRISI C. E., HOUDE R., *et al.* (1977) Accumulation of normeperidine in patients with renal failure or cancer. *Ann. Intern. Med.* **86**, 738–41.

145. TAKEMORI A. E. (1974) Determination of pharmacological constants: Use of narcotic antagonists to characterize analgesic receptors. In Braude M. C., Harris L. S., May E. L., Smith J. P. 7 Villarreal J. E. V. (eds.), *Narcotic Antagonists, Advances in Biochemical Psychopharma-*

cology, vol 8, pp. 335–44. Raven Press, New York.

146. TAMSEN A. (1981) *Patient-Controlled Analgesic therapy*, Doctoral Thesis, University of Uppsala, Sweden.

147. UTTING J. E. & SMITH J. M. (1979) Postoperative analgesia. *Anaesthesia* **34**, 320–32.

148. VERBEECK R. K., BRANCH R. A. & WILKINSON G. R. (1981) Meperidine disposition in man: Influence of urinary pH and route of administration. *Clin. Pharmacol. Ther.* **30**, 619–28.

149. VON CUBE B., TESCHEMACHER H., HERZ A., *et al.* (1970) Permeation mor-phinartic wirksamer Substanzen and den Ord der antinociceptiven Wirkung im Gehirn in Abhangigkeit von ihrer Lipo-idloslichkeit nach intravenoser und nach intraventricularer Applikation. *Naunyn-Schmiedebergs Arch. Pharmacol.* **265**, 455–73.

150. VREE T. B., HEKSTER C. A. & VAN DER KLEIJN E. (1982) Significance of ap-parent half-lives of a metabolite with a higher elimination rate than its parent drug. *Drug Intelligence and Clinical Pharmacy* **16**, 126–31.

151. WAUQUIER A., VERHEYEN J. L., VAN DEN BROECK W. A. E. & JANSSEN P. A. J. (1979) Visual and computer-based analy-sis of 24 H sleepwaking patterns in the dog. *Electroencephalography Clin. Neuro-physiol.* **46**, 33–48.

152. WAY E. L. & ADLER T. K. (1961) The biological disposition of morphine and its surrogates. *Bull. WHO* **25**, 227–62.

153. WAY W. L., COSTLEY E. C. & WAY E. L. (1965) Respiratory sensitivity of the new-born infant to meperidine and morphine. *Clin. Pharmacol. Ther.* **6**, 454–61.

154. WEDDELL S. J. & RITTER R. R. (1980) Epidural morphine: serum levels and pain relief. *Anesthesiology* **53**, s419.

155. WILKINSON G. R. & SHAND D. G. (1975) A physiological approach to hepatic drug clearance. *Clin. Pharmacol. Ther.* **18**, 377–90.

156. YANG J. C., CLARK W. C., NGAI S. H., BERKOWITZ B. A. & SPECTOR S. (1979) Analgesic action and pharmacokinetics of morphine and diazepam in man. *Anesthesiology* **51**, 495–502.

157. YOSHIMURA H., IDA S., OGURI K. & ISUKAMOTO H. (1973) Biochemical basis for analgesic activity of morphine-6-glucoride-I. Penetration of morphine-6-glucuronide in the brain of rats. *Biochem. Pharmacol.* **22**, 1423–30.

10 Ketamine

WALTER S. NIMMO and
JOHN A. CLEMENTS

Ketamine, 2-(o-chlorophenyl)-2-(methylamino)-cyclohexanone, is a non-barbiturate general anaesthetic for intravenous or intramuscular use. As well as producing general anaesthesia, it produces profound somatic analgesia, enhanced muscle tone, cardiovascular stimulation and occasionally mild respiratory depression. It has a molecular weight of 238, high lipid solubility and a pKa of approximately 7.5[10].

After intravenous use in a dose of $2 \, mg \, kg^{-1}$, onset of anaesthesia is rapid. The high lipid solubility, 5–10 times that of thiopentone[10] ensures its rapid transfer across the blood–brain barrier. The increase in cerebral blood flow that is seen in dogs almost immediately after its administration[11] may also contribute to the rapid achievement of high brain concentrations.

Brain concentrations rapidly decline in parallel with the decrease in plasma concentrations. In the rat, the central nervous system retains the drug preferentially in a ratio of 6.5:1, brain to plasma[9]. However, unconsciousness is terminated by redistribution of the drug from the brain to other tissues and consciousness returns in man 10–15 minutes after a dose of $2 \, mg \, kg^{-1}$ i.v. Complete recovery is more protracted.

The drug readily crosses the placenta and is rapidly distributed to fetal tissues. Concentrations in fetal plasma are about equal to those of maternal plasma[23]. About 12% of ketamine is bound to albumin[31].

After administration to humans, ketamine is demethylated by the hepatic microsomal enzymes to norketamine (metabolite I)[4, 12] (Fig. 10.1). It has been postulated that the cyclohexylamine ring is hydroxylated in one of two different positions to form metabolites III and IV, which can either be conjugated and excreted

235

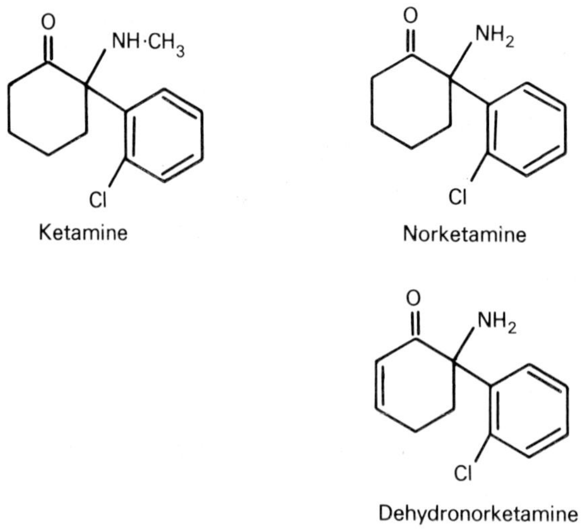

Ketamine

Norketamine

Dehydronorketamine

Fig. 10.1 Chemical structures of ketamine, norketamine (metabolite I) and dehydronorketamine (metabolite II).

or dehydrated to form dehydronorketamine (metabolite II). Ketamine may also undergo hydroxylation of its cyclohexylamine ring at one of two sites to form metabolites V or VI. These may either be conjugated and excreted or dehydrated to form metabolite VII; demethylation of this compound would produce metabolite II[12, 27, 28].

Alteration of hepatic microsomal enzyme metabolising capacity, by enzyme induction or inhibition, has no effect on the duration of loss of righting reflex in rats caused by ketamine and does not change the brain and plasma ketamine concentrations during the initial 10 minutes after intravenous administration[22]. However, the duration of ataxia and agitation is increased by enzyme inhibition and decreased by enzyme induction[10]. In animals ketamine induces its own metabolism.

In man, the mean plasma half-life of ketamine is longer in patients premedicated with diazepam or quinalbarbitone than it is after atropine premedication[20]. Diazepam is a competitive inhibitor of N-dealkylation of ketamine[2]. The half-life of ketamine is not likely to be altered by lorazepam since this benzodiazepine does not undergo N-demethylation.

In animals, halothane slows the uptake, distribution and redistribution of ketamine and metabolite I[30]. This increases the plasma and brain ketamine half-lives and prolongs the period of ataxia. These effects may be due to cardiovascular depression with reduction in hepatic blood flow or to an inhibition of ketamine biotransformation[13].

There is little information on the pharmacological activity of the metabolites in man. A potency ratio of 3:1 between ketamine and norketamine has been suggested[29], and the latter may have some analgesic action in humans[15]. Metabolite II (dehydronorketamine) has been reported to have only 1 % of the anaesthetic activity of the parent drug[6]. However, neither metabolite reaches high enough brain concentrations to contribute to the hypnotic action in rats[10]. The relationship between plasma concentrations of the drug and its metabolites and the incidence of post-hypnotic sequelae such as dreams or hallucinations in man requires further study.

It has been postulated that metabolite II (dehydronorketamine) does not exist *in vivo* and is an artifact of the extraction and analytical procedure[24]. Ketamine, norketamine and dehydronorketamine concentrations in plasma may be measured simultaneously as their heptafluorobutyryl derivatives by gas liquid chromatography with electron capture detection[3, 7].

Intravenous bolus injection

The pharmacokinetics of ketamine in both anaesthetic and analgesic doses have been studied[7, 12, 31]. After intravenous injection of anaesthetic doses (2–2.5 mg kg^{-1} body weight) ketamine distributes rapidly in body tissues. In five adult patients who received 2 mg kg^{-1} as a bolus injection we found plasma ketamine concentrations fell from 1800 ng ml^{-1} (range 1140–2770 ng ml^{-1}) at 5 minutes to 640 ng ml^{-1} (range 440–780 ng ml^{-1}) after 30 minutes (Fig. 10.2). Concentrations further declined to

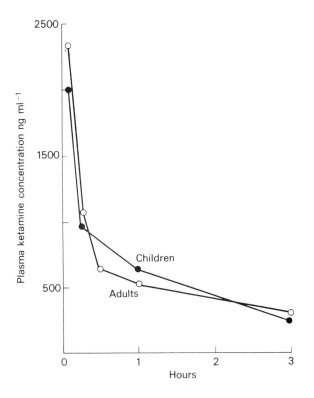

Fig. 10.2 Mean plasma ketamine concentrations up to 3 hours after administration of ketamine 2 mg kg^{-1} i.v. to 5 adults and 4 children.

150 ng ml^{-1} at 5 hours. The rapid distribution of ketamine, which is associated with its uptake into most body tissues, was largely complete after 30 minutes. Thereafter, only slow distribution into adipose tissue occurs. The concentrations of ketamine in venous blood plasma declined bi-exponentially and were adequately fitted by a two-compartment open pharmacokinetic model with elimination from the central compartment (Table 10.1). The half-times in the fast, or alpha, and slow, or beta, phases ($T^\alpha_{\frac{1}{2}}$ and $T^\beta_{\frac{1}{2}}$) were 15 minutes and 168 minutes respectively. The decline in concentration in the fast phase is largely due to distribution into tissues, whereas the slow loss in the beta phase is due to metabolism of ketamine to norketamine and other metabolites. The large value for the apparent distribution volume in the beta phase (V_β) is consistent with its uptake in adipose tissue and the high lipid solubility of ketamine. The mean pharmacokinetic values in our study are similar to those reported by Wieber and others[31]. In 8 adult male volunteers who received 2.2 mg kg^{-1} ketamine i.v., plasma ketamine concentrations at 10–15 minutes were approximately 1000 ng ml^{-1}[12]. Concentrations of 640–1000 ng ml^{-1} represent the minimum concentrations for anaesthesia[12, 17, 19].

Table 10.1 Pharmacokinetic values (mean $\pm$ s.e.m) in patients receiving ketamine by intravenous injection.

	Study	
	[7]	[31]
Number of patients	5	5
Intravenous dose (mg kg^{-1})	2	2.5
$T^\alpha_{\frac{1}{2}}$ (min)	15.5 ± 3.4	11
$T^\beta_{\frac{1}{2}}$ (min)	168 ± 18	150
V_1 (l)	84.6 ± 20.0	60.3 ± 4.1
V_B (l)	214 ± 29	214 ± 35
Clearance (ml min^{-1})	890 ± 100	1227 ± 285

Norketamine rises to measurable concentrations in plasma after 2.5–5 minutes and reaches peak concentrations of about 300 ng ml^{-1} at 30 minutes. The observation that metabolite concentrations are still increasing at the time of recovery from ketamine anaesthesia in man suggests that ketamine biotransformation does not contribute significantly to its short duration of anaesthesia.

Only small amounts (approximately 2.5% of the administered dose) of unchanged ketamine appears in the urine[31]. The cumulative excretion of norketamine in 24 hours is 1.6% and of dehydronorketamine in 72 hours is 16%. The remaining 80% of the injected dose is thought to be excreted as conjugates with glucuronic acid. Chang and others[5] administered tritium-labelled ketamine to humans and found the mean 5-day recovery in urine to be 91% of the dose, with only 3% in the faeces.

When a small dose of ketamine (0.25 mg kg^{-1} body weight) is administered by bolus intravenous injection to healthy subjects, plasma ketamine concentrations of 100–200 ng ml^{-1} occur at 5 min. The concentrations after this small dose also decline in a bi-exponential manner and can be fitted by a two-compartment pharmacokinetic model. The disposition is similar to that of anaesthetic doses in patients; initial distribution occurs very rapidly with a disposition half-life in the alpha phase of 17 min and is complete at about one hour. The subsequent slow elimination occurs largely by metabolism, with a plasma half-life of 186 min[7]. The mean total body clearance (19.1 ml min^{-1} kg^{-1}, equivalent to 1.41 l min^{-1}) is approximately equal to liver blood flow and this suggests that extensive hepatic metabolism is occurring.

The clearance value of 19.1 ml min^{-1} kg^{-1} in subjects given 0.25 mg kg^{-1} by bolus intravenous injection is significantly higher than that (13.1 ml min^{-1} kg^{-1}) in patients given 2 mg kg^{-1} by the same route. This difference may be due to the effects of halothane, administered to the patients but not to volunteers, on the distribution and metabolism of ketamine. It is known that in some individuals ketamine raises the cardiac output and may therefore increase hepatic blood flow and tissue perfusion. For a high clearance drug, such as ketamine, an increase in hepatic blood flow will increase the clearance value[32]. Halothane is known to prevent this effect of ketamine[26], and so it will reduce the clearance value in patients.

Even after injection of small doses of ketamine (0.125 mg kg^{-1} or 0.25 mg kg^{-1}) measurable quantities of the metabolite, norketamine, are found and peak plasma concentrations at 20–60 min after injection are 30–100% of the corresponding ketamine concentrations. An ischaemic exercise test in volunteers who had received small doses of ketamine showed that plasma ketamine concentrations of 100–150 ng ml^{-1} or greater were associated with elevation of pain thresholds. Thus, a range of plasma concentrations exists over which analgesia occurs without loss of consciousness. Doses of 0.125 mg kg^{-1} and 0.25 mg kg^{-1} produced analgesia lasting less than 5 minutes and between 5 and 10 minutes respectively. This short duration of analgesia is also due to the rapid distribution of ketamine.

Intramuscular administration

Absorption of ketamine from an intramuscular injection in patients is rapid and after administration of 6 mg kg^{-1} to three adult patients the mean peak concentration of 2920 ng ml^{-1} occurred at 22 min; concentrations remained above 640 ng ml^{-1} for between two and three hours. The investigation was discontinued after three patients had been studied because the 2–3 hour period of post-operative anaesthesia produced by this dose of ketamine was unacceptably long. Further studies in five patients who received a bolus intravenous injection of 2 mg kg^{-1} showed that peak concentrations of 700–1820 ng ml^{-1} (mean 1530 ng ml^{-1}) were reached at 18 min. Concentrations remained above 640 ng ml^{-1} for one hour and then slowly declined to 150 ng ml^{-1} at

5.5 hours. The terminal plasma half-life was 120 minutes and the mean clearance value was 13.3 ml min^{-1} kg^{-1}. Studies in ten patients, half of whom received ketamine by bolus intravenous injection and half by intramuscular injection, showed the bio-availability from the muscle site to be 99% (Nimmo *et al.*, unpubl. obs.).

After intramuscular injection of a small dose (0.5 mg kg^{-1}) absorption of ketamine is rapid and peak concentrations of about 240 ng ml^{-1} occur at 20 min. In a cross-over study in four volunteers the bioavailability was 93% (range 86–97%) of that of an intravenous injection; the plasma half-life was 155 min and the clearance was 23.2 ml min^{-1} kg^{-1}[7, 16]. Therefore in the small doses used in these studies the intramuscular route produces plasma ketamine concentrations similar to those after intravenous injection.

Of particular interest in this study was the observation that ketamine 0.5 mg kg^{-1} i.m. produced analgesia for a period of 30–45 minutes without impairment of consciousness.

Oral administration

Ketamine (0.5 mg kg^{-1}) given as an oral solution resulted in only very low concentrations of ketamine and the bioavailability (16.5%) was low. There was extensive first-pass metabolism and relatively high concentrations of norketamine were present[16]. The analgesic effect, recorded only at 30 minutes after administration, was less than that seen after intramuscular injection. Presumably the effect was due in part to pharmacological activity of norketamine or another unidentified metabolite. A larger dose (300 mg) taken orally has been reported to produce marked effects, including loss of consciousness[18], but the pharmacokinetics of ketamine in this dose have not been investigated in man.

Intravenous infusion

Idvall and others[17] studied ketamine infusions in 31 patients undergoing major abdominal surgery. After induction of anaesthesia with ketamine 2 mg kg^{-1} i.v., an infusion of 40 μg kg^{-1} min^{-1} was established; this was adjusted to maintain sleep and produce adequate operation conditions. The mean infusion rate required ($\pm$ SD) was 41$\pm$21 μg kg^{-1} min^{-1} and the steady-state plasma ketamine concentration was 1700–2400 ng ml^{-1}. The plasma half-life after stopping the infusion was calculated to be 79$\pm$8 minutes but blood samples were taken for 2 hours only and so this may have been an underestimate[14]. Metabolite I appeared as early as 5 minutes after injection of the loading dose and metabolite II after 20 minutes. Maximum concentrations of these metabolites were observed 3 hours after induction of anaesthesia.

In a preliminary study in patients undergoing cholecystectomy we have given a bolus dose of ketamine 1 mg kg^{-1} i.v. at the beginning of surgery followed by a constant rate infusion of $3 \mu g \, kg^{-1} \, min^{-1}$ for 24 hours in an attempt to produce analgesia without impairment of consciousness. This regime is calculated to produce a steady-state concentration of about $200 \, ng \, ml^{-1}$; preliminary results of a clinical study with the regimen are good.

Paediatrics

In a study of children aged 4–10 years undergoing minor elective surgery, ketamine in doses of $2 \, mg \, kg^{-1}$ i.v. and $6 \, mg \, kg^{-1}$ i.m. resulted in plasma ketamine concentrations which were almost identical to those observed in adult patients (Figs. 10.2 and 10.3). There was, however, a trend towards more rapid absorption in children after i.m. administration[15].

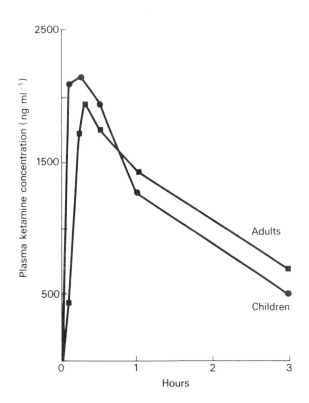

Fig. 10.3 Mean plasma ketamine concentrations up to 3 hours after administration of ketamine $6 \, mg \, kg^{-1}$ i.m. to 3 adults and 5 children.

Plasma concentrations of metabolite I in children were double those in adults although the times of peak concentrations did not differ. It is not known whether this is due to faster formation or slower elimination of metabolite I or both. Detailed pharmacokinetic analysis is not possible because ethical considerations precluded the withdrawal of more than five samples of blood from these children. After ketamine

3 mg kg^{-1} i.v. to paediatric patients, Allen and his colleagues[1] reported that the apparent volumes of distribution of the central compartment in children under 6 months of age was greater than in older children. No other differences in pharmaco-kinetic parameters were demonstrated, but blood samples were taken for only one hour.

There are reports of variation in response to ketamine with age and in particular, a suggestion that children are resistant to the effects of the drug[21, 25]. We have measured plasma ketamine concentrations in nine children upon awakening after one hour of ketamine anaesthesia[15]. There was considerable variation in concentrations and these ranged from 870 to 3780 ng ml^{-1} (mean 2250 ± 400 ng ml^{-1} ($\pm$ SEM)). The concentrations were higher than those reported in adults on awakening (640 ng ml^{-1}[17], and 700–1100 ng ml^{-1}[19]). Therefore, any increased ketamine requirements in children may result from decreased sensitivity to the drug rather than from a difference in pharmacokinetics.

Ketamine isomers

The ketamine molecule contains a chiral centre with two optical isomers or enantiomers. Almost all published studies and pharmacokinetic data relate to the racemic mixture. Recently, White and colleagues[29, 30] have reported the patterns of formation and excretion of ketamine metabolites to be similar after the administration to man of the ($+$) or ($-$) enantiomers or the racemic mixture in equi-anaesthetic doses. However, there are some important differences in the pharmacological action of the optical isomers. For example, ($+$) ketamine is a more potent anaesthetic and analgesic than ($-$) ketamine (potency ratio 3.4:1). These differences appear to be due to pharmacodynamic rather than to pharmacokinetic factors.

SUMMARY

The pharmacological action produced by ketamine depends upon the plasma ketamine concentration. Therefore the effect observed and the duration of the effect are determined by the dose and the route of administration. Anaesthesia and analgesia are associated with plasma ketamine concentrations greater than about 640 and 150 ng ml^{-1}, respectively.

The pharmacokinetics of intravenous ketamine is characterised by a very rapid initial alpha-disposition phase. This corresponds to a short period of anaesthesia after a dose of 1–2 mg kg^{-1}, or of analgesia after a dose of 0.25 mg kg^{-1}. These short periods of activity severely limit the usefulness of intravenous ketamine as an agent for maintenance anaesthesia or for analgesia. However, there is a slow decrease of plasma ketamine concentrations during the post-distribution beta phase and after anaesthetic doses the concentrations remain above 150 ng ml^{-1} for several hours, giving a useful period of pain relief.

Although absorption from an intramuscular site is rapid, relatively high doses (6 mg kg^{-1}) have been used so as to achieve an early onset of anaesthesia. However, absorption continues for a further 20–40 minutes and anaesthetic concentrations persist for 2–3 hours after injection, making post-operative recovery unacceptably protracted. In adults the lower dose of 2 mg kg^{-1} would fail to induce anaesthesia in some patients and in others the delay would be unacceptably long. Therefore the intramuscular route is not satisfactory for induction of anaesthesia in adults.

In contrast, absorption in children from an intramuscular injection (6 mg kg^{-1}) is faster than in adults receiving the same dose, and induction is very rapid. Since peak concentrations are reached earlier in children, concentrations decline faster after the peak. This behaviour, together with the observation that awakening occurs at higher concentrations in children, makes the intramuscular route very acceptable in children.

In a lower dose (0.5 mg kg^{-1}) a single intramuscular injection in adults produces analgesia for 30–45 minutes without loss of consciousness.

For post-operative pain relief ketamine may be given by intravenous infusion at a low rate (3 μg kg^{-1} min^{-1}) if preceeded by a loading dose (1 mg kg^{-1} intravenously). This infusion rate, which is much lower than those reported by other investigators, is being evaluated in patients in the post-operative period.

Acknowledgement

We are grateful to the Scottish Hospital Endowments Research Trust for financial support and to Parke-Davis & Co. for the supply of ketamine, norketamine, dehydronorketamine and the bromo-analogue of ketamine.

REFERENCES

1. ALLEN P. D., REYNOLDS R. N., MADDIE R. M. & ORSULAK P. J. (1980) The pharmacokinetics of ketamine in the pediatric surgical patient. *Anesthesiology* **53**, S333.
2. BORONDY P. E. & GLAZKO A. J. (1977) Inhibition of ketamine metabolism by diazepam. *Fed. Proc.* **36**, 938.
3. CHANG T. & GLAZKO A. J. (1972) A gas chromatographic assay for ketamine in human plasma. *Anesthesiology* **36**, 401–404.
4. CHANG T. & GLAZKO A. J. (1974) Biotransformation and disposition of ketamine. *Int. Anesth. Clin.* **12**, 157–77.
5. CHANG T., SAVORY A., ALBIN M., GOULET R. & GLAZKO A. J. (1970) Metabolic disposition of tritium-labelled ketamine in normal human subjects. *Clin. Res.* **18**, 597.
6. CHEN G. (1969) The pharmacology of ketamine. In Kreuscher (ed.), *Anesthesiology and Resuscitation*, Vol. 40, pp. 1–11. Springer-Verlag, New York.
7. CLEMENTS J. A. & NIMMO W. S. (1981) The pharmacokinetics and analgesic effect of ketamine in man. *Br. J. Anaesth.*, **53**, 27–31.

8. CLEMENTS J. A., NIMMO W. S. & GRANT
I. S. (1982) Bioavailability, pharmacokinetics and analgesic activity of ketamine in man. *J. Pharmaceut. Sci.* **71**,
539–42.

9. COHEN M. L., CHAN S. L., WAY W. L. &
TREVOR A. J. (1973) Distribution in the
brain and metabolism of ketamine in the
rat after intravenous administration.
Anesthesiology **39**, 370–6.

10. COHEN M. J. & TREVOR A. J. (1974) On
the cerebral accumulation of ketamine
and the relationship between metabolism
of the drug and its pharmacological
effects. *J. Pharmacol. Exp. Ther.* **189**,
351–8.

11. DAWSON B., MICHENFELDER J. D. &
THEYE R. (1971) Effect of ketamine on
canine cerebral blood flow and metabolism. *Anesth. Analg.* **50**, 443–7.

12. DOMINO E. F. (1980) Ketamine: isomers
and metabolites. In Rugheimer & Zindler
(eds.), *Anaesthesiology*, International
Congress Series 538, Excerpta Medica
pp. 696–699.

13. GHONEIM M. M. & KORTTILA K. (1977)
Pharmacokinetics of intravenous anaes-
thetics: implications for clinical use. *Clin.
Pharmacokin.* **2**, 344–72.

14. GIBALDI M. & WEINTRAUB H. (1971)
Some considerations as to the determination and significance of biologic half-
life. *J. Pharm. Sci.* **60**, 624–26.

15. GRANT I. S., CLEMENTS J. A., MCNICOL
L. R. & NIMMO W. S. (1983) Phar-
macokinetics of ketamine in children.
Br. J. Anaesth. (in press).

16. GRANT I. S., NIMMO W. S. & CLEMENTS
J. A. (1981) Pharmacokinetics and anal-
gesic effects of i.m. and oral ketamine. *Br.
J. Anaesth.* **53**, 805–9.

17. IDVALL J., AHLGREN I., ARONSEN K. F.
& STENBERG P. (1979) Ketamine infusions: pharmacokinetics and clinical
effects. *Br. J. Anaesth.* **51**, 1167–72.

18. JOHNSON M. (1972) The prevention of
ketamine dreams. *Anaesth. Intens. Care*
1, 70–4.

19. LITTLE B., CHANG T., CHUCOT L., DILL
W. A., ENRILE L., GLAZKO A. J., JASSINI
M., KRETCHMER H. & SWEET A. Y.
(1972) A study of ketamine as an ob-
stetrical anaesthetic agent. *Am. J. Obstet.
Gynaecol.* **113**, 247–60.

20. LO J. L. & CUMMING J. F. (1975)
Interaction between sedative premedi-
cants and ketamine in man and in isolated
perfused rat livers. *Anesthesiology* **43**,
307–12.

21. LOCKHART C. H. & NELSON W. L. (1974)
The relationship of ketamine requirement to age in pediatric patients. *Anesthesiology* **40**, 507–510.

22. MARIETTA M. P, WHITE P. F., PUDWILL
C. R., WAY W. L. & TREVOR A. J. (1976)
Biodisposition of ketamine in the rat: self
induction of metabolism. *J. Pharm. Exp.
Ther.* **196**, 536–44.

23. MIRKIN B. L. (1973) Drug distribution in
pregnancy. In Boreus (ed.) *Fetal Pharmacology*, pp. 1–26. Raven Press, New
York.

24. STENBERG P. & IDVALL J. (1981) Does
ketamine metabolite II exist in vivo? *Br.
J. Anaesth.* **53**, 778.

25. SUSSMAN D. R. (1974) A comparative
evaluation of ketamine anaesthesia in
children and adults. *Anesthesiology* **40**,
459–62.

26. VICKERS M. D., WOOD-SMITH F. G. &
STEWART H. C. (1978) In *Drugs in
Anaesthetic Practice*, 5th edition, p 48.
Butterworth, London.

27. WHITE P. F., HAM J., WAY W. L. &
TREVOR A. J. (1980a) Pharmacology of
ketamine isomers in surgical patients. In
Rugheimer & Zindler (eds.) *Anaesthesiology*, International Congress Series
538, Excerpta Medica pp. 732–4.

28. WHITE P. F., HAM J., WAY W. L. &
TREVOR A. J. (1980b) Pharmacology of
ketamine isomers in surgical patients.
Anaesthesiology **52**, 231–9.

29. WHITE P. F., JOHNSTON R. R. & PUDWILL
C. R. (1975) Interactions of ketamine and
halothane in rats. *Anesthesiology* **42**,

179–86.

30. WHITE P. F., MARIETTA M. P., PUDWILL C. R., WAY W. L. & TREVOR A. J. (1976) Effect of halothane anaesthesia on the biodisposition of ketamine in rats *J. Pharm. Exp. Ther.* **196**, 545–55.

31. WIEBER J., GUGLER R., HENGSTMANN J. H. & DENGLER H. J. (1975) Pharmacokinetics of ketamine in man. *Anaesthetist* **24**, 260–3.

32. WILKINSON G. R. & SHAND D. G. (1975) A physiological approach to hepatic clearance. *Clin. Pharm. Therap.* **18**, 377–90.

11 Pharmacokinetics of Muscle Relaxants and their Antagonists

RONALD D. MILLER

Pharmacokinetics refer to the rates of distribution, metabolism and excretion of a drug and/or its metabolites. Pharmacodynamics describe the relationship between the blood concentration of a drug and its effect. The pharmacokinetics and pharmacodynamics of muscle relaxants and their antagonists have been recently reviewed by the author of this chapter[36] and by Hull[25], and Cronnelly and Morris[6]. These reviews served as the basis for this manuscript. The precise relationship between the dose of drug and the time-course of effect is dependent on both pharmacokinetic and pharmacodynamic factors.

One of the problems in attempting to derive a more accurate dosage regimen for muscle relaxants and a more meaningful interpretation of drug concentration relative to neuromuscular blockade has been the inability to measure concentrations of muscle relaxants at their sites of action. To help solve this problem, the technique of compartmental analysis has come into use. Feldman, however, argues that making mathematical models to represent the complexities of the human body is seldom worthwhile[19]. Confusion probably occurs when one views a compartment as a specific anatomical entity, because this is rarely appropriate.

A compartment is simply a theoretical entity defined kinetically in terms of the rate of change in its drug concentration relative to the drug concentration in plasma, the biological specimen most readily available for pharmacokinetic studies. A compartment may represent many different types of tissues and organs that have in common the rate at which the particular drug under discussion enters and leaves them. In fact, it is impossible to assign with certainty a given organ or tissue to a particular pharmacokinetic compartment until one actually measures the change of drug concentrations in that tissue or organ over time and in relation to plasma concentrations measured simultaneously. Nevertheless, it is useful to construct theoretical pharmacokinetic models in order to summarise the disposition of a dose of that drug in the body and to predict the consequences of different dosage regimens. To the extent that the model fails to provide accurate predictions, it will have to undergo revision. Once the predictive function is realised, the model can serve its function in allowing the anaesthesiologist and the investigator to use drugs more efficiently and rationally; that is, to produce and to maintain the desired effects with a minimum of toxicity for the patient, and to produce and to maintain steady state conditions for investigations of drug actions. These objectives can and have been achieved with the help of pharmacokinetic models even though the anatomical and physiological significance of their compartments were uncertain. The amount of muscle relaxant in a compartment as a function of time can be assessed without knowing where that compartment is physically located in the body[48].

More physiologically- and anatomically-based models may be easier for clinicians to accept. However, the development of such models is limited because they require the analysis of drug concentrations in a very large number of tissue samples, certainly beyond the realm of possibility for human investigations. Furthermore, average organ size and blood flows must be assumed.

A simpler approach is to characterise drug distribution and elimination using only the dose, plasma concentrations and time. Despite Feldman's reservations, a pharmacokinetic analysis can be extremely important. For example, Katz has described the variability in the responses of patients to muscle relaxants[27]. Much of the variability can be explained by differences among patients in the pharmacokinetics of muscle relaxants. Undoubtedly, diseases and physiological changes alter the rate at which the muscle relaxants are distributed to tissues by the circulatory system and are eliminated from the body (e.g. renal failure). Many of the drugs anaesthetists administer may alter the pharmacokinetics of muscle relaxants and their antagonists (e.g. inhaled anaesthetics). If all these factors were known, muscle relaxant dose could be more precise and much of the variability among patients, and even within the same patient under different conditions, could be avoided.

Of course, drugs, diseases and physiological changes may also alter the sensitivity of the neuromuscular junction to relaxants (e.g. myasthenia gravis). But here again, pharmacokinetics can be useful in the design of studies intended to measure differences in sensitivity, and pharmacokinetics can assist in calculating the dosage adjustments indicated by the altered sensitivity to relaxants.

ANALYTICAL TECHNIQUES

Until recently, pharmacokinetic data have not been available because analytical methods to measure muscle relaxant concentrations in blood and other body tissues were limited in sensitivity and specificity for the active (unchanged) form of the relaxant. However, in the last nine years, assays for all nondepolarising muscle relaxants and their antagonists have been developed. Horowitz and Spector developed a radioimmunoassay for +-tubocurarine that was later modified to measure metocurine concentrations in body tissues[24, 30]. This technique had the advantage over the previously developed fluorimetric method of being more sensitive and it did not require extraction of the drug from biological fluids. Sensitive and specific assays for neostigmine, pyridostigmine and edrophonium have been developed using high pressure liquid chromatography[10]. Pancuronium has proven to be a difficult compound to assay. Virtually all the pharmacokinetic studies of pancuronium have used the fluorimetric method developed by Kersten *et al.*[28]. This method can estimate concentrations above 1.5 μg, but is not specific, that is, the assay does not distinguish between unchanged pancuronium and its metabolites[1]. Recently, Paanakker and Van der Laar (in prep.) developed a high pressure liquid chromatographic method to analyse pancuronium. This technique is specific, but unfortunately is not especially sensitive (50 ng ml^{-1}). We recently developed a mass spectrometric method for analysing pancuronium and vecuronium (ORG NC 45), a new short-acting nondepolarising muscle relaxant[41]. Although this technique is time-consuming and tedious, it is sensitive in that it will detect concentrations of 1 ng ml^{-1} or more. Although the methods are not yet applicable to routine clinical practice, the reader should be aware of the problems and limitations of these assays, without which a pharmacokinetic analysis is impossible.

PHARMACOKINETICS IN NORMAL SUBJECTS

The general factors which govern the pharmacokinetics of muscle relaxants are nicely summarised by Crankshaw and Cohen[4]. Basically, they can be subdivided into two groups:

1 Factors which influence the amount of free drug in the blood stream;
2 Factors which influence the transfer of muscle relaxants between the blood stream and the neuromuscular junction.

The amount of free muscle relaxant in the bloodstream is the crucial factor dictating the amount of muscle relaxant that ultimately reaches the neuromuscular junction. Once a muscle relaxant is administered intravenously, the concentration of the relaxant in the bloodstream will be determined by the volume and the dose of the drug injected, the rate at which the drug is injected, and the blood circulation time. Dispersion of the bolus of drug will only be complete after a number of recirculations. Another important factor is the amount of neuromuscular blocking drug bound to plasma proteins. Obviously when a drug is highly bound to proteins only a very small amount of it is readily available for diffusion out of capillaries and into the neuromuscular junction.

There are three primary processes by which the muscle relaxants are removed from the bloodstream. First is biotransformation. Suxamethonium is the only muscle relaxant which is extensively metabolised and it occurs mainly in plasma. Pancuronium and fazadinium are metabolised to a lesser extent in the liver. Conversely, +-tubocurarine, metocurine and gallamine appear to be eliminated completely unchanged. Excretion into urine by the kidney or into bile and gut by the liver are the other two processes by which drug is removed from the blood stream and ultimately from the body. These primary elimination factors will be summarised below. However, there are other routes of elimination from the blood stream, which probably include various exocrine glands, particularly the salivary glands, and loss of drug into inactive tissue depots. The extent to which the muscle relaxants are eliminated by extrarenal and extrahepatic organs and distributed to inactive tissue depots has never been determined in man.

There are several factors which determine how rapidly the muscle relaxant is transferred from the blood stream to the neuromuscular junction. The neuromuscular junction apparently is perfused with blood at a much greater rate than muscle as a whole. There is minimal resistance to the transfer of skeletal muscle relaxants from blood plasma to the neuromuscular junction, the site of action of these drugs. Drug access to the postjunctional membrane, and perhaps to the motor nerve terminal, requires only distribution in the extracellular space and not passage across cellular membranes.

The rate of disappearance of muscle relaxant from plasma is characterised by a rapid initial phase followed by a slower one (Fig. 11.1). Distribution to tissues is the major cause of the initial decrease, whereas the slower decay is due to excretion primarily in urine and bile. Because muscle relaxants are highly ionised, they do not readily cross cellular membranes and, therefore, have a limited volume of distribution. The initial distribution volume is 80–140 ml kg^{-1}, and the distribution volume at steady-state (V_D^{ss}) usually is 200–450 ml kg^{-1}. This indicates that muscle relaxants do

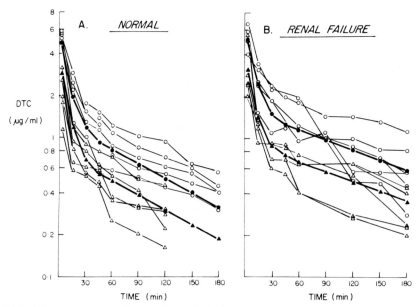

Fig. 11.1 Plasma concentration vs. time relationship of +-tubocurarine in patients with and without renal failure. The solid, dark line represents the estimated mean population response for the dose and the type of patient. The circles represent a dose of $0.5\,\text{mg kg}^{-1}$, and the triangles represent a dose of $0.3\,\text{mg kg}^{-1}$[48].

not distribute uniformly throughout the body, and it is in contrast to lipid soluble drugs (e.g. fentanyl, thiopental) which have a V_D^{ss} in excess of $2\,\text{l kg}^{-1}$. Tables 11.1–11.3 summarise the kinetic and dynamic data available in the literature.

FACTORS AFFECTING PHARMACOKINETICS

Renal failure

Because all of the nondepolarising muscle relaxants currently available for clinical use are dependent in large part on the kidney for their elimination, renal failure can profoundly affect their pharmacokinetics. Gallamine and decamethonium are entirely dependent on renal excretion for their elimination, and it is obvious that they should not be used in patients with impaired renal function. We believe that +-tubocurarine is the preferred nondepolarising muscle relaxant for patients with decreased renal function, for the reasons given below. However, one should keep in mind some of the limitations of the presently available data.

Recent studies in man indicate that +-tubocurarine is less dependent than pancuronium on renal excretion[25, 31]. Pancuronium disappeared from plasma at a much slower rate than +-tubocurarine in patients with renal failure; this finding is in

Table 11.1 Pharmacokinetic and pharmacodynamic data for pancuronium.

Investigators	Number of patients	Age (y)	Anaesthetic	$T_{\frac{1}{2}}^{\beta}$ (h)	Cl (ml kg^{-1} min^{-1})	V_D (ml kg^{-1})	C_P^0 (μg ml^{-1})
Normal							
McLeod et al.[34]	6	20–47	N$_2$O-halothane + narcotic	1.7	1.0	148	—
Somogyi et al.[49]	7	26–75	N$_2$O-halothane	2.2	1.8*	261	0.17 (80%)°
Duvaldestin et al.[11]	12	—	N$_2$O-narcotic	1.9	1.9	279	—
Miller et al.[37]	5	48±5	N$_2$O-narcotic	1.6	1.8	241	—
Somogyi et al.[52]	16	22–76	N$_2$O-halothane	—	1.9	304	0.21 (77%)°
Shanks et al.[47]	8	40–84	N$_2$O-narcotic	—	—	—	0.20 (50%)°
Hull et al.[26]				1.7	1.0	130	0.30 (50%)°
Westra et al.[58]				2.4	1.8	280	—
Duvaldestin et al.[15]	43	25–60	N$_2$O-narcotic	1.8	1.8	275	0.22 (70%)°
Cromnelly et al.[5]	4	—	N$_2$O-halothane	2.1	1.8	263	0.08 (50%)°
Aged							
McLeod et al.[33]	7	74–86	N$_2$O-narcotic	—	0.79	240	—
Duvaldestin et al.[15]†	28	75–86	N$_2$O-narcotic	3.4	1.2	320	0.20 (70%)°
Cirrhosis							
Duvaldestin et al.[11]†	14	36–64	N$_2$O-narcotic	3.5	1.5	416	—
Cholestasis							
Somogyi et al.[50]	9	52–80	N$_2$O(−)halothane	4.5	0.97	307	—
Westra et al.[58]†				3.7	1.5	430	—
Renal failure							
McLeod et al.[34]†	7	32–53	N$_2$O-halothane + narcotic	8.2	0.31	236	—
Somogyi et al.[51]	10	35–69	N$_2$O-halothane	4.3	0.8*	296	—

C_P^0 is the plasma concentration at which muscle twitch tension was depressed to the degree indicated in parenthesis (% depression from control).

* Data converted from ml min^{-1} to ml kg^{-1} min^{-1} by assuming a body weight of 70 kg.

† Compare the data to that from the same study for normal patients.

Table 11.2 Pharmacokinetic and pharmacodynamic data for +-tubocurarine.

Investigators	Number of patients	Age (y)	Anaesthetic	$T_{\frac{1}{2}}^{\beta}$ (h)	Cl (ml kg^{-1} min^{-1})	V_D (ml kg^{-1})	C_p^0 50 (μg ml^{-1})
Normal							
Matteo et al.[32]	48	16–72	N$_2$O-halothane or narcotic	—	—	—	0.45
Stanski et al.[53]	14	34±10	N$_2$O-narcotic	2.0	2.3	300	0.60
	7	40±13	N$_2$O-halothane (0.4–0.7%)	1.7	2.5	290	0.36
	7	32±6	N$_2$O-halothane (1–1.2%)	1.4	2.6	300	0.22
Matteo et al.[31]	18	—	N$_2$O-halothane	2.8	1.8	420	—
Ramzan et al.[43]	12	17–72	N$_2$O-narcotic	2.9	2.7	159	1.43 (60%)
Stanski et al.[54]	7	38±12	N$_2$O-enflurane	1.7	2.1	250	0.52
Ham et al.[23]	7	44±6	N$_2$O-narcotic	1.3	3.8	292	0.57
Renal failure							
Miller et al.[38, 48]	10	—	N$_2$O-halothane	2.2	1.5	250	0.38
Sheiner et al.[48]							
Hypothermia (31°C)							
Ham et al.[23]*	10	45±5	N$_2$O-narcotic	1.4	2.5	236	0.46

C_p^0 50 is the plasma concentration at which muscle twitch tension was depressed by 50% from control.
* Compare the data to that from the same study for normothermic patients.

Table 11.3 Pharmacokinetic and pharmacodynamic data for other nondepolarising relaxants.

Investigators	Number of patients	Age (y)	Anaesthetic	$T_{\frac{1}{2}}^{\beta}$ (h)	Cl (ml kg⁻¹ min⁻¹)	V_D (m kg⁻¹)	C_P^0 50 (μg ml⁻¹)
FAZADINIUM							
Normal							
Duvaldestin et al.[14]	10	20–52	N₂O-narcotic	1.3	2.1	234	—
Duvaldestin et al.[12]	11	—	N₂O-narcotic	1.4	(91)*	287	—
Cirrhosis							
Duvaldestin et al.[16]	8	42–61	N₂O-narcotic	2.6	(75)*	448	—
Cholestasis							
Duvaldestin et al. [16]	8	40–65	N₂O-narcotic	1.7	(82)*	350	—
Renal failure							
Duvaldestin et al.[12]	14	20–57	N₂O-narcotic	2.3	(65)*	310	—
GALLAMINE							
Normal							
Ramazn et al.[44]				2.3	1.2	210	5.82
Westra et al.[58]				2.7	1.2	240	—
Cholestasis							
Ramzan et al.[45]	7	35–67	N₂O-narcotic	2.7	1.2	247	—
Westra et al.[58]				3.7	0.9	260	—
Renal failure							
Ramzan et al.[46]				12.5	0.24	280	—
METUBINE							
Normal							
Mejer et al.[35]	5	—	N₂O-narcotic	3.6	1.4†	422	—
Brotherton & Matteo[2]				5.8	1.2	570	—
Renal failure							
Brotherton & Matteo[2]				11.6	0.38	480	—

Table 11.3 (Contd.)

Investigators	Number of patients	Age (y)	Anaesthetic	$T_{\frac{1}{2}}^{\beta}$ (h)	Cl (ml kg^{-1} min^{-1})	V_D (ml kg^{-1})	C_P^0 50 (μg ml^{-1})
VECURONIUM							
Normal							
Fahey et al.[17]	4	20–55	N$_2$O-halothane	1.3	3.2	194	—
Cronnelly et al.[5]	5	—	N$_2$O-halothane	1.1	5.3	268	0.09
Renal failure							
Fahey et al.[17]	4	20–55	N$_2$O-halothane	1.6	2.5	239	—

C_P^0 50 is the plasma concentration at which muscle twitch tension is depressed by 50% from control.

* Clearance reported as ml min^{-1} m^{-2} body surface area.

† Data converted from ml min^{-1} to ml kg^{-1} min^{-1} by assuming a body weight of 70 kg.

contrast to that in normal patients in which the rate of disappearance of both drugs was nearly the same (Fig. 11.2). However, it should be noted that the apparently slow elimination of pancuronium in patients with renal failure may in part represent the accumulation of relatively inactive metabolites which are dependent on the kidney for their elimination and are indistinguishable from the parent drug by the fluorometric assay used in this study[34]. (The radioimmunoassay for +-tubocurarine is specific for the unchanged drug[38]). Also, it is noteworthy that some investigators have not found such a marked prolongation of the elimination half-life of pancuronium, even though they used the same fluorometric assay[51]. All investigators agree that there is much greater variability in the elimination of muscle relaxants by patients with renal failure than by those with normal renal function. This probably reflects the varying degree of renal impairment as well as the presence of associated diseases, such as diabetes mellitus or anaemia, which conceivably affect drug disposition.

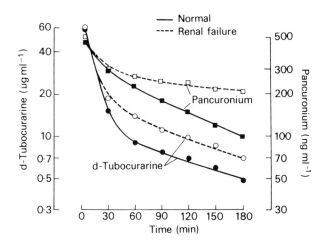

Fig. 11.2 Rates at which the plasma concentrations of +-tubocurarine and pancuronium decrease in patients with and without renal failure[34, 48]. Note that the decay rate for +-tubocurarine is about the same in patients with normal renal function. However, the decay rate for pancuronium is much slower in patients with renal failure.

+-tubocurarine also appears to be less dependent than metocurine on renal function for its elimination[35]. Brotherton and Matteo examined the pharmaco-kinetics of metocurine in anephric patients during and following renal transplantation[1]. In comparison to patients with normal renal function preoperatively and anaesthetised in a similar manner for a craniotomy, the patients with renal failure exhibited a markedly lower clearance, reduced urinary excretion (< 3 % vs. 43 % of the dose in 24 hours), and a prolonged elimination half-life (Table 11.3). The distribution volume of metocurine was somewhat lower and excretion in bile slightly higher (7 % vs. 2 % of the dose in 24 hours). The net effect was the retention of 22 % of the metocurine dose (0.3 mg kg^{-1}, i.v.) in the body (vs. 0.05 % in patients with normal kidneys) up to 24 hours after its injection. Fortunately, the neuromuscular blocking effects could be antagonised with neostigmine. Interestingly, the patients with renal failure appeared to be less sensitive to metocurine; they had a plasma concentration of 1.05 ng ml^{-1} at

90 % inhibition of the evoked compound electromyographic response, a concentration 2.3 times greater than that found in patients with normal kidneys[1].

What is the best way to determine the extent to which a drug is dependent on the kidney for its elimination? One method is simply to measure the percentage of the injected dose that is excreted in urine. However, only about 50 % of an injected dose of any of the nondepolarising relaxants is usually recovered in the urine of normal patients[1, 2, 12, 16, 31, 38]. Somewhat greater recoveries have been achieved for gallamine and pancuronium from patients with an indwelling urinary bladder catheter, but even then, about 30 % of the dose remains unaccounted for[16]. What happens to it? Although nondepolarising relaxants other than gallamine are probably excreted in bile, it seems improbable that this route alone can account for the unrecovered dose. Rather, it is likely that the relaxants are stored in body tissues for prolonged periods and are only excreted in very small quantities (analytically still undetectable) over a period of weeks. For example, + -tubocurarine binds to cartilage, and some have suggested this tissue represents a substantial pool for the drug[42]. Also, + - tubocurarine is taken up very rapidly by lysosomes. Lysosome-bound + -tubocurarine is not available for biliary excretion and remains in the lysosomes even when the concentration in the cytosol decreases to very low levels[56]. This may represent another site for prolonged storage of + -tubocurarine.

Perhaps a more appropriate method to determine the influence of renal failure on the pharmacokinetics of muscle relaxants is simply to compare the rate at which these drugs are cleared from the plasma of patients in the presence and absence of renal function. When this kind of analysis is performed, the more rapid clearance of D-tubocurarine makes it preferable to either metocurine or pancuronium in the patient with impaired renal function. However, if the anaesthetist follows the concept that the muscle relaxant least dependent on renal excretion for its elimination should be used when anaesthetising patients with impaired or absent renal function, suxamethonium appears to be the drug of choice. Although this author commonly utilises suxamethonium in patients with renal failure, it obviously is not suitable for longer cases because of the development of a profound phase II blockade.

Two new short-acting nondepolarising neuromuscular blocking drugs are currently in use in several countries. One or both may prove to be minimally dependent on the kidney for elimination from the body. Only 15–20 % of an injected dose of vecuronium (ORG NC 45) is eliminated in the urine of patients[17]. Although not confirmed in man, the major route of vecuronium's elimination from rats appears to be via the bile[55]. The other short-acting muscle relaxant, atracurium, may not be dependent on the kidney or liver for its excretion because of Hoffman elimination, a form of spontaneous breakdown of the quaternary ammonium groups at an alkaline pH. This mechanism of metabolism of atracurium remains to be proven. Also, current clinical studies of atracurium in patients with impaired renal or hepatic function indicate no increased duration of blockade in these types of patients.

Biliary tract or liver disease

Pancuronium and fazadinium are the only nondepolarising muscle relaxants which have been extensively studied from a pharmacokinetic point of view in patients with biliary or liver disease (Tables 11.1 and 11.3). Both the neuromuscular blockade and the elimination half-lives were prolonged in patients with extrahepatic biliary obstruction[16, 51, 58]. The prolonged elimination half-life has been attributed to an increased volume of distribution and to an increase in the plasma concentration of bile salts which inhibit the hepatic uptake of pancuronium (and also vecuronium)[57, 58]. Also, in patients with hepatic cirrhosis, the volumes of distribution of pancuronium and fazadinium were increased and their elimination half-lives prolonged[11]. The increased distribution volume could not be explained by a reduced binding of either drug to serum proteins as measured *in vitro*[13]. Under circumstances in which pancuronium is distributed to a larger volume, a larger dose may well be required to achieve a given degree of neuromuscular blockade. However, once that level of blockade has been achieved, it should last longer because of the slower elimination of pancuronium. Monitoring and recording the degree of neuromuscular blockade in patients with impaired hepatic function should demonstrate whether or not these predictions based on pharmacokinetics are correct.

Age

Only two reports examine the clinical impression that ageing alters the pharmaco-kinetics and pharmacodynamics of neuromuscular blocking drugs. McLeod *et al.* found that ageing decreased the clearance of pancuronium from plasma (Table 11.1)[33]. Unfortunately, neuromuscular blockade *per se* was not monitored and it is not possible to determine the effect of the decreased clearance from plasma on the intensity and duration of neuromuscular blockade by pancuronium. More recently, Duvaldestin *et al.* concluded that, because of the prolonged elimination half-life, elderly patients (75–86 y) had a duration of neuromuscular blockade from pan-curonium nearly twice as long as their younger counterparts (25–60 y)[15].

At the other end of the age scale, Fisher *et al.* attempted to perform a pharmacokinetic and dynamic analysis of +-tubocurarine in children[20]. They concluded that neonates and infants have an increased sensitivity to +-tubocurarine (lower blood concentration to achieve a given degree of neuromuscular blockade) compared with adult patients. However, because of a larger volume of distribution in neonates and infants, the initial dose required for the same degree of blockade did not differ from that required in adults. Because of a longer elimination half-life, the duration of +-tubocurarine neuromuscular blockade is probably prolonged in children compared to adults.

Hypothermia

In cats, hypothermia was found to prolong both +-tubocurarine and pancuronium-induced neuromuscular blockade [21, 37]. The blockade induced by either relaxant was prolonged because of delayed urinary and biliary excretion. With pancuronium, the block may have also been prolonged because of decreased metabolism to inactive metabolites [37]. More moderate degrees of hypothermia (31.8–35.8°C) had little effect on the pharmacokinetics of +-tubocurarine in man (Table 11.2) [23]. A larger temperature differential equivalent to that used in animal studies might have produced a temperature-dependent change in +-tubocurarine pharmacokinetics. Despite the apparent lack of influence of hypothermia on the pharmacokinetics of +-tubocurarine in man, recovery time (25–75% recovery of control twitch) was prolonged 82% by hypothermia as measured by twitch tension, but not by electromyography (Fig. 11.3) [23]. That mechanical recovery of neuromuscular blockade was prolonged by hypothermia, and electrical recovery was not, suggests that neuromuscular transmission *per se* was not significantly affected by hypothermia, at least within the moderately low temperature range studied. These results suggest that hypothermia affects the mechanical properties of the muscle itself. In fact, one patient had a marked prolongation of D-tubocurarine neuromuscular blockade which could not be fully antagonised by neostigmine and necessitated mechanical ventilation after operation until body temperature returned near normal. Also there was a tendency for the rate of equilibrium of D-tubocurarine concentrations between serum and the neuromuscular junction to be prolonged by hypothermia (Fig. 11.4) [23]. This suggests that hypothermia reduced blood flow to the neuromuscular junction and delayed the onset

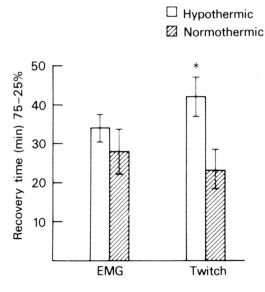

Fig. 11.3 The time (minutes, mean ± standard error) for spontaneous recovery of neuromuscular function from 75% to 25% depression of twitch tension [23]. EMG indicates the electromyographic response.

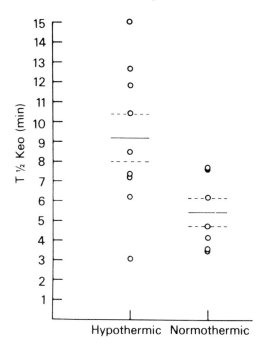

Fig. 11.4 The half-life for equilibrium of the serum concentration and the degree of paralysis as determined by the pharmacodynamic model. The solid line represents the mean and the dashed line represents the standard error[23].

of paralysis after administration of + -tubocurarine. However, other than the delayed half-life for equilibrium, the decrease in body temperature to 31.9° C did not significantly alter the pharmacokinetics of + -tubocurarine.

General anaesthetics

Despite differing effects on renal and liver function, the choice of general anaesthetic has little or no influence on the pharmacokinetics of + -tubocurarine. Although this is the only muscle relaxant to have been studied in this regard, the conclusions for + -tubocurarine may well apply to other nondepolarising muscle relaxants [53, 54]. In comparison to nitrous oxide-narcotic anaesthesia, halothane affects the pharmacodynamics of + -tubocurarine in two ways. First, it prolongs the time required for equilibrium between plasma concentrations and pharmacological effect, which is presumably due to decreased muscle perfusion during halothane anaesthesia. Secondly, halothane decreases the plasma concentration of + -tubocurarine required for neuromuscular blockade, which presumably means that the sensitivity of the neuromuscular junction to + -tubocurarine is increased during halothane anaesthesia (Fig. 11.5 and Table 11.2) [53]. Also, the neuromuscular blockade from + -tubocurarine is more variable in magnitude during nitrous oxide-narcotic anaesthesia, as compared to halothane anaesthesia (Fig. 11.5). From an investigative point of view, anaesthesia with halothane may be preferable to nitrous oxide-narcotic anaesthesia in order to

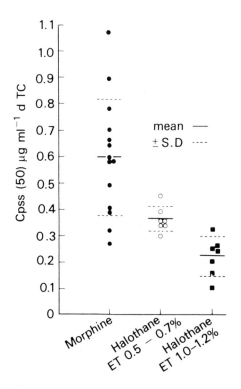

Fig. 11.5 Differences in sensitivity to +-tubocurarine (dTC) under different anaesthetic conditions. CP$_{ss}$ [50] is the steady-state plasma concentration that produces a 50% blockade of neuromuscular function. Lower plasma concentrations are required (i.e. greater sensitivity to dTC) during halothane-N$_2$O anaesthesia than during morphine-N$_2$O anaesthesia. Note the greater variability with the morphine-nitrous oxide technique[53].

decrease the variability of response in studies of muscle relaxants. From a clinical point of view, the variability emphasises the need to monitor the effect of muscle relaxants with a peripheral nerve stimulator, especially during nitrous oxide-narcotic anaesthesia.

Unlike halothane, the ability of enflurane to enhance a +-tubocurarine neuromuscular blockade was time-dependent. Despite a constant blood level of +-tubocurarine, paralysis increased at a rate of 9 ±4% per hour[54]. This finding has been confirmed by Fahey *et al.* in unpublished studies. It is thought that halothane achieves its maximum effect rapidly because it acts on neural tissue (e.g. central nervous system) where blood flow is high. Enflurane not only acts on the central nervous system, but also acts on the neuromuscular junction and skeletal muscle, where the rate of blood flow is less. Thus, a longer time is required for enflurane to achieve its maximal enhancement of a nondepolarising neuromuscular blockade.

Size of the initial dose

It has been popular among anaesthetists to administer an initial dose of muscle relaxant far exceeding that required to produce a 95–99% depression of twitch tension. Feldman [18] has proposed that a single large bolus of muscle relaxant given at the start of anaesthesia will produce prolonged, adequate paralysis with a relatively low plasma concentration of muscle relaxant at the end of anaesthesia. He further postulated that the use of frequently repeated small doses of muscle relaxant that are just sufficient to produce adequate paralysis will result in a higher post-operative concentration of muscle relaxant. With a higher concentration of muscle relaxant at the end of surgery, antagonism of this neuromuscular blockade would be more difficult[18]. Only Ham *et al.*[22] have examined the validity of this hypothesis. No difference was evident in the pharmacokinetics and pharmacodynamics of +-tubocurarine in a comparative study of three groups of patients given the drug by three dosage protocols: (a) 34 mg/70 kg as a large intravenous bolus; (b) repetitive smaller doses of about 8 mg/70 kg; (c) a continuous infusion of +-tubocurarine at a rate necessary to maintain a 90 % depression of twitch tension. There was also no difference in the ability of neostigmine to antagonise +-tubocurarine after any of the three dosage schedules[22]. Clearly these findings do not support Feldman's predictions.

If there is no advantage to administering a large overdose of muscle relaxant initially, why is it done? Certainly administering a large dose of muscle relaxant has its advantages. The onset of paralysis is more rapid after a larger dose, and this allows suxamethonium and pancuronium to be used for a rapid sequence of anaesthetic induction and endotracheal intubation. A large dose also provides excellent surgical conditions rapidly and mitigates the necessity of precisely regulating the anaesthetic dose. Nevertheless, this author believes that the use of small, frequent doses or a continuous infusion of muscle relaxant while monitoring neuromuscular function with a peripheral nerve stimulator may have advantages over the large bolus technique. For example, the duration of neuromuscular blockade needed for a surgical procedure is not always predictable in advance. The large dose technique may result in 100 % blockade, which cannot always be antagonised with anticholinesterase agents; with smaller doses or a continuous infusion, the extent of neuromuscular blockade can be varied more readily with changing surgical needs.

BIOTRANSFORMATION

Pancuronium

About 15–40 % of an injected dose of pancuronium is deacetylated to 3-OH, 17-OH, or 3,17-OH pancuronium derivatives. The metabolites have been studied individually in anaesthetised patients (Fig. 11.6)[37]. The 3-OH metabolite is the most prominent quantitatively in plasma after a dose of pancuronium and it is the most potent. It is half as potent as pancuronium (Fig. 11.7). Although the 3-OH metabolite has a duration of action similar to that of pancuronium and has similar pharmacokinetics, several questions remain. Is the block from the metabolite easily antagonised? Do the metabolites accumulate in patients with renal failure? With the development of the new

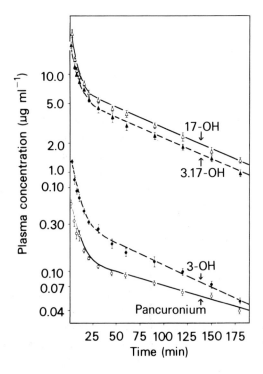

Fig. 11.6 Correlation between time and plasma concentration of pancuronium and its 3-OH, 17-OH, or 3,17-OH derivatives. The symbols and brackets represent the mean ± standard error. The lines were computed from pharmacokinetic data obtained in man[37].

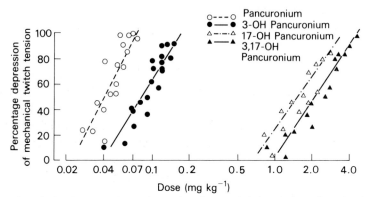

Fig. 11.7 Correlation between dose of muscle relaxant and depression of mechanical twitch tension. The lines represent the analysis of linear regression for pancuronium and its 3-OH, 17-OH and 3,17-OH derivatives, respectively[37].

mass spectrometry assay, answers to these questions will hopefully soon appear. There is little doubt that the metabolism of pancuronium is clinically important.

Suxamethonium

Few studies are available on the pharmacokinetics of the depolarising muscle relaxant, suxamethonium (succinylcholine). Only Dal Santo has actually measured the plasma concentrations of suxamethonium[9]. Suxamethonium is primarily metabolised by pseudocholinesterase to succinylmonocholine (a very weak blocking agent) and subsequently to succinic acid and choline. A common misconception is that the neuromuscular blockade from suxamethonium is terminated by its metabolism. In fact, metabolism in plasma dictates the amount of suxamethonium that actually reaches the neuromuscular junction. Dal Santo has shown that once paralysis occurs, it is the diffusion of suxamethonium away from the neuromuscular junction that is responsible for the dissipation of its neuromuscular blockade.

The short duration of the paralysing effect coincides with the rapid disappearance of suxamethonium from plasma as a result of both its biotransformation and its rapid passage into extravascular compartments. Urinary excretion of suxamethonium represents less than 10% of the dose and does not affect the kinetics of elimination significantly. Specifically, Dal Santo found in dogs that 80% of radioactive suxamethonium disappeared from the plasma and only 10% was found in the urine within five minutes after its administration. Seven hours later, 1.4% of the suxamethonium dose was still in plasma, but 70% of the radioactivity had been eliminated in the urine and 29% was untraced. The elimination products in urine consisted of primarily succinylmonocholine and choline; only small amounts of succinyldicholine were recovered. Unfortunately, pharmacokinetic studies of suxamethonium have not been performed in man.

FACTORS AFFECTING PHARMACODYNAMICS

Burn injuries

Recently, Martin *et al.* reported that the plasma concentration of + -tubocurarine necessary to produce a given neuromuscular blockade was markedly increased in patients who have been burned (Fig. 11.8)[29]. The apparent increase in the need for + -tubocurarine may be related to the increased number of receptors present at the neuromuscular junction when patients have been burned, bedridden, or have denervated tissue. An increased number of receptors may also account for the massive hyperkalaemic response to suxamethonium.

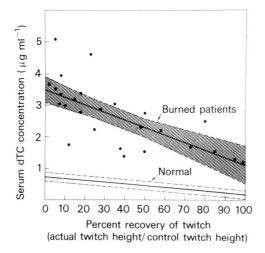

Fig. 11.8 Correlation between serum concentration of +-tubocurarine (dTC) and percent depression of twitch tension in patients with and without burn injuries. Note that the burn patients appear to be relatively resistant to +-tubocurarine[29].

PHARMACOKINETICS OF THE ANTAGONISTS

In the past five years, the pharmacokinetics of neostigmine, pyridostigmine and edrophonium have been determined while antagonising nondepolarising neuromuscular blockade in anaesthetised patients[8, 39, 40]. Edrophonium, 0.5 mg kg^{-1}, has a duration of action similar to that of neostigmine, 0.07 mg kg^{-1}. This is because neostigmine, pyridostigmine and edrophonium differ little in their pharmacokinetics and equivalent doses can be expected to have a similar duration of action (Table 11.4). The initial and steady state volumes of distribution for these drugs exceed normal plasma and extracellular volumes, as well as the distribution volumes of +-tubocurarine and pancuronium[35, 51]. These large volumes are remarkable since quaternary amines are not expected to cross cellular membranes easily, and the drugs are not highly bound to protein. Nevertheless, they appear to undergo extensive uptake by some tissue.

The effects of renal failure and kidney transplantation on the pharmacokinetics of the anticholinesterase drugs are important since they are used to antagonise the residual effects of nondepolarising muscle relaxants which are more slowly excreted and longer lasting in the absence of renal function. The pharmacokinetics of anticholinesterase drugs injected in patients one hour after receiving a renal transplant from a living relative are similar to those in patients with normal renal function[7, 8, 39, 40]. If, however, renal function is severely impaired or absent, elimination of these antagonists is decreased and their half-lives are prolonged (Table 11.4). The decrease in anticholinesterase clearance from plasma in anephric patients exceeds that reported for pancuronium and +-tubocurarine[35, 38, 51]. Reports of 'recurarisation' in anephric patients are, therefore, probably not the result of the muscle relaxant outlasting the antagonist. Rather the 'recurarisation' may involve interactions between

Table 11.4 Pharmacokinetic variables for anticholinesterase drugs in anaesthetised patients with and without renal function.

Drug	Kidney status	$T_{\frac{1}{2}}^{\beta}$ (min)	Cl (ml kg^{-1} min^{-1})	V_D^{ss} (l kg^{-1})
Neostigmine[8] (0.07 mg kg^{-1})	normal	80	9.0	0.70
	anephric	183	3.4	0.78
Pyridostigmine[7] (0.35 mg kg^{-1})	normal	112	8.6	1.10
	anephric	379	2.1	1.00
Edrophonium[39] (0.5 mg kg^{-1})	normal	110	9.6	1.10
	anephric	206	2.7	0.68

antibiotics or diuretics with the residual muscle relaxant. Such interactions are not well antagonised by anticholinesterase drugs and muscle weakness could occur even in the presence of an antagonist in a normally adequate concentration.

Edrophonium (Tensilon) antagonism of a nondepolarising neuromuscular blockade was formerly thought to be unreliable and too short in duration. However, by increasing the dose from 10 mg/70 kg to 30–70 mg/70 kg, a prompt and sustained antagonism has been found[39]. Pharmacokinetic analysis indicates that edrophonium lacks significant pharmacokinetic differences from neostigmine (Table 11.4), and that the short duration of action after small doses is due to a rapid decline of its concentrations to less than the minimum required during the distribution phase. Larger doses allow effective concentrations to remain after the distribution phase is completed. In the latter case, the duration of action is determined by the slower elimination phase.

Since the pharmacokinetics and duration of action of edrophonium, 35–70 mg/70 kg, appear to be similar to those of neostigmine, 5 mg/70 kg, which drug should be used? Although neostigmine is the traditional choice, I believe that edrophonium's quicker onset of antagonism and lesser muscarinic side-effects represent advantages over pyridostigmine and neostigmine. In fact, edrophonium requires half the amount of atropine than does an equivalent dose of neostigmine[7].

GLOSSARY

Generic		Trade
British	American	
Atracurium		
Fazadinium		
Metocurine		Metubine
Pancuronium		Pavulon
Suxamethonium	Succinylcholine	Anectine
+-Tubocurarine		
Vecuronium (ORG NC 45)		

REFERENCES

1. AGOSTON S., VERMEER G. A., KERSTEN U. W. & MEIJER D. K. F. (1973) The fate of pancuronium bromide in man. *Acta Anaesthesiol. Scand.* **17**, 267–75.

2. BROTHERTON W. P. & MATTEO R. S. (1981) Pharmacokinetics and pharmacodynamics of metocurine in humans with and without renal failure. *Anesthesiology* **55**, 273–6.

3. BUZELLO W. & AGOSTON S. (1978) Pharmacokinetics of pancuronium in patients with normal and impaired renal function. *Anaesthesist* **27**, 291–97.

4. CRANKSHAW D. P. & COHEN E. N. (1975) Uptake, distribution and elimination of skeletal muscle relaxants. In Katz R. L. (ed.), *muscle relaxants*, p. 125, Excerpta Medica, Amsterdam.

5. CRONNELLY R., FISHER D. M., MILLER R. D., GENCARELLI P., NGUYEN-GRUENKE L. & CASTAGNOLI N. JR. (1983) Pharmacokinetics and pharmacodynamics of vecuronium (ORG NC 45) and pancuronium in anesthetized man. *Anesthesiology* **58**, 405–8.

6. CRONNELLY R. & MORRIS R. B. (1982) Antagonism of neuromuscular blockade. *Br. J. Anaesth.* **54**, 183–94.

7. CRONNELLY R., STANSKI D. R., MILLER R. D. & SHEINER L. B. (1980) Pyridostigmine kinetics with and without renal function. *Clin. Pharmacol. Ther.* **28**, 78–81.

8. CRONNELLY R., STANSKI D. R., MILLER R. D., SHEINER L. B. & SOHN Y. J. (1979) Renal function and the pharmacokinetics of neostigmine in anesthetized man. *Anesthesiology* **51**, 222–6.

9. DAL SANTO G. (1968) Kinetics of distribution of radioactive labeled muscle relaxants. *Anesthesiology* **29**, 435–43.

10. DE RUYTER M. G. M., CRONNELLY R. & CASTAGNOLI N. JR. (1980) Reversed-phase ion-pair liquid chromatography of quaternary ammonium compound. *J. Chromatograph.* **183**, 193–201.

11. DUVALDESTIN P., AGOSTON S., HENZEL E., KERSTEN U. W. & DESMONTS J. M. (1978) Pancuronium pharmacokinetics in patients with liver cirrhosis. *Br. J. Anaesth.* **50**, 1131–5.

12. DUVALDESTIN P., BERTRAND J. C., CONCINA D., HENZEL D., LARENG L. & DESMONTS J. M. (1979) Pharmacokinetics of fazadinium in patients with renal failure. *Br. J. Anaesth.* **51**, 943–6.

13. DUVALDESTIN P. & HENZEL D. (1982) Binding of tubocurarine, fazadinium, pancuronium and ORG NC 45 to serum proteins in normal man and in patients with cirrhosis. *Br. J. Anaesth.* **54**, 513.

14. DUVALDESTIN P., HENZEL D.,

DEMETRIOU M. & DESMONTS J. M. (1978) Pharmacokinetics of fazadinium in man. *Br. J. Anaesth.* **50**, 773–7.

15. DUVALDESTIN P., SAADA J., BERGER J. L., D'HOLLANDER, A. & DESMONTS J. M. (1982) Pharmacokinetics, pharmacodynamics, and dose-reponse relationship of pancuronium in control and elderly subjects. *Anesthesiology* **56**, 36–40.

16. DUVALDESTIN P., SAADA J., HENZEL D. & SAUMON G. (1980) Fazadinium pharmacokinetics in patients with liver disease. *Br. J. Anaesth.* **52**, 789–94.

17. FAHEY M. R., MORRIS R. B., MILLER R. D., NGUYEN T. L. & UPTON R. A. (1981) Pharmacokinetics of ORG NC 45 (Norcuron) in patients with and without renal failure. *Br. J. Anaesth.* **53**, 1049–53.

18. FELDMAN S. A. (1973) The rational use of muscle relaxants. In Feldman, *Muscle Relaxants*, 1st edition, p. 149, W. B. Saunders, London.

19. FELDMAN S. A. (1980) (Letter to the editor) *Surv. Anesth.* **24**, 266.

20. FISHER D. M., O'KEEFE C., STANSKI D. R., CRONNELLY R., MILLER R. D. & GREGORY G. A. (1982) Pharmacokinetics and pharmacodynamics of d-tubocurarine children and adults. *Anesthesiology* **57**, 203–8.

21. HAM J., MILLER R. D. & BENET L. Z. (1978) Pharmacokinetics and pharmacodynamics of d-tubocurarine hypothermia in the cat. *Anesthesiology* **49**, 324–9.

22. HAM J., MILLER R. D., SHEINER L. B. & MATTEO R. S. (1979) Dosage-schedule independence of d-tubocurarine pharmacokinetics and pharmacodynamics, and recovery of neuromuscular function. *Anesthesiology* **50**, 528–33.

23. HAM J., STANSKI D. R., NEWFIELD P. & MILLER R. D. (1981) Pharmacokinetics and dynamics of d-tubocurarine during hypothermia in humans. *Anesthesiology* **55**, 631–5.

24. HOROWITZ P. E. & SPECTOR S. (1973) Determination of d-tubocurarine concentration by immunoassay. *J. Pharm.*

Exp. Ther. **185**, 94–100.

25. HULL C. J. (1982) Pharmacodynamics of non-depolarizing neuromuscular blocking agents. *Br. J. Anaesth.* **54**, 169–82.

26. HULL C. J., ENGLISH M. J. M. & SIBBALD A. (1980) Fazadinium and pancuronium: A pharmacodynamic study. *Br. J. Anaesth.* **52**, 1209–21.

27. KATZ R. L. (1971) Clinical neuromuscular pharmacology of pancuronium. *Anesthesiology* **34**, 550–6.

28. KERSTEN U. W., MEIJER D. K. F. & AGOSTON S. (1973) Fluorimetric and chromatographic determination of pancuronium bromide and its metabolites in biological materials. *Clin. Chim. Acta* **44**, 59–66.

29. MARTIN J. A. J., SZYNFELBEIN K., ALI H. H., MATTEO R. S. & SAVARESE J. J. (1980) Increased d-tubocurarine requirement following major thermal injury. *Anesthesiology* **52**, 352–5.

30. MATTEO R. S. & KHAMBATTA H. J. (1979) Relation of serum metocurine concentration to neuromuscular blockade in man. *Anesthesiology* **57**, S287.

31. MATTEO R. S., NISHITATENO K., PUA E. K. & SPECTOR S. (1980) Pharmacokinetics of d-tubocurarine in man: Effect of an osmotic diuretic on urinary excretion. *Anesthesiology* **52**, 335–8.

32. MATTEO R. S., SPECTOR S. & HOROWITZ P. E. (1974) Relationship of serum d-tubocurarine concentration to neuromuscular blockade in man. *Anesthesiology* **41**, 440–3.

33. MCLEOD K., HULL C. J. & WATSON M. J. (1979) Effects of ageing on the pharmacokinetics of pancuronium. *Br. J. Anaesth.* **51**, 435–8.

34. MCLEOD K., WATSON M. J. & RAWLINS M. D. (1976) Pharmacokinetics of pancuronium in patients with normal and impaired renal function. *Br. J. Anaesth.* **48**, 341–5.

35. MEIJER D. K. F., WEITERING J. G., VERMEER G. A. & SCAF A. H. J. (1979) Comparative pharmacokinetics of d-

tubocurarine and metocurine in man. *Anesthesiology* **51**, 402–7.

36. MILLER R. D. (1982) Pharmacokinetics of competitive muscle relaxants. *Br. J. Anaesth.* **54**, 161–7.

37. MILLER R. D., AGOSTON S., BOOIJ L. H. D. J., KERSTEN U. W., CRUL J. F. & HAM J. (1978) The comparative potency and pharmacokinetics of pancuronium and its metabolites in anesthetized man. *J. Pharmacol. Exp. Ther.* **207**, 539–43.

38. MILLER R. D., MATTEO R. S., BENET L. Z. & SOHN Y. J. (1977) The pharmacokinetics of d-tubocurarine in the man with and without renal failure. *J. Pharmacol. Exp. Ther.* **202**, 1–7.

39. MORRIS R. B., CRONNELLY R., MILLER R. D., STANSKI D. R. & FAHEY M. R. (1981) Pharmacokinetics of edrophonium and neostigmine when antagonizing d-tubocurarine neuromuscular blockade in man. *Anesthesiology* **54**, 399–402.

40. MORRIS R. B., CRONNELLY R., MILLER R. D., STANSKI D. R. & FAHEY M. R. (1981) Pharmacokinetics of edrophonium in anephric and renal transplant patients. *Br. J. Anaesth.* **53**, 1311–15.

41. NGUYEN T. L., GRUENKE L. D., UPTON R. A., CASTAGNOLI N. JR. & MILLER R. D. (1983) Quantitative analysis in biological fluids of the quaternary ammonium salts, pancuronium and norcuron (ORG NC 45) by direct insertion CIMS. *Biomed. Mass Spec.* (in press).

42. OLSEN G. D., CHAN E. M. & RIKER W. K. (1975) Binding of d-tubocurarine di(methyl-^{14}C) ether iodide and other amines to cartilage, chondroitin sulfate and human plasma proteins. *J. Pharm. Exp. Ther.* **195**, 242–50.

43. RAMZAN M. I., SHANKS C. A. & TRIGGS E. J. (1980) Pharmacokinetics of tubocurarine adminstered by combined i.v. bolus and infusion. *Br. J. Anaesth.* **52**, 893–9.

44. RAMZAN M. I., TRIGGS E. J. & SHANKS C. A. (1980) Pharmacokinetic studies in man with gallamine triethiodide: I. Single

and multiple clinical doses. *Eur. J. Clin. Pharm.* **17**, 135–43.

45. RAMZAN M. I., SHANKS C. A. & TRIGGS E. J. (1981) Pharmacokinetics and pharmacodynamics of gallamine triethiodide in patients with total biliary obstruction. *Anesth. Analg.* **60**, 289–96.

46. RAMZAN M. I., SHANKS C. A. & TRIGGS E. J. (1981) Gallamine disposition in surgical patients with chronic renal failure. *Br. J. Clin. Pharmacol.* **12**, 141–7.

47. SHANKS C. A., SOMOGYI A. A. & TRIGGS E. J. (1979) Dose-response and plasma concentration-response relationships of pancuronium in man. *Anesthesiology* **51**, 111–18.

48. SHEINER L. B., STANSKI D. R., VOZEH S., MILLER R. D. & HAM J. (1979) Simultaneous modeling of pharmacokinetics and pharmacodynamics: Application to d-tubocurarine. *Clin. Pharmacol. Ther.* **25**, 358–71.

49. SOMOGYI A. A., SHANKS C. A. & TRIGGS E. J. (1976) Clinical pharmacokinetics of pancuronium bromide. *Eur. J. Clin. Pharmcol.* **10**, 367–72.

50. SOMOGYI A. A., SHANKS C. A. & TRIGGS E. J. (1977) Disposition kinetics of pancuronium bromide in patients with total biliary obstruction. *Br. J. Anaesth.* **49**, 1103–8.

51. SOMOGYI A. A., SHANKS C. A. & TRIGGS E. J. (1977) The effects of renal failure on the disposition and neuromuscular blocking action of pancuronium bromide. *Eur. J. Clin. Pharmacol.* **12**, 23–9.

52. SOMOGYI A. A., SHANKS C. A. & TRIGGS E. J. (1978) Combined i.v. bolus and infusion of pancuronium bromide. *Br. J. Anaesth.* **50**, 575–82.

53. STANSKI D. R., HAM J., MILLER R. D. & SHEINER L. B. (1979) Pharmacokinetics and pharmacodynamics of d-tubocurarine during nitrous oxide-narcotic and halothane anesthesia in man. *Anesthesiology* **51**, 235–41.

54. STANSKI D. R., HAM J., MILLER R. D. & SHEINER L. B. (1980) Time-dependent

increase in sensitivity to d-tubocurarine during enflurane anesthesia in man. *Anesthesiology* **52**, 483–7.

55. UPTON R. A., NGUYEN T. L., MILLER R. D. & CASTAGNOLI N. JR (1982) Renal and biliary elimination of vecuronium (ORG NC 45) and pancuronium in rats. *Anesth. Analg.* **61**, 313–6.

56. WEITERING J. G., LAMMERS W., MEIJER D. K. F. & MULDER G. J. (1977) Localization of d-tubocurarine in rat liver lysosomes: Lysosomal uptake, biliary excretion and displacement by quinacrine in vivo. *Arch. Pharm.* **299**, 277–81.

57. WESTRA P., HOUWERTJES M. C., WESSELING H. & MEIJER D. K. F. (1981) Bile salts and neuromuscular blocking agents. *Br. J. Anaesth.* **53**, 407–15.

58. WESTRA P., VERMEER G. A., DE LANGE A. R., SCAF A. H. J., MEIJER D. K. F. & WESSELING H. (1981) Hepatic and renal disposition of pancuronium and gallamine in patients with extrahepatic cholestasis. *Br. J. Anaesth.* **53**, 331–8.

59. WINGARD L. B. & COOK D. R. (1976) Pharmacodynamics of tubocurarine in humans. *Br. J. Anaesth.* **48**, 839–45.

12 Pharmacokinetics of Local Anaesthetic Drugs

BENJAMIN G. COVINO

ABSORPTION PHASE
Site of injection
Dose of local anaesthetic
Addition of a vasoconstrictor
Pharmacological characteristics of local anaesthetic agents

DISTRIBUTION PHASE

ELIMINATION PHASE

PLACENTAL TRANSMISSION

FACTORS INFLUENCING PHARMACOKINETICS
Age
Acid–base status
Physiological status of the patient

CLINICAL SIGNIFICANCE OF LOCAL ANAESTHETIC PHARMACO-
    KINETICS

GLOSSARY

The kinetics of drug absorption, distribution, and elimination are important determinants of both clinical efficacy and potential toxicity. Most therapeutically useful agents are administered at a distance from their intended site of action. The rate and degree of absorption from the site of administration, the rate of delivery to and removal from the target organ will determine the ultimate effects of a particular agent. On the other hand, local anaesthetic drugs are usually administered close to their intended site of action, i.e. some specific portion of the peripheral or central nervous system. The effectiveness of local anaesthetic drugs will be influenced to some extent by the rate at which they disappear from the site of injection. However, the absorption, distribution and elimination of local anaesthetic drugs are major determinants of their systemic toxicity. The primary toxicity of local anaesthetic agents involves the central nervous system[16] and secondarily the cardiovascular system[50]. Most clinicians are familiar with the classical signs of local anaesthetic toxicity, i.e. CNS excitation followed by overt convulsive activity and systemic hypotension secondary to peripheral vasodilation and myocardial depression. These effects on the central nervous and cardiovascular systems are related to the concentrations of the local anaesthetic in the brain, peripheral vascular smooth muscle, and the heart, and in turn, to its concentration in plasma. The plasma and tissue levels of a particular local anaesthetic are determined by its pharmacokinetics, and these differ considerably among the local anaesthetics currently used in clinical practice.

The most common cause of toxic reactions to local anaesthetics is their accidental rapid intravascular injection. The intravenous toxicity of local anaesthetic agents is related primarily to their intrinsic anaesthetic potency[14]. However, the duration of a toxic reaction is related primarily to the distribution and elimination kinetics of the various drugs.

The toxicity of extravascularly administered local anaesthetic drugs is related in part to their local anaesthetic potency, but more importantly to their rate of vascular absorption, tissue redistribution, and elimination. The purpose of this chapter is to review the absorption, distribution and elimination kinetics of the various local anaesthetics and the factors which influence their pharmacokinetics. A clear understanding of the pharmacokinetics of local anaesthetic agents should be beneficial in the prevention of toxic reactions during the performance of regional anaesthesia.

ABSORPTION PHASE

The absorption of local anaesthetic agents is related primarily to the site of injection, dose, presence of a vasoconstrictor in the local anaesthetic solution, and the pharmacological profile of the specific local anaesthetic.

Site of injection

The rates of absorption of local anaesthetic agents from different anatomical sites vary markedly. In general, intercostal nerve blockade is associated with the most rapid rate of absorption and the highest plasma levels regardless of which agent is used[8, 51, 62]. The paracervical area and the caudal canal also represent sites of relatively rapid absorption[18, 21]. Higher plasma levels are seen following caudal and paracervical blocks as compared to lumbar epidural injections. Peripheral nerve blocks such as those of the brachial plexus and sciatic-femoral nerves result in slower absorption and lower plasma levels than occur following intercostal or epidural blocks[33, 62]. Finally, the slowest rate of absorption and the lowest plasma levels occur following subcutaneous and subarachnoid administration[26, 48]. For example, for every 100 mg of lignocaine injected into an adult human, a peak venous plasma level of approximately 1.5 μg ml^{-1} is attained following intercostal nerve blocks, 1.2 μg ml^{-1} following paracervical and caudal blocks, 1.0 μg ml^{-1} following injection into the

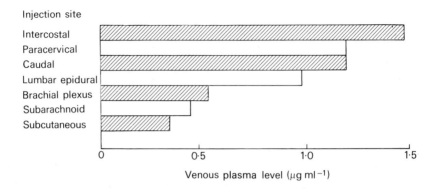

Injection site

Intercostal
Paracervical
Caudal
Lumbar epidural
Brachial plexus
Subarachnoid
Subcutaneous

0   0·5   1·0   1·5

Venous plasma level (μg ml⁻¹)

Fig. 12.1 Effect of injection site on peak venous plasma levels of lignocaine in adult humans.

lumbar epidural space, 0.6 μg ml^{-1} following brachial plexus block and approximately 0.3–0.4 μg ml^{-1} following subcutaneous and subarachnoid administration[62] (Fig. 12.1).

The differences in plasma levels following administration into various anatomical sites are related to a multiplicity of factors. The high plasma concentration following paracervical block is probably related to the great vascularity of this area. Intercostal nerve blockade requires multiple injections; thus, the local anaesthetic solution is exposed to a larger vascular surface area, resulting in a greater rate and degree of absorption. The higher plasma levels obtained following caudal anaesthesia as compared to lumbar epidural administration may reflect the greater vascularity of the bony tissue in the caudal canal. The lumbar epidural space contains considerable adipose tissue which serves as a depot site for local anaesthetic agents, thereby retarding their vascular absorption. Significant levels of lignocaine and etidocaine have been found in the epidural fat of sheep following epidural administration of these agents. Moreover, etidocaine, which is considerably more lipid soluble than lignocaine, was found to accumulate in epidural fat to a greater extent than lignocaine and also had a slower rate of absorption resulting in lower plasma levels.

This relationship of administration site to rate of drug absorption has obvious clinical implications, since the same dose of a local anaesthetic agent may be potentially more toxic in one injection area than in others. For example, average peak plasma levels in excess of 6 μg ml^{-1} have been reported with the use of 300 to 500 mg of lignocaine or mepivacaine for paracervical and intercostal nerve blockade as compared to average peak plasma levels of 3–5 μg ml^{-1} when the same dose of either drug was employed for lumbar epidural anaesthesia. Since adverse effects become manifest when the plasma level of lignocaine or mepivacaine exceeds 5 μg ml^{-1}, the potential for systemic toxicity is significantly greater following paracervical or intercostal nerve blockade compared to lumbar epidural anaesthesia, despite the use of the same total dose of local anaesthetic agent for both procedures.

The rate of local anaesthetic absorption differs for different muscular injection sites. A significantly higher peak plasma level occurs following administration of lignocaine into the deltoid muscle as compared to injection into the vastus lateralis and gluteus maximus[11, 37, 49]. The greater absorption from the deltoid muscle appears to reflect its greater blood flow[22]. Extremely low plasma levels of lignocaine following injection into the gluteus maximus may result from this region's greater adiposity, which tends to retard vascular absorption.

Absorption and toxicity from topical use of local anaesthetic agents also differ according to site of application. In general, absorption occurs most rapidly following intratracheal administration[3]. Systemic absorption and toxicity are less following intranasal instillation and administration into the urethra and urinary bladder[3]. These differences are due, in part, to the inherent variations in vascularity of the different anatomical sites and to the properties of the pharmaceutical preparations utilised for topical anaesthesia. For example, rapid absorption from the tracheo-bronchial tree is undoubtedly related not only to the vascularity of this area, but also to the use of anaesthetic sprays which tend to disperse the anaesthetic solution over a wide surface area. On the other hand, local anaesthetic agents are commonly applied to mucous membranes or instilled into the urethra in the form of an ointment or gel which tend to delay vascular absorption.

Intratracheal administration is a common practice prior to insertion of endo-tracheal tubes. Plasma levels varying from 2 to 5 μg ml^{-1} have been observed following the intratracheal administration of 200 mg of lignocaine in a spray form. Tetracaine appears to be absorbed very rapidly from the trachea; its LD_{50} is similar for intratracheal and intravenous administration. Several deaths have followed the use of intratracheal tetracaine.

The variability in the rate of absorption as a function of the injection site renders useless the concept of a single maximum dose of a local anaesthetic. For example, lignocaine concentrations above 5 μg ml^{-1} of plasma are associated with signs of CNS toxicity. Based on the rate of vascular absorption from various injection sites, the maximum dose of lignocaine should be approximately 350 mg for intercostal nerve blocks, 400 mg for paracervical blocks, 500 mg for lumbar epidural anaesthesia, 800 mg for brachial plexus blocks, and greater than 1000 mg for subcutaneous infiltration. At present, 200–300 mg is considered the maximum dose of lignocaine for any procedure. Clearly the practice of establishing the maximum recommended dose of a local anaesthetic in terms of its potential toxicity without considering the site of injection has little clinical relevance.

Chapter 12

Dose of local anaesthetic

There is a direct proportion between the total dose and the rate of absorption or peak plasma concentration of local anaesthetic (Table 12.1). There appears to be no significant correlation between body weight and the concentration resulting from a given dose in adult humans[63]. No studies of children or obese patients have yet been reported.

Table 12.1 Peak venous plasma levels of various local anaesthetics (without epinephrine) following lumbar epidural administration.

	Peak venous blood level (μg ml^{-1})							
Dose (mg)	100	150	200	300	400	500	600	900
Lidocaine	—	—	3.3	—	4.3	—	7.3	—
Prilocaine	—	—	1.7	—	2.7	—	4.5	5.2
Mepivacaine	—	—	—	—	—	—	5.6	—
Bupivacaine	0.8	1.3	—	—	—	—	—	—
Etidocaine	—	—	1.0	1.3	—	—	—	—

Some investigators have noted a non-linear relationship between the lumbar epidural dose of bupivacaine or etidocaine and their peak levels in venous plasma[14]. Others found a linear relationship in the range of doses (100 vs. 150 mg) used clinically (J. van Kleef & A. Burm, pers. commun.). Non-linearity for these very lipid-soluble drugs theoretically could reflect saturation of epidural lipids at very high concentrations, so that more of the dose remains free and available for systemic absorption. Also, the administration of large volumes or more concentrated solutions of these drugs may result in a greater degree of vasodilation, which would again favour a more rapid absorption.

The peak anaesthetic plasma level during regional anaesthesia is a function of the total dose of drug administered. Alterations in volume and concentration of lignocaine, prilocaine, and etidocaine within the clinical range do not influence the rate of absorption and subsequent peak venous blood level provided the total dose remains the same[33, 51]. Studies in animals originally suggested that the toxicity of certain local anaesthetics such as lignocaine increased as the concentration of local anaesthetic solution was increased[28]. However, the intramuscular injection of 2–64% lidocaine in rabbits showed little difference in the LD$_{50}$ provided the total dosage was kept constant[R. Boyes, pers. commun.].

Local anaesthetic agents do differ with regard to their peripheral vascular effects. Mepivacaine possesses less vasodilator activity than lignocaine and may exert a vasoconstrictor action in certain vascular beds[1]. Low concentrations of mepivacaine may result in a relatively slow rate of vascular absorption due to minimal effects on vascular tone in the area of injection. As the concentration of mepivacaine is increased, the vasodilator effect becomes dominant, resulting in an increased rate of vascular absorption.

Addition of a vasoconstrictor

A variety of vasoconstrictor drugs have been added to local anaesthetic solutions in an effort to decrease the rate of vascular absorption and thereby reduce the potential of systemic toxicity and prolong the duration of regional anaesthesia[51, 62]. Differences in the effectiveness of this approach exist among the local anaesthetics, the types of regional anaesthesia and the vasoconstrictors employed. For infiltration procedures, a significantly longer duration of anaesthesia occurs if epinephrine is added to any local anaesthetic solution. However, the duration of intradermal anaesthesia produced by lignocaine is prolonged to a greater degree than that of bupivacaine by the addition of epinephrine[12, 59].

With regard to peripheral nerve blocks, all of the currently available local anaesthetic agents appear to benefit from the addition of epinephrine (Table 12.2). Studies involving the interscalene approach to the brachial plexus in patients have shown approximately a 50% reduction in the peak venous plasma concentrations of lignocaine, prilocaine, etidocaine, and bupivacaine when these agents were administered in solutions containing epinephrine[68].

Table 12.2 Effect of epinephrine (5 μg ml^{-1}) on peak venous plasma levels (μg ml^{-1}) of various local anaesthetic agents.

	Lumbar epidural block			Brachial plexus block		
	Venous plasma concentration (μg ml^{-1})			Venous plasma concentration (μg ml^{-1})		
	Dose (mg)	Without epinephrine	With epinephrine	Dose (mg)	Without epinephrine	With epineprhine
Lidocaine	400	4.3	3.0	450	4.5	3.6
Prilocaine	400	2.7	2.2	450	2.3	1.2
Mepivacaine	500	5.0	3.2	500	3.7	3.0
Bupivacaine	100	0.79	0.74	150	2.2	1.2
Etidocaine	300	1.3	1.2	150	1.3	0.9

Differences exist concerning the effect of epinephrine in reducing the rate of vascular absorption (Table 12.2) and prolonging the duration of anaesthesia following central neural blocks. The addition of epinephrine to lignocaine or mepivacaine is associated with a significant prolongation in the duration of lumbar epidural anaesthesia and a significant decrease in the rate of vascular absorption[51, 62]. The addition of epinephrine to prilocaine has considerably less effect, and it has minimal if any influence on the duration of action and absorption of epidural bupivacaine or etidocaine[33, 63].

The effect of vasoconstrictors on the rate of absorption and duration of action of local anaesthetic agents administered intrathecally is unclear[40]. Both epinephrine and phenylephrine are believed to prolong the duration of spinal anaesthesia produced by tetracaine[35]. Epinephrine has been reported to exert little influence on the duration of spinal anaesthesia by lignocaine or bupivacaine[10] (D. B. Scott, pers. commun.). There was no retardation of vascular absorption of bupivacaine from the subarachnoid space of dogs when epinephrine was added to the anaesthetic solution[H. Feldman, pers. commun.]. These apparently conflicting results for tetracaine compared to the other local anaesthetics have not been adequately explained.

Epinephrine is the most commonly employed vasoconstrictor in local anaesthetic solutions. In the lumbar epidural space, a $1 : 80\,000$ concentration of epinephrine did not cause significantly greater reduction in the peak plasma level of lidocaine than a $1 : 200\,000$ concentration[8]. Injections into the gingival mucosa suggest that a $1 : 100\,000$ concentration of epinephrine $(10\ \mu\mathrm{g}\ \mathrm{ml}^{-1})$ is optimal in potentiating the anaesthetic activity of lignocaine[5]. Other vasoconstrictors such as phenylephrine, norepinephrine and felypressin have been added to local anaesthetic solutions. Theoretically, alpha-adrenergic receptor agonists such as phenylephrine or direct vascular smooth muscle stimulants such as felypressin should be more advantageous than a mixed alpha- and beta-agonist such as epinephrine. However, neither norepinephrine nor phenylephrine in concentrations of $1 : 20\,000$ appear to be as effective in reducing the rate of absorption of lidocaine and mepivacaine as epinephrine $1 : 200\,000$[17, 56]. On the other hand, phenylephrine appears to prolong the duration of spinal and epidural anaesthesia to a greater extent than does epinephrine[35, 56].

Pharmacological characteristics of local anaesthetic agents

The rate of absorption of local anaesthetic agents is also determined by the properties of the specific drugs. A comparison of agents of equivalent anaesthetic potency reveals that lidocaine and mepivacaine showed similar peak venous plasma concentrations while the peak levels of prilocaine were significantly lower following administration of identical doses of these agents for either epidural or brachial plexus anaesthesia (Table 12.2)[51, 68]. A comparison of the two more potent local anaesthetic agents, bupivacaine and etidocaine, reveals that the peak plasma level of etidocaine was significantly lower than that of bupivacaine following the lumbar epidural or interscalene administration of equal doses[33, 68]. The basis of these differences among equivalent anaesthetics is not clear.

DISTRIBUTION PHASE

Plasma concentrations of local anaesthetics following absorption from the injection site are a function of:

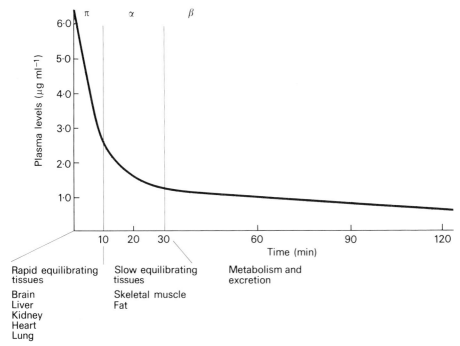

Fig. 12.2 Typical disappearance curve of local anaesthetic agents in plasma. Separation of disappearance curve into various compartments which represent fast (π) and slow (α) tissue distribution and elimination (β) by metabolism and excretion (β).

1 The rate of distribution from the vascular to tissue compartments; and
2 The rate elimination via metabolic and excretory pathways (Fig. 12.2).

The kinetics of the systemic disposition local anaesthetics are most easily determined following their intravenous administration. A bi- or triphasic decline of local anaesthetic concentration in plasma over time is evident for all agents (Fig. 12.2)[6, 63, 64]. The pi (π) phase represents the initial, fast disappearance of the drug from plasma into rapidly equilibrating tissues, i.e. highly perfused tissues. A second, slower distribution phase (alpha-phase) reflects drug distribution to slowly equilibrating tissues. The final or beta-phase is representative of the ultimate elimination of the drug from the body via metabolic and excretory ways. Keep in mind that all three phases begin concurrently as soon as the drug reaches the systemic circulation, and that the elimination or beta-phase continues after the effect of the distribution phases is minimised by (pseudo) equilibrium of the drug between plasma and the tissues.

The characteristics of the distribution phases of the amino-amide local anaesthetics appear to be related to the intrinsic lipophilicity of these agents and the relative amount of free drug in plasma. The latter is a function of the pKa and the degree of plasma protein binding. Prilocaine is the least protein-bound of the amide local anaesthetics[65]. Approximately 45 % of prilocaine exists in the free form in plasma which probably accounts for its short $T_{\frac{1}{2}}^{\pi}$, 29 seconds. Etidocaine and bupivacaine are highly bound to plasma proteins (95 %)[65]. Etidocaine possesses a shorter $T_{\frac{1}{2}}^{\pi}$ (129 seconds) than bupivacaine (162 seconds), although only 7–9 % of both agents exists in the free form in plasma. This more rapid rate of tissue distribution of etidocaine is undoubtedly related to its more lipophilic nature.

The $T_{\frac{1}{2}}^{\pi}$ is related to the rate of uptake of local anaesthetic agents by vessel-rich tissues, such as lung, brain, heart, liver and kidney. The lung, in particular, appears to play an important role in the removal of local anaesthetics from the circulation during the very early portion of the distribution phase. Tucker and Boas determined the plasma concentrations of lignocaine in the pulmonary artery and a peripheral artery following tourniquet release in subjects undergoing intravenous regional anaesthesia[66]. Pulmonary vs. peripheral arterial differences of 4–8 μg ml^{-1} were observed 15 seconds following cuff deflation, which indicated a 30 % uptake of lignocaine by lung tissue. Studies in pigs and man showed that 25 % of lignocaine was taken up by the lung within seconds following intravenous administration[45]. The percentage of local anaesthetic extracted by the lung is dose-related[31]. Forty percent of lignocaine was taken up by lung tissue of pigs immediately following i.v. injection of 0.5 mg kg^{-1}. At a dose of 2 mg kg^{-1} the maximum uptake fell to 25 % indicating that the ability of the lung to absorb local anaesthetics is limited. Human studies have shown that 80–90 % of the injected dose of lignocaine was extracted during the first passage through the lungs[32]. The site of uptake in the lungs is not known. Post and Lewis have reported that nortryptyline causes a 50 % reduction in the uptake of lignocaine by the lung[46].

Differences exist regarding the degree of accumulation of various local anaesthetic agents by the lung[14]. Measurements of prilocaine, lignocaine and etidocaine in lung tissue 10 minutes following subcutaneous injection in guinea pigs revealed significantly higher lung/plasma concentration ratios for prilocaine compared to the other agents. The ratios for lignocaine, in turn, were greater than those for etidocaine. The results suggest that plasma protein binding may be the most important determinant of lung uptake, since prilocaine, which is least protein bound, was concentrated to the greatest extent in the lung, while etidocaine, which is highly protein bound, showed the lowest levels.

Local anaesthetic agents are distributed throughout all body tissues, but the relative concentration in different tissues varies as a function of time after injection. The more highly perfused organs show higher concentrations than less well perfused organs immediately following drug administration. One minute following the intravenous injection of lignocaine, approximately 70 % of the injected dose was found in vessel-rich tissues[4]. Within 4 minutes approximately 30 % of the total injected dose of lignocaine was present in skeletal muscle. Although the concentration per gram of muscle tissue was not large, skeletal muscle is the largest mass of tissue in the body and serves as the greatest reservoir for local anaesthetic agents. Differences exist between the tissue levels of various local anaesthetic agents, for example, Sung and Truant observed higher levels of lignocaine compared to procaine in fat tissue and liver of rats[58]. Mepivacaine showed a distribution pattern similar to that of lignocaine, with a rapid accumulation in liver, kidney, salivary glands and brain[55]. A comparison of the tissue levels of etidocaine and bupivacaine in guinea pigs demonstrated a greater accumulation of etidocaine in adipose tissue[14].

The volume of distribution (V_D) is a calculated kinetic term representing the total distributive proterites of a drug. V_D does not represent a true physiological space, but is indicative of the extent to which a drug is taken up by body tissues. Drugs which are highly lipid soluble, such as etidocaine, and poorly bound to plasma proteins, such as prilocaine, tend to accumulate in various tissue compartments and so appear to have a large volume of distribution (Table 12.3). Calculation of the volume of distribution of various amide local anaesthetic agents reveals values which vary from 666 litres for etidocaine to values of 150–380 litres for mepivacaine, prilocaine, lignocaine and bupivacaine[63, 64].

Table 12.3 Pharmacokinetic properties of amide local anaesthetic agents.

	Lidocaine	Mepivacaine	Prilocaine	Bupivacaine	Etidocaine
V_D extrap (litres)	212	150	380	209	666
$T_{\frac{1}{2}}^{\pi}$ (s)	57	43	29	162	129
$T_{\frac{1}{2}}^{\beta}$ (min)	96	114	93	210	156
Cl (l/min)	0.95	0.78	2.84	0.47	1.22
Hepatic ext. (%)	63	52	189*	31	81

* A percentage greater than 100 indicates that prilocaine is being removed from blood by both hepatic and extrahepatic sites; see text.

ELIMINATION PHASE

The terminal elimination or beta-phase represents elimination of the injected local anaesthetic from the body by metabolism and excretion (Fig. 12.2). Metabolism of local anaesthetic agents is dependent on the chemical structure of the various drugs. The amino-esters, e.g. procaine, are hydrolysed in plasma by cholinesterase enzymes. The amino-amides such as lidocaine are metabolised primarily in the liver by microsomal enzymes. The rate of hydrolysis of amino-esters varies markedly. *In vitro* studies have shown that chloroprocaine has the most rapid rate of hydrolysis ($4.7\ \mu mol\ ml^{-1}\ hr^{-1}$) while a rate of $1.1\ \mu mol\ ml^{-1}\ hr^{-1}$ was observed for procaine and $0.3\ \mu mol\ ml^{-1}\ hr^{-1}$ for tetracaine[24]. The very rapid rates of hydrolysis of the amino-esters makes it difficult to obtain precise pharmacokinetic data. Half-lives of 21–25 seconds have been reported for chloroprocaine compared to values of 39–43 seconds for procaine[63]. A correlation does exist between the hydrolysis rates and the $T_{\frac{1}{2}}^{\beta}$ of these agents.

Some of the metabolites formed by the hydrolysis of the various esters have been identified. For example, procaine is hydrolysed to para-aminobenzoic acid and diethylamino ethanol. Para-aminobenzoic acid is excreted in the urine whereas diethylamino ethanol may undergo further metabolism.

The elimination kinetics of amino-amides have been studied extensively (Table 12.3)[64]. Prilocaine, a secondary amine, has a short $T_{\frac{1}{2}}^{\beta}$. The remaining amino-amides are tertiary amines with elimination half-lives ranging from 1.6 hours for lignocaine to 3.5 hours for bupivacaine. Sung and Truant incubated lignocaine with various rat tissue slices and found the liver to be the most active organ for metabolising this agent[58]. Similar *in vitro* studies with mepivacaine have shown that this agent is readily metabolised by rat liver slices incubated under aerobic conditions. Although prilocaine is also readily metabolised by rat liver slices, some degradation occurs when this agent is incubated with kidney slices. Isolated liver perfusion studies with bupivacaine and etidocaine have revealed that these compounds also undergo hepatic degradation.

In vivo studies have confirmed that the liver is the primary site of metabolism for local anaesthetic agents of the amide-type. Hepatectomy resulted in substantially higher tissue levels of lignocaine in rats and an increase in the anaesthetic activity and duration of toxic symptoms produced by this agent[58]. The rate of disappearance of lignocaine from blood was decreased in hepatectomised dogs and in patients whose liver had been removed during the course of liver transplantation[2].

Simultaneous measurements of arterial and hepatic venous concentrations of lidocaine along with determinations of hepatic blood flow demonstrated that approximately 70% of lignocaine in the arterial blood was removed and presumably metabolised in normal subjects[57]. These observations are concordant with systemic clearance values for lignocaine; that is, 0.95 l/min is approximately 70% of normal liver blood flow (Table 12.3). The systemic clearance and hepatic extraction of mepivacaine and etidocaine are close to those of lignocaine. The very high clearance of prilocaine (exceeding liver blood flow and producing an apparent hepatic extraction in excess of 100%) indicates that it is biotransformed in both the liver and at other sites in the body (e.g. kidney; see above). There are indications that the hepatic extraction of bupivacaine is concentration-dependent; during continuous infusion, the extraction declined from approximately 80% to less than 50%[67]. A concentration-dependent, saturable process of elimination would explain the higher systemic clearance estimates found in humans after spinal anaesthetic doses (i.e. low plasma concentrations) than after much larger epidural doses producing higher plasma concentrations (A. G. L. Burm, pers. comm.).

The complete spectrum of metabolic products of the amino-amides has not been elucidated. The metabolism of lignocaine has been studied most extensively. Hollunger originally proposed that the initial step in the metabolism of lignocaine involved oxidative de-ethylation to monoethylglycinexylidide and acetaldehyde[29]. Mono-ethylglycinexylidide subsequently was hydrolysed to xylidine and monoethylglycine. Xylidine itself underwent further oxidation to some unknown product. Keenaghan and Boyes summarised the information available concerning the metabolism of lignocaine in various animals species and demonstrated considerable species variability[30]. Significant amounts of monoethylglycinexylidide and xylidine were recovered from guinea pig urine. Rats formed large quantities of the meta-hydroxy derivatives of both lignocaine and monoethylglycinexylidide, and the conjugates of these two metabolites underwent extensive enterohepatic recirculation in rats. However, these metabolites and evidence of enterohepatic circulation were essentially lacking in dogs and men. Hydroxyxylidine was the major metabolic product of lignocaine found in canine and human urine. The dog and human were similar in terms of lignocaine metabolism, whereas the rat appeared to be quite different.

N-demethylation appears to be the initial step in the degradation of mepivacaine in mice and rats[60]. Hydroxylation of mepivacaine also occurs in rats and man. Approximately 60% of the dose of mepivacaine administered to rats is excreted as an aromatic hydroxy derivative. In man, conjugates of these hydroxy metabolites of mepivacaine account for 25–40% of the administered dose[60]. In addition, three neutral metabolites of mepivacaine have been identified in human urine. Only 50% of the administered mepivacaine has been receovered in studies reported thus far.

The metabolism of prilocaine differs significantly from that of lignocaine and mepivacaine, due apparently to the lack of one methyl group on the aromatic portion of the molecule. O-toluidine and N-propylamine have been identified as metabolites of prilocaine[25]. Hydroxylation also appears to be an important route of metabolism because Mather has reported recovery of 18% of the injected dose of prilocaine as the 4-hydroxy and 6-hydroxy derivatives of 2-methylamine[34].

Detailed data are not available on the newer amide-type of local anaesthetic agents, i.e. bupivacaine and etidocaine. Preliminary studies by Reynolds revealed that 5% of the dose of bupivacaine was recovered in human urine as the N-dealkylated metabolite, pipecoloxylidine[47]. Goehl and associates observed that the rat excreted substantial quantities of bupivacaine as an aromatic hydroxy metabolite, whereas the monkey excreted over 50% of the dose as the hydrolysis product, pipecolic acid[27].

Metabolic studies of etidocaine have shown that only 1.1% of the administered dose was recovered in guinea pig urine as the secondary amine metabolite, whereas 14.9% of lignocaine was identified as the secondary amine metabolite[7]. The excretion of 2,6-xylidine in guinea pigs was also considerably lower following etidocaine (2.2%) than following lignocaine administration (16.2%). The presence of the branched alkyl chain in etidocaine probably results in metabolic products which are markedly different from those of lignocaine. Although 20 metabolites of etidocaine have been found in human urine, these account for only 40% of the injected dose[63].

The kidney is the main excretory organ for local anaesthetics and their metabolites. Among local anaesthetic esters, procaine is hydrolysed almost completely in plasma and less than 2% of unchanged drug is excreted by the kidney. Approximately 90% of para-aminobenzoic acid, the primary metabolite of procaine, is found unchanged in the urine, whereas only one-third of diethylamino alcohol, the other metabolite, is excreted unchanged. Similarly, only small amounts of unchanged chloroprocaine and tetracaine are found in urine.

Only small amounts of the amide-type local anaesthetic agents are excreted unchanged via the kidneys[63]. Of an intravenous dose of lignocaine, less than 10% was found in the urine of human volunteers as the unchanged drug and approximately 80% was recovered in the form of various metabolites. From 1–16% of administered mepivacaine appears as unchanged drug in human urine, whereas 25–40% is excreted as degradation products. Unchanged bupivacaine accounts for only 16% of the drug recovered from human urine. Less than 1% of etidocaine has been found in urine as the unchanged drug.

A comparative study of the renal clearance of prilocaine and lidocaine in man by Eriksson and Granberg indicated a substantially higher clearance value for prilocaine, which they believed to be related to the lower protein binding of prilocaine[20]. The renal clearance of both prilocaine and lignocaine was found to be inversely proportional to the pH of urine; at a lower pH, more of the local anaesthetic is ionised and less is reabsorbed from the glomerular filtrate by the renal tubule.

The elimination kinetics of local anaesthetics are summarised most easily by comparing the elimination half-times and calculated clearance values for the various drugs (Table 12.3). Elimination (β) half-time ($T_{\frac{1}{2}}^{\beta}$) is directly proportional to the volume of distribution and inversely proportional to the clearance of the individual compounds. Prilocaine has the shortest $T_{\frac{1}{2}}^{\beta}$ and the greatest clearance (in excess of liver blood flow). Although lignocaine's clearance is slower, its distribution volume is less than that of prilocaine, so its ultimate elimination from the body occurs at the same rate (i.e. the $T_{\frac{1}{2}}^{\beta}$ is the same for lignocaine as for prilocaine). On the other hand, the higher clearance of etidocaine compared to lignocaine is offset by a much larger distribution volume, so the half-time for elimination of etidocaine is longer than that of lignocaine. A large distribution volume means low plasma concentrations of the drug, and therefore less of the dose is brought to the liver per unit time for metabolic elimination.

The prolonged half-time of bupivacaine is associated with a low clearance and hepatic extraction, both indicating a limited ability of the liver to metabolise this local anaesthetic.

PLACENTAL TRANSMISSION

Like most drugs, local anaesthetics traverse the placenta by passive diffusion of the free, unionised form[53, 54]. The rate of transmission thus depends on the concentration gradient of this form of the drug between maternal and fetal plasma. The extent of fetal accumulation of the drug depends on the duration of a maternal–fetal concentration gradient. As is true in the adult, most of the drug entering the fetal circulation is distributed to fetal tissues outside the vasculature. This distribution process tends to lower fetal plasma levels and the transmission of drug from mother to fetus will continue until all of the following equilibria are satisfied:

Placenta

Fetal tissues $\leftrightharpoons$ Fetal plasma $\rightleftharpoons$ Maternal plasma

There are important implications of these general principles. The higher the maternal plasma level and the longer it is maintained, the more rapid and extensive will be the transfer of drug to the fetus. As a consequence, all those factors tending to produce higher and longer lasting drug levels in maternal plasma will also tend to increase the transfer of local anaesthetic to the fetus. Thus, injection into a well-perfused maternal site of a high dose of a slowly eliminated (long $T_{\frac{1}{2}}^{\beta}$) local anaesthetic that is minimally bound to plasma protein would be expected to result in considerable transfer of the anaesthetic to the fetus. Since all of these factors vary somewhat independently, it is not always possible to predict the outcomes of specific cases.

Umbilical vein/maternal plasma concentration ratios (UV/M) are often measured and frequently misinterpreted or at least incompletely understood. The UV/M describes the relative concentrations of drug, both free and protein-bound, in fetal and maternal plasma. Since it is the free drug that diffuses across the placenta and equilibrates between maternal and fetal plasma, it is important to recognise the following implications of UV/M values.

1   Measurements made during the maternal drug distribution phase (high maternal plasma levels) will reflect the potential rate of drug transfer which can be expected to be lower for drugs more highly bound to maternal plasma protein. This, in fact, appears to be the case (Table 12.4). Of course, other factors affecting drug diffusion across biological membranes may also be important (e.g. lipid solubility, degree of ionisation).

2   Since passive diffusion is the mechanism of placental transfer, the UV/M value at equilibrium should be independent of the actual concentrations. Thus, although the maternal plasma levels of mepivacaine differed by more than twofold in two independent investigations (2.9 vs. 6.9 $\mu g\,ml^{-1}$), the UV/M values were virtually identical (0.69 vs. 0.71 respectively)[39, 41].

3   UV/M values at equilibrium (or during the pseudoequilibrium after completion of drug distribution phases) primarily reflect differences in the amount of protein-bound drug in maternal and fetal plasma. Local anaesthetic binding to proteins in fetal plasma

Table 12.4 Relationship between plasma protein binding capacity and placental transfer of
amide local anaesthetics.

	Plasma protein- binding capacity (%)	Umbilical vein/maternal blood (UV/M) ratio
Prilocaine	55	1.0 –1.18
Lidocaine	64	0.52–0.69
Mepivacaine	77	0.69–0.71
Bupivacaine	95	0.31–0.44
Etidocaine	99	0.14–0.35

is approximately 50% less than their binding to maternal plasma proteins. Thus, the
UV/M values tend to be less than unity at equilibrium.

4   UV/M values do *not* indicate the total amount of drug transferred to the fetus. The
total amount is that in fetal plasma plus a much larger amount in extravascular tissues.

Although the patterns of distribution of lignocaine in maternal and fetal tissues are
generally similar, certain differences do exist[23]. Significantly higher levels of
lignocaine were found in fetal liver than in adult liver. This may be indicative of poorly
developed enzyme systems in the fetus such that amide-type local anaesthetic drugs
may not be metabolised as rapidly in fetal liver. Studies comparing etidocaine and
lignocaine revealed a greater uptake by fetal brain of etidocaine than of lidocaine.
Etidocaine tends to accumulate in peripheral fat in adults. The lack of peripheral fat
depots in the fetus could result in relatively higher plasma concentrations and greater
uptake of this agent by other lipid organs such as brain.

Those drugs which demonstrate the highest degree of protein binding also tend to
be more lipid soluble, so that the rate of placental transfer and tissue uptake of the
unbound drug is enhanced. Thus, the maternal/fetal anaesthetic blood concentrations
may differ markedly between agents, but the total amount of drug transferred across
the placenta may be similar for agents that are more or less extensively bound to plasma
proteins. It was originally postulated that agents which possess a high protein-binding
capacity should be potentially less toxic for the fetus. However, if the rate of fetal tissue
uptake is greater for drugs of high protein binding and high lipid solubility, then the
potential fetal toxicity would be similar for all of the local anaesthetic compounds.

FACTORS AFFECTING PHARMACOKINETICS

Age

Morishima and colleagues studied the pharmacokinetics of lignocaine and etidocaine
in adult sheep, newborn lambs and fetal sheep *in utero*[42, 43]. Following intravenous
administration, the half-life of lignocaine in plasma was shortest in the fetus *in utero*,

due most likely to the low degree of plasma protein-binding of lignocaine in the fetus and its rapid retrograde diffusion across the placenta to the mother. The $T_{\frac{1}{2}}^{\beta}$ of lignocaine and etidocaine in the newborn lamb and the adult ewe were similar, but the similarity in elimination half-times is deceiving. The newborn lamb showed a much higher volume of distribution (V_D) and the renal excretion of the unchanged drug was 9 times greater in the newborn lamb than in the adult ewe. These differences may reflect a lower plasma protein binding of lignocaine and etidocaine in the newborn lamb which would result in greater availability of free drug for tissue uptake and for clearance (Cl) by the kidney. The elimination half-time is the same since $T_{\frac{1}{2}}^{\beta} = V_D/Cl$. It is interesting to note that there was little difference in the hepatic clearance of lignocaine in the newborn lamb and the adult ewe.

Studies of the kinetics of lignocaine and mepivacaine in human neonates following subcutaneous administration of these drugs showed a significant prolongation of the elimination half-life of both drugs[36, 38]. The elimination half-life of lignocaine averaged 2.3 hours in the neonate compared to 1.6 hours in adults. Mepivacaine showed an elimination half-life of 8.7 hours in neonates and 1.9–2.3 hours in adults. The prolonged elimination times are related in part to the greater tissue accumulation of lignocaine and mepivacaine in neonates (i.e. larger V_D), which again may reflect decreased plasma protein binding. The renal excretion of unchanged lignocaine and mepivacaine in the human neonate was approximately 8 times greater than that in adults, but this was insufficient to offset the increase in V_D; hence the $T_{\frac{1}{2}}^{\beta}$ was longer in the human neonate than in the adult.

A comparative pharmacokinetic study of lignocaine in adults whose mean age was approximately 65 years, compared to adults with a mean age of approximately 25 years revealed a significant prolongation of the elimination half-life in the elderly population[44]. This appears related to a significantly greater volume of distribution in the older age group. No other pharmacokinetic difference was observed between the two groups. The greater percentage of adipose tissue and the sometimes lower levels of plasma proteins in an elderly population may contribute to the larger distribution volume of lignocaine[28a].

Acid–base status

Hypercapnia and acidosis are known to increase the toxicity of local anaesthetic agents[19]. Changes in their pharmacokinetics in the presence of hypercarbia and acidosis may account in part for the enhanced toxicity. An inverse correlation has been reported between hydrogen ion concentration and the degree of plasma protein-binding of lignocaine[9]. Thus, acidosis results in a greater free fraction of the drug in plasma, making more drug available for diffusion into tissues. Indeed, higher tissue levels of lignocaine have been observed in acidotic animals compared to non-acidotic animals[43].

Increased tissue levels of local anaesthetics in the presence of acidosis may also occur as a consequence of ion trapping within cells to the extent that the intracellular pH declines to a greater degree than extracellular pH. A decrease in intracellular pH favours the conversion of local anaesthetics from unionised base form to the cationic form. Since the cationic form does not diffuse readily across cell membranes, it will tend to be trapped within the cell and ionised molecules will tend to accumulate. Indeed, fetal acidosis has been reported to lead to ion trapping of local anaesthetic agents, which results in a greater uptake of these agents by the fetus[15].

Physiological status of the patient

Any change in physiological status which influences drug distribution and elimination will alter the pharmacokinetics of local anaesthetics and their potential toxicity. For example, among the amino-esters the rate of elimination is related to the rate of hydrolysis by plasma pseudocholinesterase. Patients with atypical plasma cholinesterases or decreased levels of plasma cholinesterases (e.g. hereditary deficiency, liver disease) will tend to hydrolyse amino-esters more slowly and to exhibit a decreased rate of elimination of these compounds. The *in vitro* half-time for hydrolysis of procaine was 138 seconds in plasma taken from patients with liver disease, compared to 39 seconds in plasma from normal subjects[63].

Alterations in hepatic blood flow or hepatic metabolism will markedly influence the rate of degradation and the elimination half-time of the amino-amides. There is a direct relationship between hepatic blood flow and hepatic extraction of lignocaine from plasma[57]. Patients with cardiac disease resulting in passive congestion of the liver and decreased hepatic blood flow show a significant prolongation in the elimination half-time of lignocaine[61]. Pharmacological agents altering hepatic blood flow also affect the hepatic extraction of agents such as lignocaine. The concomitant administration of isoproterenol during a continuous infusion of lignocaine decreased the steady state arterial level of lignocaine, presumably due to an increase in hepatic blood flow (i.e. increased cardiac output and decreased splanchnic vascular resistance). On the other hand, the administration of norepinephrine, which decreases hepatic blood flow, decreased the clearance and increased the steady state plasma levels of lignocaine during its continuous infusion[4].

Studies performed in patients during and following recovery from acute hepatitis have revealed marked differences in the elimination half-times of lignocaine[69]. During the active phase of hepatitis, the half-life of a 100 mg i.v. dose was approximately 160 minutes. Several months following recovery, a normal half-life of 80 minutes was observed in the same subjects. An abnormally high venous plasma level of lignocaine (13 μg ml^{-1}) was observed in a patient with severe hepatic dysfunction due to chronic alcoholism[52]. Finally, it has been demonstrated that both in animals and man the rate of disappearance of lignocaine from plasma is markedly decreased during hepatectomy.

The pharmacokinetics of lignocaine have been investigated in patients with renal failure[13]. Renal failure does not influence the pharmacokinetics of the parent compound, but the rate of disappearance from plasma of glycinexylidide, a secondary metabolite of lignocaine that depends on renal excretion for its elimination, was markedly decreased. No change in the elimination half-time of monoethylglycine-xylidine was found in these patients, since this primary metabolite of lignocaine is cleared from plasma by the liver.

CLINICAL SIGNIFICANCE OF LOCAL ANAESTHETIC PHARMACOKINETICS

Although the distribution and elimination of local anaesthetics can influence to some degree their clinical utility, the major clinical importance of their pharmacokinetics involves their potential toxicity to the central nervous and cardiovascular systems. Both CNS and cardiovascular reactions to local anaesthetics are dependent on the concentration of the agent in plasma and the corresponding levels achieved in the brain and heart. The plasma and tissue levels are a function of the rate of absorption, the rate of distribution to tissues and organs, and the rate of elimination (Fig. 12.3). Any factors which increase the rate of absorption from the injection site, increase the rate and extent of distribution to the CNS and heart, or decrease the rate of elimination tend to increase their potential toxicity. It is important to recognise that differences exist between the various agents with regard to the basic pharmacokinetic properties which influence their potential for toxic reactions. For example, chloroprocaine undergoes the most rapid rate of hydrolysis in plasma and is the least toxic of the amino-ester local anaesthetics. On the other hand, tetracaine is hydrolysed most slowly and is potentially the most toxic member of this class. Among the amino-amide compounds, prilocaine shows the most favorable pharmacokinetic properties in terms of rapid tissue distribution and rapid rate of elimination; it is clearly the least toxic of the amino-amide

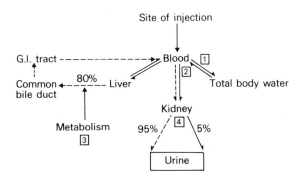

Fig. 12.3 Summary of physiological disposition of local anaesthetic agents. 1 = tissue redistribution phase; 2 = site of hydrolysis of ester local anaesthetic agents; 3 = hepatic metabolism of amide local anaesthetic agents; 4 = renal excretion of parent compound (solid line) and metabolites (dashed line).

compounds. On the other hand, bupivacaine is cleared most slowly from the body and potentially is the most toxic of the amino-amides. In general, correlations exist between the anaesthetic potency of various agents, their pharmacokinetic profile, and their potential toxicity. Although tetracaine and bupivacaine are potentially the most toxic, they are also the most potent so that smaller doses are required to produce adequate regional anaesthesia. Comparative studies of the doses required for adequate regional anaesthesia and the plasma level necessary to produce toxic reactions indicates that little difference exists between the therapeutic ratio or margin of safety of the various local anaesthetics if they are employed in their appropriate equivalent anaesthetic doses. Thus, knowledge of the pharmacokinetics of local anaesthetics is essential to the effective and safe practice of regional anaesthesia with any of these drugs.

GLOSSARY

	Generic	Trade
British	American	
Lignocaine	Lidocaine	Xylocaine
Bupivacaine		Marcaine
Mepivacaine		Carbocaine
Prilocaine		Citanest
Etidocaine		Duranest
Amethocaine	Tetracaine	Pontocaine

REFERENCES

1. ÅBERG G. & DHUNÉR K-G. (1972) Effect of mepivacaine (Carbocaine®) on femoral blood flow in the dog. *Acta Pharm. Toxicol.* **31**, 262–72.
2. ALDRETE J. A., HOMATAS J., BOYES R. N. & STARZL T. E. (1970) Effects of hepatectomy on the disappearance rate of lidocaine from blood in man and dog. *Anesth. Analg.* **49**, 687–90.
3. ÅSTRÖM A. & PERSSON N. H. (1961) The toxicity of some local anaesthetics after application on different mucous membranes and its relation to anesthetic action on the nasal mucosa of the rabbit. *Pharm. Exp. Ther.* **132**, 87–90.
4. BENOWITZ N. L. (1974) Clinical applications of the pharmacokinetics of lido-

caine. *Cardiovasc. Clin.* **6**, 77–101.
5. BJORN H. & HULDT S., IV. (1947) The efficiency of Xylocaine as a dental terminal anesthetic compared to that of procaine. *Svensk. Tandlak. Tidskr.* **40**, 831–51.
6. BOYES R. N., Scott D. B., JEBSON P. J., GODMAN M. J. & JULIAN D. G. (1971) Pharmacokinetics of lidocaine in man. *Clin. Pharmacol. Ther.* **12**, 105–16.
7. BOYES R. N. (1975) A review of the metabolism of amide local anaesthetic agents. *Br. J. Anaesth.* **47**, 225–30.
8. BRAID D. P. & SCOTT D. B. (1965) The systemic absorption of local analgesic drugs. *Br. J. Anaesth.* **37**, 394–404.
9. BURNEY R. G., DiFAZIO C. A. & FOSTER

J. A. (1978) Effects of pH on protein binding of lidocaine. *Anesth. Analg.* **57**, 478–80.

10. CHAMBERS W. A., LITTLEWOOD D. G., LOGAN M. R. & SCOTT D. B. (1981) Effect of added epinephrine on spinal anesthesia with lidocaine. *Anesth. Analg.* **60**, 417–20.

11. COHEN L. S., ROSENTHAL J. E., HORNER D. W., ATKINS J. M., MATTHEWS O. A. & SARNOFF S. J. (1972) Plasma levels of lidocaine after intramuscular administration. *Am. J. Card.* **29**, 520–3.

12. COLLEY P. S. & HEAVNER J. E. (1981) Blood levels of bupivacaine after injection into the scalp with and without epinephrine. *Anesthesiology* **54**, 81–4.

13. COLLINSWORTH K. A., STRONG J. M., ATKINSON JR A. J., WINKLE R. A., PERLROTH F. & HARRISON D. C. (1975) Pharmacokinetics and metabolism of lidocaine in patients with renal failure. *Clin. Pharmacol. Ther.* **18**, 59–64.

14. COVINO B. G. & VASSALLO H. D. (1976) *Local Anesthetics: Mechanisms of Action and Clinical Use.* Grune and Stratton, New York.

15. DATTA S., BROWN JR W. U., OSTHEIMER G. W., WEISS J. B. & ALPER M. H. (1981) Epidural anesthesia for cesarean section in diabetic parturients: Maternal and Neonatal acid-base status and bupivacaine concentration. *Anesth. Analg.* **60**, 574–87.

16. DE JONG R. H., HEAVNER J. E. & DE OLIVEIRA L. F. (1972) Effects of nitrous oxide on the lidocaine seizure threshold and diazepam protection. *Anesthesiology* **37**, 299–303.

17. DHUNÉR K-G. & LEWIS D. H. (1966) Effect of local anaesthetics and vasoconstrictors upon regional blood flow. *Acta Anaesth. Scand. (Suppl)* **23**, 347–52.

18. DIGIOVANNI A. J. (1971) Inadvertent intraosseous injection—a hazard of caudal anesthesia. *Anesthesiology* **34**, 92–4.

19. ENGLESSON S. (1973) The influence of acid-base changes on central nervous system toxicity of local anaesthetic agents. Doctoral thesis, University of Uppsala, Sweden.

20. ERIKSSON E. & GRANBERG P-O. (1965) Studies on the renal excretion of Citanest® and Xylocaine®. *Acta Anaesth. Scand. (Suppl)* **16**, 79–85.

21. EVANS J. A., CHASTAIN G. M. & PHILLIPS J. M. (1969) The use of local anesthetic agents in obstetrics. *South. Med. J.* **62**, 519–24.

22. EVANS E. F., PROCTOR J. D., FRATKIN M. J., VELANDIA J. & WASSERMAN A. J. (1975) Blood flow in muscle groups and drug absorption. *Clin. Pharmacol. Ther.* **17**, 44–7.

23. FINSTER M., MORISHIMA H. O., BOYES R. N. & COVINO B. G. (1972) The placental transfer of lidocaine and its uptake by fetal tissues. *Anesthesiology* **36**, 159–63.

24. FOLDES F. F., DAVIDSON G. M., DUNCALF D. & KUWABARA S. (1965) The intravenous toxicity of local anesthetic agents in man. *Clin. Pharmacol. Ther.* **6**, 328–35.

25. GEDDES I. C. (1965) Studies of the metabolism of Citanest ^{14}C. *Acta Anaesth. Scand. (Suppl)* **16**, 37–44.

26. GIASI R. M., D'AGOSTINO E. & COVINO B. G. (1979) Absorption of lidocaine following subarachnoid and epidural administration. *Anesth. Analg.* **58**, 360–3.

27. GOEHL T. J., DAVENPORT J. B. & STANLEY M. J. (1973) Distribution, biotransformation and excretion of bupivacaine in the rat and the monkey. *Xenobiotica* **3**, 761–72.

28. GOLDBERG L. (1974) Studies on local anesthetics. III. Pharmacological properties of xylocaine. *Svensk. Tandlak. Tidskr.* **40**, 819–30.

28a. GREENBLATT D. J., SELLERS E. M. & SCHRADER R. I. (1972) Drug disposition in old age. *New Engl. J. Med.* **306**, 1081–8.

29. HOLLUNGER G. (1960) On the metabolism of lidocaine. I. The properties of the enzyme system responsible for the oxidative metabolism of lidocaine. II. The biotransformation of lidocaine. *Acta Pharmacol. Toxicol.* **17**, 356–64.

30. KEENAGHAN J. B. & BOYES R. N. (1972) The tissue distribution, metabolism and excretion of lidocaine in rats, guinea pigs, dogs and man. *J. Pharmacol. Exp. Ther.* **180**, 454–63.

31. LÖFSTRÖM J. B., ALM B-E., BERTLER Å., JORFELDT L., LEWIS D. & POST C. (1978) Lung uptake of lidocaine. *Acta Anaesth. Scand. (Suppl)* **70**, 80–2.

32. LÖFSTRÖM J. B. (1978) Tissue distribution of local anaesthetics with special reference to the lung. *Int. Anesthesiol. Clin.* **16**, 53–71.

33. LUND P. C., BUSH D. F. & COVINO B. G. (1975) Determinants of etidocaine concentration in the blood. *Anesthesiology* **42**, 497–503.

34. MATHER L. E. & TUCKER G. T. (1978) Pharmacokinetics and biotransformation of local anesthetics. *Int. Anesthesiol. Clin.* **16**, 23–51.

35. MEAGHER R. P., MOORE D. C. & DEVRIES J. C. (1966) Phenylephrine: The most effect potentiator of tetracaine spinal anesthesia. *Anesth. Analg.* **45**, 134–9.

36. MEFFIN P., LONG G. J. & THOMAS J. (1973) Clearance and metabolism of mepivacaine in the human neonate. *Clin. Pharmacol. Ther.* **14**, 218–25.

37. MEYER M. B. & ZELECHOWSKI K. (1971) Intramuscular lidocaine on normal subjects. In D. B. Scott and D. G. Julian (eds.), *Lidocaine in the Treatment of Ventricular Arrhythmias.* E & S Livingstone, Edinburgh.

38. MIHALY G. W., MOORE R. G., THOMAS J., TRIGGS E. J., THOMAS D. & SHANKS C. H. (1978) The pharmacokinetics and metabolism of the anilide local anaesthetics in neonates. I. Lignocaine. *Eur. J. Pharmacol.* **13**, 143–52.

39. MOORE D. C., BRIDENBAUGH L. D., BAGDI P. A. & BRIDENBAUGH P. O. (1968) Accumulation of mepivacaine hydrochloride during caudal block. *Anesthesiology* **29**, 585–8.

40. MORCH E. T., ROSENBERG M. K. & TRUANT A. T. (1957) Lidocaine for spinal anaesthesia. A study of the concentration in the spinal fluid. *Acta Anaesth. Scand.* **1**, 105–15.

41. MORISHIMA H. O., DANIEL S. S., FINSTER M., POPPERS P. J. & JAMES S. (1966) Transmission of mepivacaine hydrochloride (Carbocaine) across the human placenta. *Anesthesiology* **27**, 147–54.

42. MORISHIMA H. O., FINSTER M., PEDERSEN H., FUKUNAGA A., RONFELD R. A., VASSALLO H. G. & COVINO B. G. (1979) Pharmacokinetics of lidocaine in fetal and neonatal lambs and adult sheep. *Anesthesiology* **50**, 431–6.

43. MORISHIMA H. O., PEDERSEN H., FINSTER M., SAKUMA K., BRUCE S. L., GUTSCHE B. B., STARK R. I. & COVINO B. G. (1981) Toxicity of lidocaine in adult, newborn, and fetal sheep. *Anesthesiology* **55**, 57–61.

44. NATION R. L., TRIGGS E. J. & SELIG M. (1977) Lignocaine kinetics in cardiac patients and aged subjects. *Br. J. Clin. Pharmacol.* **4**, 439–48.

45. POST C. (1979) Studies on the pharmacokinetic function of the lung with special reference to lidocaine. *Acta Pharmacol. Toxicol.* **44**, 1–53.

46. POST C. & LEWIS D. H. (1979) Displacement of nortriptyline and uptake of ^{14}C-lidocaine in the lung after administration of ^{14}C-lidocaine to nortriptyline intoxicated pigs. *Acta Pharmacol. Toxicol.* **45**, 218–24.

47. REYNOLDS F. (1971) A comparison of the potential toxicity of bupivacaine, lignocaine and mepivacaine during epidural blockade for surgery. *Br. J. Anaesth.* **43**, 567–71.

48. SCHWARTZ M. L., COVINO B. G.,

NARANG R. M., SETHI V., THOLPADY S. S., KUANGPARICHAT M., GIORDANO C. & MEYER M. B. (1974) Blood levels of lidocaine following subcutaneous administration prior to cardiac catheterization. *Am. Heart J.* **88**, 721–3.

49. SCHWARTZ M. L., MEYER M. B., COVINO B. G., NARANG R. M., SETHI V., SCHWARTZ A. J. & KAMP P. (1974) Antiarrhythmic effectiveness of intramuscular lidocaine: Influence of different injection sites. *J. Clin. Pharm.* **14**, 77–83.

50. SCOTT D. B. (1981) Toxicity caused by local anaesthetic drugs. *Br. J. Anaesth.* **53**, 553–4.

51. SCOTT D. B., JEBSON P. J. R., BRAID D. P., ORTENGREN B. & FRISCH P. (1972) Factors affecting plasma levels of lignocaine and prilocaine. *Br. J. Anaesth.* **44**, 1040–9.

52. SELDEN R. & SASAHARA A. A. (1967) Central nervous system toxicity induced by lidocaine. *J. Am. Med. Assoc.* **202**, 908–9.

53. SHNIDER S. M. & WAY E. L. (1968) The kinetics of transfer of lidocaine (Xylocaine®) across the human placenta. *Anesthesiology* **20**, 944–50.

54. SHNIDER S. M. & WAY E. L. (1968) Plasma levels of lidocaine (Xylocaine®) in mother and newborn following obstetrical conduction anesthesia. *Anesthesiology* **20**, 951–8.

55. SJOSTRAND U. & WIDMAN B. (1973) Distribution of bupivacaine in the rabbit under normal and acidotic conditions. *Acta Anaesthesiol. Scand. (Suppl)* **50**, 5–24.

56. STANTON-HICKS M., BERGES P. U. & BONICA J. J. (1973) Circulatory effects of peridural block: IV. Comparison of the effects of epinephrine and phenylephrine. *Anesthesiology* **39**, 308–14.

57. STENSON R. E., CONSTANTINO R. T. & HARRISON R. C. (1971) Interrelationships of hepatic blood flow, cardiac output, and blood levels of lidocaine in man. *Circulation* **43**, 205–11.

58. SUNG C. Y. & TRUANT A. P. (1954) The physiological disposition of lidocaine and its comparison in some respects with procaine. *J. Pharmacol. Exp. Ther.* **112**, 432–43.

59. SWERDLOW M. & JONES R. (1970) The duration of action of bupivacaine, prilocaine and lignocaine. *Br. J. Anaesth.* **42**, 335–9.

60. THOMAS J. & MEFFIN P. (1972) Aromatic hydroxylation of lidocaine and mepivacaine in rats and humans. *J. Med. Chem.* **15**, 1046–9.

61. THOMSON P. D., MELMON K. L., RICHARDSON J. A., COHN K., STEINBRUNN W., CUDIHEE R. & ROWLAND M. (1973) Lidocaine pharmacokinetics in advanced heart failure, liver disease, and renal failure in humans. *Ann. Intern. Med.* **78**, 499–508.

62. TUCKER G. T., MOORE D. C., BRIDENBAUGH P. O., BRIDENBAUGH L. D. & THOMPSON G. E. (1972) Systemic absorption of mepivacaine in commonly used regional block procedures. *Anesthesiology* **37**, 277–87.

63. TUCKER G. T. & MATHER L. E. (1979) Clinical pharmacokinetics of local anaesthetics. *Clin. Pharmacokinet.* **4**, 241–78.

64. TUCKER G. T. & MATHER L. E. (1975) Pharmacokinetics of local anaesthetic agents. *Br. J. Anaesth.* (Suppl) **47**, 213–24.

65. TUCKER G. T., BOYES R. N., BRIDENBAUGH P. O. & MOORE D. C. (1970) Binding of anilide-type local anesthetics in human plasma: II. Implications *in vivo*, with special reference to transplacental distribution. *Anesthesiology* **33**, 304–14.

66. TUCKER G. T. & BOAS R. A. (1971) Pharmacokinetic aspects of intravenous regional anesthesia. *Anesthesiology* **34**, 538–49.

67. WIKLUND L. & BERLIN-WAHLEN A. (1977) Splanchnic elimination and systemic toxicity of lupinicaine and etido-

caine in man. *Acta Anaesth. Scand.* **21**, 521–8.

68. WILDSMITH J. A. W., TUCKER G. T., COOPER S., SCOTT D. B. & COVINO B. G. (1977) Plasma concentrations of local anaesthetics after interscalene brachial plexus block. *Br. J. Anaesth.* **49**, 461–6.

69. WILLIAMS R. L., BLASCHKE T. F., MEFFIN P. J., MELMON K. L. & ROWLAND M. (1976) Influence of viral hepatitis on the disposition of two compounds with high hepatic clearance: Lidocaine and indocyanine green. *Clin. Pharmacol. Ther.* **20**, 290–9.

13 Kinetics and Dynamics of Beta-adrenoceptor Agonists

C. PRYS-ROBERTS

Beta-adrenoceptor antagonists, colloquially referred to as 'beta-blockers', are perhaps the most important drugs acting on the cardiovascular system which are commonly found in the pre-operative medications of patients presenting for surgery. They are also widely used during and after anaesthesia for the suppression of undesirable effects of sympathetic nervous activity on the heart. Considerable misunderstanding has occurred in the past as to the degree of beta-adrenoceptor antagonist activity in patients presenting for cardiac surgery and its influence on ventricular performance after cardiopulmonary bypass[45, 53]. In this respect, confusion between pharmacokinetic profile and pharmacodynamic effect of the drug has been the cause of such misunderstanding.

In this chapter, the pharmacokinetics of a number of beta-adrenoceptor antagonists will be placed in perspective with their pharmacodynamic effects. Firstly, in the context of pre-operative therapy and the desirability for its maintenance in the post-operative period; and secondly in the context of intravenous administration of the drugs, during anaesthesia or in the intensive care situation, either by intermittent injection or continuous infusion.

GENERAL PHARMACOLOGY OF BETA-ADRENOCEPTOR ANTAGONISTS

The differentiation by Ahlquist[3] of the effects of natural transmitters and synthetic sympathomimetic amines according to simple receptor subtypes, α and β, was a major step forward in pharmacology. Subsequent studies of sympathomimetic agonists and antagonists have revealed further sub-groups of this simple classification[4, 24] designated $\beta1$ and $\beta2$ receptors (Table 13.1). It is worth emphasising that this classification antedated the recognition of pre-synaptic ($\alpha2$) and post-synaptic ($\alpha1$) subtypes of the corresponding α-adrenoceptors[48]. The pre-synaptic $\alpha2$ receptors have been shown to play an important part in the regulation of neurotransmission, in that noradrenaline, or other drugs such as clonidine, exciting the pre-synaptic $\alpha2$ receptors inhibit further release of noradrenaline from the nerve ending. Conversely, stimulation of presynaptic β-receptors leads to an increase of noradrenaline release, whereas their blockade by β-receptor antagonists inhibits noradrenaline release.

Ariens[4] proposed that $\beta1$ receptors represented those which responded to noradrenaline released as a neurotransmitter, whereas $\beta2$ receptors represented those

Table 13.1   Classification of β-adrenoceptor agonists and antagnoists.

	$\beta1$-selective	Non-selective	$\beta2$-selective
Agonist	Prenalterol	Isoprenaline Dobutamine	Solbutamol Terbutaline
Antagonist	Practolol Atenolol Metoprolol Acebutalol	Propranolol Exprenolol Alprenolol Labetalol Pindolol	Butoxamine

which responded to humorally mediated sympathomimetic amines. This concept is consistent with the finding that noradrenaline has the highest relative affinity for β1 receptors, while adrenaline has the highest relative affinity for β2 receptors[9].

The agonist–antagonist interaction is defined by the dose-response curve to an agonist, e.g. isoprenaline, and its rightwards displacement by an antagonist. This relationship (Fig. 13.1) defines the primary pharmacological effects of β-receptor antagonists, but these drugs also have a variety of secondary characteristics (Table 13.2).

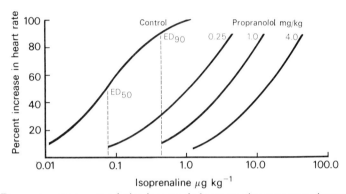

Fig. 13.1 Dose-response curves relating increase in heart rate in response to increasing doses of isoprenaline, and their modification by three doses of propranolol.

Table 13.2 Secondary characteristics of β-adrenoceptor antagonists.

Decrease maximal rate of depolarisation of excitable cardiac cells (quinidine-like action)
Local anaesthetic action (membrane stabilisation)
Partial agonism (intrinsic sympathomimetic activity)
Tissue or organ selectivity
Associated α-adrenoceptor antagonism

Receptor selectivity

This property of *selective affinity* for β1 or β2 receptors is consistent with radio-ligand binding studies[9, 19, 31] which can identify the homogeneity of binding sites for either β1 or β2 antagonists, or heterogeneity of binding sites (non-linear Hofstee plot) indicating mixed β1 and β2 receptors in a tissue[55].

Intrinsic sympathomimetic activity (ISA)

Many β-adrenoceptor antagonists increase heart rate, decrease diastolic arterial pressure, and increase plasma glucose and free fatty acid concentrations in catecholamine-depleted animals[18]. In this respect the drugs act as partial agonists.

Local anaesthetic activity

Many, but not all, β-adrenoceptor antagonists can act as local anaesthetics when applied to intact nerves or surface mucous membranes, an effect which is independent of their receptor activity[14]. This membrane stabilising effect has been likened to that of quinidine, also a local anaesthetic, and some myocardial depressant effects have been attributed to this property. However, the term 'quinidine-like' activity should be reserved for the antidysrhythmic property referred to below[51].

Antidysrhythmic activity

In common with some other drugs which exert local anaesthetic effects (quinidine, procainamide, phenytoin, lignocaine) β-adrenoceptor antagonists decrease the rate of rise of the initial depolarisation wave of the cardiac action potential[52].

The general factors which influence the action of any drug given by mouth are:
1   Dose and dose interval
2   Rate and extent of absorption
3   Bioavailability
4   Distribution and binding
5   Elimination

Absorption

Fig. 13.2 shows the mode of absorption and fate of β-adrenoceptor antagonists which are eliminated by hepatic metabolism. Most of the drugs in this class are rapidly and completely absorbed from the gastrointestinal tract and the more lipophilic drugs, such as propranolol, oxprenolol and alprenolol, undergo 'first-pass' metabolism in the liver. Consequently, the amount of the drug ingested which is available for distribution to the tissues, 'the bioavailability', is variable. Drugs which are hydrophophilic, such as atenolol, nadolol and sotalol are absorbed more slowly than the lipophilic drugs, but the difference is of little clinical significance. However, both types of drug can be formulated in slow-release preparations which are less rapidly absorbed than the standard preparation. This allows a delay in the achievement of a lower peak plasma concentration, and prolongation of therapeutic concentrations over a 24-hour period (Fig. 13.3).

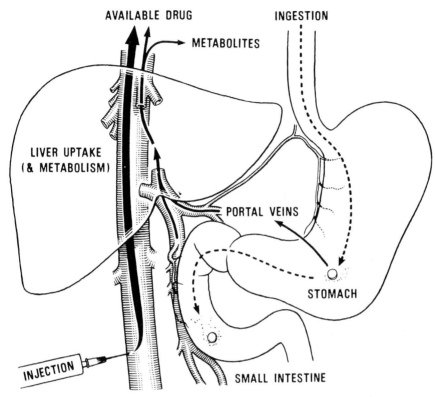

Fig. 13.2 Representation of gastric absorption of propranolol, and the effects of 'first-pass metabolism' in the liver.

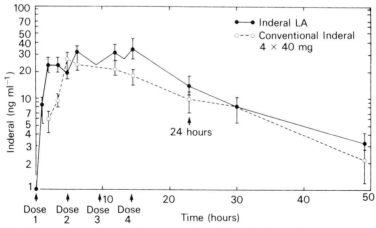

Fig. 13.3 Whole blood propranolol concentrations (Inderal) in 12 subjects after acute dosing with Inderal LA and with conventional Inderal tablets (4×40 mg). By courtesy of ICI Pharmaceuticals Division, Alderley Park, Cheshire, U.K.

Bioavailability

Fig. 13.2 indicates that a variable amount of an ingested dose is available for redistribution. Fig. 13.4 shows that the plasma concentrations following intravenous administration of 5 mg metoprolol exceed those after the same dose taken by mouth. The rate at which the drug is eliminated, the half-life of the decay of plasma concentration is approximately the same in both cases. The ratio of the area under the oral curve to the intravenous curve represents the bioavailability of the drug. Table 13.3 shows data on the bioavailability and pharmacokinetic profiles of a number of β-adrenoceptor antagonists. Ingestion of food can markedly affect the absorption of some drugs, particularly those which are incompletely absorbed from the gastro-intestinal tract. When atenolol or metoprolol were given with a meal the bioavailability was increased by up to 30 %[42]. The absorption of atenolol has also been shown to be reduced by 33 % when the drug was administered with an antacid[42]. These factors must be taken into account when prescribing these drugs to be taken pre-operatively without food.

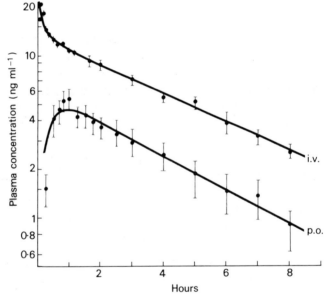

Fig. 13.4   Plasma concentration curves after 5 mg metoprolol administered intravenously (i.v.) or orally (p.o.). (After Johnsson *et al.*[22]).

Distribution

The distribution half-lives of most β-adrenoceptor antagonists are short (5–10 minutes) indicating a rapid distribution betwen blood and tissues, and the large volumes of distribution (1–11 l kg^{-1}) imply that the drugs are extensively distributed to extravascular sites, leaving only 1–2 % of the drug located in the blood.

Protein binding

Propranolol (93 %) and oxprenolol (80 %) are strongly bound to plasma proteins, but metoprolol (12 %), atenolol (0 %) and sotalol (0 %) are carried in the blood as free drug. Other drugs such as labetalol and pindolol are about 50 % protein bound. In assessing the pharmacodynamic effects of these drugs, the degree of protein binding must be taken into account as only the 'free' drug is effective. During cardiopulmonary bypass, the protein binding of propranolol has been shown to decrease to such an extent that the free fraction of propranolol was increased from 6.6 % to 13.5 %. These changes were considered to be related to the increase of free fatty acid concentrations consequent on heparin administration, and to a lesser extent due to haemodilutional effects of the pump prime[56]. These changes were effectively reversed by the effects of protamine.

Elimination

The liver and the kidney both play an important part in the elimination of β-adrenoceptor antagonists. Highly polar, hydrophilic drugs such as atenolol, practolol, nadolol and sotalol are almost entirely eliminated through the kidneys, and the clearance of these drugs approximates the glomerular filtration rate ($0.1–0.2\,l\,min^{-1}$) resulting in long (5–12 h) elimination half-lives (Table 13.3).

By contrast the most lipophilic drugs, propranolol, alprenolol and labetalol are extensively metabolised during their 'first pass' through the liver, and their clearance approximates the hepatic blood flow ($1–2\,l\,min^{-1}$). Because such a small amount of these drugs is carried in the blood, hence a large volume of distribution ($3–5\,l\,kg^{-1}$ body weight); despite the high hepatic uptake, the elimination of half-lives of these drugs are moderately long (3–4 h). This contrasts with many intravenous anaesthetics such as alphaxalone and di-isopropyl phenol which have high clearance, but much shorter half-lives (1–1.5 h).

Active metabolites

Propranolol, acebutalol and alprenolol are all degraded to active metabolites which may contribute to the pharmacological effect of the parent drug[12].

Effect of liver disease on metabolism

Because of its extensive hepatic metabolism, propranolol has usually been used as the model for the effects of liver dysfunction on drug metabolism[6, 7]. In cirrhotic patients the bioavailability of propranolol, metoprolol and labetalol is increased, the elimination half-lives are prolonged to almost double the values in normal patients and the clearances are diminished [6, 7, 20, 42].

Table 13.3 Bioavailability and pharmacokinetic characteristics of β-adrenoceptor antagonists classified according to route of elimination.

	Bioavailability (% ingested dose)	Protein-binding (%)	Distribution volume ($l\,kg^{-1}$)	Elimination $T_{\frac{1}{2}}$ (h)	Total body clearance ($l\,min^{-1}$)
Hepatic clearance					
Labetalol	30	50	11.0	3–4	2.4
Alprenolol	10*	85	3.3	2–3†	1.2
Propranolol	30*	93	3.6	3–4†	1.0
Metoprolol	50	12	5.0	3–4	1.1
Acebutalol	50*	25	2.3	3–4	0.6
Oxprenolol	30	80	1.2	2–3	0.4
Hepatic and renal clearance					
Pindolol	50–100	50	1.2	3–4	0.4
Nadolol	25‡	30	2.0	10–12	0.2
Renal clearance					
Sotalol	100	0	1.4	10–15	0.1
Atenolol	50	0	0.7	5–7	0.1

* dose-dependent bioavailability.
† active metabolites formed.
‡ biliary excretion without hepatic metabolism.

Effect of renal disease on metabolism

Impaired renal function has little effect on the elimination of those drugs which are mainly metabolised in the liver, although concurrent liver disease may be associated with raised plasma concentrations of the drugs[5, 23, 26]. By contrast, the elimination of atenolol, pindolol, acebutalol or sotalol has been shown to be substantially lengthened in patients with renal failure[25, 35, 37, 50, 54].

PHARMACODYNAMICS

The occupancy of β-adrenoceptors by antagonist drugs is dependent on the free fraction of the relevant drug in the plasma which determines the extracellular fluid distribution. This agonist–antagonist interaction can be demonstrated by one of two methods, namely inhibition of exercise-induced tachycardia, or demonstration of a rightwards shift of the dose-response curve to a suitable agonist, usually isoprenaline.

Inhibition of exercise-induced tachycardia

While a decrease of resting heart rate is consistent with adequate β-adrenoceptor blocking effect, only an inhibition of tachycardia induced by β-adrenoceptor activation can be used for quantitative estimation of adequate antagonism. Exercise-induced tachycardia may be quantitated by graded bicycle ergometry[47], graduated treadmill exercise[8] or by a simple fixed work step test involving a consistent step-height and rate and duration of stepping[34]. These tests are non-invasive and perfectly adequate for use in pharmacology laboratories, out-patient clinics or in the medical ward. The heart rate response to glyceryl trinitrate (0.5 mg sublingual) has also been described[16].

The normal index used is the percentage decrease of exercise-induced tachycardia, and this can be modified for determining equipotent doses (and equivalent plasma concentrations) of drugs which produce a predefined percentage decrease (20–25%). Table 13.4 shows the relationship between dose and plasma concentration required to inhibit exercise-induced tachycardia by 20–25%.

Isoprenaline dose-response curves

The construction of response curves relating increase of heart rate (or other variables) to increasing bolus doses or infusion rates of isoprenaline, enables dose-response curves to be constructed (Fig. 13.1). From these, the degree of blockade can be measured as the increased dose of isoprenaline required to produce a given response. Correct pharmacological practice would demand that the ED_{50}, the mid-point of the dose-response curve, should be used. However, this creates unacceptable constraints in human studies and in practice an increase of heart rate by 25 beats per minute (CD_{25}) is

Table 13.4 Oral and intravenous dosage of β-adrenoceptor antagonists in relation to plasma concentrations required to cause 20% inhibition of exercise tachycardia.

	Reference	Oral dose (mg)	Intravenous dose (mg)	Plasma concentration (ng ml^{-1})
Practolol	[2, 17]	200	20–40	750–1000
Propranolol	[11, 12, 44]	80	10–20	50–70
Metoprolol	[22, 23]	100	50	100
Labetalol	[30]	200	50–100	180
Alprenolol	[1]	100	10	50–60
Atenolol	[, 54]	100	40–50	200–500
Sotalol	[19]	300	—	20
Oxprenolol	[19]	80	25	80–100
Acebutalol	[32, 35]	200	50–100	1200
Pindolol	[25, 47]	5–12	5	16
Nadolol		80–160		
Timolol		20		

normally accepted[10], as this coincides with the straight part of the log dose-response relationship. In normal healthy volunteers[10] aged between 21 and 32 years the CD_{25} for isoprenaline was 0.9 μg (range 0.4–2.5 μg), and in a group of 11 patients aged between 50 and 65 during anaesthesia the CD_{25} was 4.5 μg (range 1.3–8.6 μg)[13].

Receptor theory (see Chapter 2) would predict[11] that:

$$(DR - 1) = KaPc$$

where DR is the ratio of the doses of isoprenaline required for a given response (CD_{25}), Ka is the association rate constant, and Pc is the plasma concentration of the antagonist. Fig. 13.5 shows that for propranolol (DR – 1) shows a linear correlation with Pc[43], and a similar relationship was also demonstrated by the same authors for free propranolol concentration.

According to receptor theory, when antagonism is expressed as the decrease of a given response (R), then:

$$\frac{R}{1 - R} = \frac{Pc}{Ka}$$

Expressed as a plot of R against log Pc, this gives a linear relationship of 20–80% of the maximal response[28, 43]. Thus comparisons can be made between results derived from exercise testing and those obtained from isoprenaline dose-response studies. The latter have obvious advantages for the assessment of β-adrenoceptor blockade in the anaesthetised or unconscious patient who cannot perform exercise.

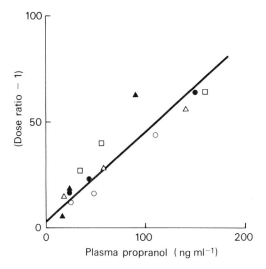

Fig. 13.5 Relationship between plasma propranolol concentration and the antagonism of isoprenaline-induced tachycardia (DR − 1). Each point represents a different subject given 20 mg propranolol, with samples being taken at 15 min, 3 h and 6 h. (After Shand *et al.*[43]).

INTRAVENOUS ADMINISTRATION

Intravenous administration of a β-adrenoceptor antagonist is more commonly used during anaesthesia and in the intensive therapy unit than in general medical practice, and ensures virtually complete bioavailability of the injected dose. For a given single dose administered, much higher plasma concentrations will be achieved more rapidly, ensuring maximal pharmacodynamic effect within a minute or two of drug adminis-tration. The decay of plasma concentration follows the same time-constant as that following oral administration (Fig. 13.4), and the degree of β-adrenoceptor blockade is dependent on the free fraction plasma concentration at any given time.

Most studies of the pharmacokinetics of intravenously administered β-adrenoceptor antagonists have been performed following doses predicted to produce average plasma concentrations and effects comparable to those achieved after therapeutic oral doses (Table 13.4). In most cases these doses are much higher than those normally employed by anaesthetists for the suppression of tachycardia or dysrhythmia.

An example of this relationship relevant to clinical anaesthesia concerns the response, and its duration, to a single intravenous dose of 20 mg practolol. This was the dose administered to hypertensive patients to protect them from the undesirable responses to the noxious stimulation of laryngoscopy and intubation[40]. This was based on the results of pharmacokinetic studies which showed that a 20 mg i.v. dose of practolol maintained plasma concentrations of practolol in excess of 1.5 μg ml^{-1} for 10 minutes. This plasma concentration was equivalent to that obtained by oral dosing with 150 mg twice daily, and was associated with 30% inhibition of exercise-induced tachycardia[2].

PHARMACODYNAMICS OF BETA-ADRENOCEPTOR ANTAGONISTS DURING ANAESTHESIA

Following intravenous injections of propranolol ($0.4\ \mathrm{mg\,kg^{-1}}$) or practolol[41] in dogs under nitrous oxide/oxygen halothane anaesthesia, dose-response curves for both chronotropic and inotropic responses were shifted by 1.2 orders of magnitude. However, no measurements of plasma concentration of either of these antagonists were made during these studies.

In studies of patients receiving very high oral doses of propranolol ($10\text{--}36\ \mathrm{mg\,kg^{-1}\,day^{-1}}$) or alternative antagonists, for the treatment of severe hypertension secondary to renal artery occlusion[38, 39] very marked shifts of the isoprenaline dose-response curve (CD_{25}: 540 μg isoprenaline) were observed during surgery, four hours after the previous oral dose (Fig. 13.6). These high doses were necessary to control the severe renin-dependent hypertension at a time before the introduction of angiotensin converting-enzyme inhibitors such as captopril.

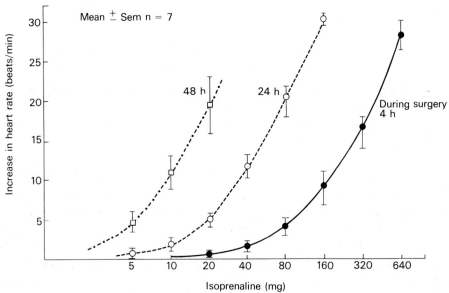

Fig. 13.6 Isoprenaline dose-response curves for 13 renal hypertensive patients receiving between 10 and $36\ \mathrm{mg\,kg^{-1}\,day^{-1}}$ propranolol. Curves were derived during surgery (approximately 4 hours after last dose of propranolol), and 24 hours and 48 hours after surgery and the last dose of propranolol. From Prys-Roberts[39], by courtesy of the Editor, *Acta Anaesthesiologica Scandinavica*.

24-hours after the previous dose the isoprenaline dose-response curve had shifted leftwards (CD_{25}: 120 μg isoprenaline) and even after 48-hours the CD_{25} (32 μg isoprenaline) had not returned to the normal range for patients in this age group.

These findings contrast with those of Nattel[36] who studied 9 patients receiving a median dose of 240 mg propranolol per day (range 160–320 mg) who showed a CD_{25} of

4.8 μg (range 1.0–10.9 μg) on the second day after withdrawal of propranolol, and a CD_{25} of 2.8 μg (range 1.5–6.4 μg) two weeks after drug withdrawal. Nattel's group found evidence of transient supersensitivity to the chronotropic effects of isoprenaline, maximal six days after propranolol withdrawal (CD_{25} 1.2 μg, range: 0.3–3.4 μg).

Earlier studies[15] on only three patients showed that during dosage with 80–240 mg day^{-1} of propranolol the CD_{25} ranged between 34 and 42 μg and had decreased to normal values (< 1.0 μg) within a 24–48-hour period. Patients presenting for surgery showed CD_{25} values of 44 μg (range 13–80 μg) while on atenolol 100 mg daily, and 49 μg (range 22–93 μg) while on labetalol 200 mg three times a day[13].

These various studies indicate that in patients taking propranolol and other β-adrenoceptor antagonists up to the day of surgery, the degree of receptor blockade is related to both the dose and the plasma concentration of propranolol, and that the time required for the regression of blockade is dependent on the pre-existing dose of the antagonist. If patients are receiving less than 240 mg per day of propranolol the regression of blockade may be complete within 24 hours, whereas for patients taking more than 2 g per day the regression may take much longer than 48-hours.

CONTINUOUS INFUSION OF BETA-ADRENOCEPTOR ANTAGONISTS

In normal therapeutic practice these drugs can conveniently be administered by mouth or down a nasogastric tube. However, for patients who cannot absorb drugs from the gastrointestinal tract because of ileus, and who need to be maintained in a state of β-adrenoceptor blockade, the drugs must be administered intravenously.

Those drugs which have a high hepatic and total body clearance are particularly suitable for administration by infusion[27]. The daily requirement for intravenous or intramuscular replacement for oral therapy can be calculated theoretically from the known bioavailability data (Table 13.3). In practice, replacement on this basis almost always results in higher plasma concentrations, and greater degrees of blockade than those found on standard oral therapy. This is mainly because regular intravenous increments at short intervals, or a continuous infusion, results in relatively constant plasma concentrations of the antagonist. Oral dosage on a twice- or thrice-daily basis results in higher peak concentrations within one hour of taking the drug, but lower concentrations for the rest of the period until the subsequent dose.

Let us consider replacement therapy for a patient with severe coronary artery disease receiving 240 mg propranolol daily (3×80 mg) by mouth, and presenting for surgery which can be predicted to cause ileus for at least 48-hours. From Table 13.3 the bioavailability data (30%) would suggest that a daily intravenous dose of 72 mg would be required. This dose (3 mg h^{-1}) was infused for more than 24-hours in 13 patients following major abdominal surgery[46] and produced a mean plasma concentration of 80 ng ml^{-1} (SEM ± 4.5 ng ml^{-1}). Apart from the tedium of cracking 72 ampoules containing 1 mg propranolol each, the consequent degrees of β-adrenoceptor blockade achieved would be far more than necessary. In practice, a daily dose of 24 mg (1 mg h^{-1} by infusion) achieves adequate blockade.

Following coronary artery surgery, plasma propranolol concentrations of about 50 ng ml^{-1} have been associated with a fourfold shift to the right of the isoprenaline dose-response curve[29].

Continuous infusion of labetalol

Despite its large volume of distribution (Table 13.3) the high total body clearance of this non-selective β-adrenoceptor antagonist, which also has α-adrenoceptor antagonist properties, makes it the most suitable drug for continuous infusion. Studies of its bioavailability[30] indicated a wide variation in the calculated values; 38 % (range 11–86 %) after a dose of 100 mg, and 28 % (range 19–49 %) after a dose of 200 mg. The distribution volume after intravenous administration was smaller (5.1 l kg^{-1}) than after oral administration, and this would account for higher plasma concentrations, and greater pharmacological effect, observed after intravenous administration.

In the management of acute hypertension complicating myocardial infarction, infusions of labetalol at a mean dose of 60 mg h^{-1} have been described[33, 49], but no pharmacokinetic data were described, nor was the degree of β-adrenoceptor blockade assessed.

In a series of 8 patients receiving β-adrenoceptor antagonists for hypertension or coronary artery disease, and presenting for aortic replacement surgery, the author [13] studied the effects of an infusion of labetalol during and after anaesthesia. Based on bioavailability data, the predicted infusion rate was 20 mg h^{-1}. However, this infusion rate produced unacceptable arterial hypotension, and infusion rates of 5–10 mg h^{-1} were found to produce adequate β-adrenoceptor blockade (CD$_{25}$ for isoprenaline: 124 μg; range 100–150 μg) without unacceptable hypotension. This degree of blockade was achieved at plasma concentrations of between 80 and 158 ng ml^{-1}.

REFERENCES

1. ÅBLAD B., BORG K. O., JOHNSSON G., REGÅRDH C-G. & SÖLVELL L. (1974) Combined pharmacokinetic and pharmacodynamic studies on alprenolol and 4-hydroxy alprenolol in man. *Life Sci.* **14**, 693.

2. AELLIG W. H., PRICHARD B. N. C. & SCALES B. (1970) Blood levels of practolol following intravenous administration. *Br. J. Pharmacol.* **40**, 573P.

3. AHLQUIST R. P. (1948) Study of the adrenotropic receptors. *Am. J. Physiol.* **153**, 586.

4. ARIENS È. J. & SIMONIS A. M. (1976) Receptors and receptor mechanisms. In P. R. Saxena & R. P. Forsyth (eds.), *Beta-adrenoceptor blocking agents*. North Holland-American Elsevier, New York.

5. BIANCHETTI G., GRAZIANI G., BRANCACCIO D., MORGANTI A., LEIONETTI G. et al. (1976) Pharmacokinetics and effects of propranolol in terminal uraemic patients and in patients undergoing regular dialysis treatment. *Clin. Pharmacokin.* **1**, 373.

6. BRANCH R. A., JAMES J. & READ A. E.

(1976) A study of factors influencing drug disposition in chronic liver disease using the model drug (+) propranolol. *Br. J. Clin. Pharmacol.* **3**, 243.

7. BRANCH R. A. & SHAND D. G. (1976) Propranolol disposition in chronic liver disease: a physiological approach. *Clin. Pharmacokin.* **1**, 264.

8. BRUCE R. A. (1974) Progress in exercise cardiology. In P. N. Yu & J. F. Goodwin (eds.), *Progress in Cardiology* **3**, 113. Lea & Febiger, Philadelphia.

9. CARLSSON E., DAHLÖFF C-G., PERSSON H. & TÅNGSTRAND B. (1977) Differentiation of cardiac chronotropic and inotropic effects of beta-adrenoceptor agonists. *Naunyn Schmiedebergs Arch. Pharmacol.* **300**, 100.

10. CLEAVELAND C. R., RANGNO R. E. & SHAND D. G. (1972) A standardized isoproterenol sensitivity test. *Arch. Int. Med.* **130**, 47.

11. CLEAVELAND C. R. & SHAND D. G. (1972) Effect of route of administration on the relationship between beta-adrenergic blockade and plasma propranolol level. *Clin. Pharmacol. Ther.* **13**, 181.

12. COLTART D. H. & SHAND D. G. (1970) Plasma propranolol levels in the quantitative assessment of beta-adrenergic blockade in man. *Br. Med. J.* **3**, 731.

13. DAGNINO J. & PRYS-ROBERTS C. (1983) Evaluation of beta-adrenoceptor responsiveness during anaesthesia in humans. *Anesth. Analg.* **62**, 245.

14. DAVIS W. G. (1970) A comparison of the local anaesthetic, quinidine-like and adrenergic *β*-blocking activities of five beta receptor antagonists. *J. Pharm. Pharmacol.* **22**, 284.

15. FAULKNER S. L., HOPKINS J. T., BOERTH R. C., YOUNG J. L., JENNETT L. B. *et al.* (1973) Time required for complete recovery from chronic propranolol therapy. *New Engl. J. Med.* **289**, 607.

16. FITZGERALD J. D. (1970) A new test of the degree of adrenergic beta-receptor blockade. *Int. J. Clin. Pharmacol.* **4**, 125.

17. FITZGERALD J. D. & SCALES B. (1968) Effect of a new adrenergic beta-blocking agent (ICI 50,172) on heart rate in relation to its blood levels. *Int. J. Clin. Pharmacol.* **1**, 467.

18. FITZGERALD J. D., WALE J. L. & AUSTIN M. (1972) The haemodynamic effects of (±) propranolol, dexpropranolol, oxprenolol, practolol and sotalol in anaesthetized dogs. *Eur. J. Pharmacol.* **17**, 123.

19. FRISHMAN W. (1979) Clinical pharmacology of the new beta-adrenergic blocking drugs. Part 1. Pharmacokynamic and pharmacokinetic properties. *Am. Heart J.* **97**, 663.

20. HEDBERG A., MINNEMAN K. P. & MOLINOFF P. B. (1980) Differential distribution of $beta_1$ and $beta_2$-adrenoceptors in cat and guinea pig heart. *J. Pharmacol. Exp. Ther.* **212**, 503.

21. HOMEIDA M., JACKSON L. & ROBERTS C. J. C. (1978) Decreased first-pass metabolism of labetalol in chronic liver disease. *Br. Med. J,* **2**, 1048.

22. JOHNSSON G., REGÅRDH C-G. & SOLVELL L. (1975) Combined pharmacokinetic and pharmacodynamic studies in man of the adrenergic $beta_1$-receptor antagonist metoprolol. *Acta Pharmacol. Toxicol.* (Copenhagen). **36**, suppl 5, 31.

23. JORDÖ L., ATTMAN P. O., AURELL M., JOHANSSON L., JONSSON G. & REGÄRDH C-G. (1980) Pharmacokinetic and pharmacodynamic properties of metoprolol in patients with imparied renal function. *Clin. Pharmacokin.* **5**, 169.

24. LANDS A. M., ARNOLD A., MCAULIFF J. P., LUDUENA F. P. & BROWN T. G. (1967) Differentiation of receptor systems activated by sympatho-mimetic amines. *Nature (Lond.)* **214**, 597.

25. LEVENE D., WEISS Y. A., SAFAR M. E., LERIA Y., AGERUS N., GEORGES D. & MILLIEZ P. L. (1977) Pharmacokinetics and hepatic extraction ratio of pindolol in hypertensive patients with normal and impaired renal function. *J. Clin. Pharmacol.* **17**, 501.

26. LOWENTHAL D. T., BRIGGS W. A., GIBSON T. P., NELSON H. & CIRKSENA J. (1974) Pharmacokinetics of oral propranolol in chronic renal disease. *Clin. Pharmacol. Ther.* **16**, 761.

27. MCALLISTER R. G. (1976) Intravenous propranolol administration: a method for rapidly achieving and sustaining desired plasma levels. *Clin. Pharmacol. Ther.* **20**, 517.

28. MCDEVITT D. G. (1977) The assessment of β-adrenoceptor blocking drugs in man. *Br. J. Clin. Pharmacol.* **4**, 413.

29. MCDONALD D. H., JARMAN R. H., KAPLAN J. A. & HUG C. C. JR. (1977) Abstract: American Society of Anesthiologists Annual Meeting.

30. MCNEIL J. J., ANDERSON A. E., LOUIS W. J. & MORGAN D. J. (1978) Pharmacokinetics and pharmacodynamic studies of labetalol in hypertensive subjects. *Br. J. Clin. Pharmacol.* **8**, 157S.

31. MAGUIRE M. E., ROSS E. M. & GILMAN A. G. (1977) Beta-adrenergic receptor: ligand binding properties and the interaction with adenylate cyclase. *Cyclic Nucleotide Res.* **8**, 1.

32. MARTIN M. A., PHILIPS F. C., TUCKER G. T. & SMITH A. J. (1978) Acebutalol in hypertension: relationship between drug concentration and effects. *Eur. J. Clin. Pharmacol.* **14**, 383.

33. MARX P. G. & REID D. S. (1979) Labetalol infusion in acute myocardial infarction with systemic hypertension. *Br. J. Clin. Pharmacol.* **8**, 9.

34. MASTER A. M. & GELLER A. J. (1969) The extent of completely asymptomatic coronary artery disease. *Am. J. Cardiol.* **23**, 173.

35. MEFFIN P. J., WINKLE R. A., PETERS F. A. & HARRISON D. C. (1977) Acebutalol disposition after intravenous administration. *Clin. Pharmacol. Ther.* **22**, 557.

36. NATTEL S., RANGNO R. E. & VAN LOON G. (1979) Mechanism of propranolol withdrawal phenomenon. *Circulation* **59**, 1158.

37. OHNHAUS E. E., NUESCHE E., METER J. & KALBERER F. (1974) Pharmacokinetics of unlabelled and ^{14}C-labelled pindolol in uraemia. *Eur. J. Clin. Pharmacol.* **7**, 25.

38. PRYS-ROBERTS C. (1979) Hemodynamic effects of anesthesia and surgery in renal hypertensive patients receiving large doses of beta-receptor antagonists. *Anesthesiology* **51**, S122.

39. PRYS-ROBERTS C. (1982) Interactions of Anaesthesia and High Pre-operative Doses of β-receptor Antagonists. *Acta Anaesth. Scand.* **26**, Suppl 76, 447–53.

40. PRYS-ROBERTS C., FOËX P., BIRO G. P. & ROBERTS J. G. (1973) Studies of anaesthesia in relation to hypertension V. Adrenergic beta-receptor blockade. *Br. J. Anaesth.* **45**, 671.

41. PRYS-ROBERTS C., ROBERTS J. G., CLARKE T. N. S., FOËX P., BENNETT M. J. & RYDER W. A. (1976) Interaction of anesthesia, beta-receptor blockade and blood loss in dogs with induced myocardial infarction *Anesthesiology* **45**, 326.

42. REGÅRDH C-G. (1980) Pharmacokinetics of β-adrenoceptor antagonists. In Poppers P. J., van Dijk B. & van Elzakker A. H. M. (eds.), *β-blockade and Anaesthesia*, pp. 29–44. Rijswijk, Astra Pharmaceutica.

43. SHAND D. G., FRISK-HOLMBERG M., MCDEVITT D., SHERMAN K. & HOLLIFIELD J. (1975) A dual antihypertensive mechanism for propranolol based on plasma level/response relationships. In Berglund G., Hansson L. & Werko L. (eds.), *Pathophysiology and Management of Arterial Hypertension*, p. 175. Molndal, Astra Pharmaceuticals.

44. SHANKS R. G., NEILL J. D., LEAHY W. J. & VARMA M. P. S. (1979) Observations on some properties of a long-acting preparation of propranolol. *Clinical Sci.* **57**, 409s.

45. SLOGOFF S., KEATS A. S., HIBBS C. W., EDMONDS C. H. & BRAGG D. A. (1977) Failure of general anesthesia to potentiate propranolol activity. *Anesthesiology* **47**, 504.

46. SMULYAN H., WEINBERG S. E. & HOWANITZ P. J. (1982) Continuous propranolol infusion following abdominal surgery. *J. Am. Med. Assoc.* **247**, 2539.

47. SOWTON E., DAS GUPTA D. S. & BAKER I. (1975) Comparative effects of beta-adrenergic blocking drugs. *Thorax* **30**, 9.

48. STARKE K. (1977) Regulation of noradrenaline release by presynaptic receptor systems. *Rev. Physiol. Biochem. Pharmacol.* **77**, 1.

49. TIMMIS A. D., FOWLER M. B., JAGGARAO N. S. V. & CHAMBERLAIN D. A. (1980) Labetalol infusion for the treatment of hypertension in acute myocardial infarction. *Eur. Heart J.* **1**, 413.

50. TJANDRAMAGA T. B., THOMAS J., CERBEECK R., VERBESSELT R., VERBEEKMOES R. & DE SCHEPPER P. J. (1976) The effect of end stage renal failure and haemodialysis on the elimination kinetics of sotalol. *Br. J. Clin. Pharmacol.* **3**, 259.

51. VAUGHAN WILLIAMS E. M. (1958) The mode of action of quinidine in isolated rabbit atria interpreted from intracellular records. *Br. J. Pharmacol.* **13**, 276.

52. VAUGHAN WILLIAMS E. M. (1966) Mode of action of beta receptor antagonists on cardiac muscle. *Am. J. Cardiol.* **18**, 399.

53. VILJOEN J. F., ESTAFANOUS G. & KELLNER G. A. (1972) Propranolol and cardiac surgery. *J. Thorac. Cardiovasc. Surg.* **64**, 826.

54. WAN S. H., KODA R. T. & MARONDE R. F. (1979) Pharmacokinetics, pharmacology of atenolol and effect of renal disease. *Br. J. Clin. Pharmacol.* **7**, 569.

55. WILLIAMS L. T. & LEFKOWITZ R. J. (1978) *Receptor binding studies in adrenergic pharmacology*, Chapter 7, pp. 83–109. Raven Press, New York.

56. WOOD M., SHAND D. G. & WOOD A. J. J. (1979) Propranolol binding in plasma during cardiopulmonary bypass. *Anesthesiology* **51**, 512.

14 Sodium Nitroprusside—Distribution, Metabolism and Causes of Toxicity

P. J. SIMPSON

Nitroprusside and red cell metabolism
Metabolism and excretion
Tachyphylaxis (acute tolerance)
Toxicity

Sodium nitroprusside ($Na_2Fe(CN)_5.NO.2H_2O$; SNP) is widely used as a vasodilator both in anaesthesia and intensive care. SNP was first administered to animals in 1886 by Hermann[9], who gave the first indication of its potential toxicity. The first definitive work on the actions and toxicology of the drug was published by Johnson in 1929[12]. He noted a rapid well-sustained fall in arterial blood pressure accompanied by tachycardia in response to intravenous nitroprusside and concluded that the vasodepressor action of the drug was due solely to peripheral vasodilation, independent of innervation. In 1951, Page[23] first used SNP clinically in the treatment of hypertension, but chronic oral administration proved unreliable. Intravenous SNP for the production of elective hypotension under anaesthesia was suggested in 1962 by Moraca et al.[20] for a variety of conditions, and since then its use has spread to neuro- and cardiac surgery as well as intensive care.

The ready availability of the drug in qualitative chemical analysis led to widespread use before the establishment of controlled trials to assess its safety, efficacy and pharmacokinetics. More recently, the availability of a lyophyllised commercial preparation, Nipride (Roche) has provided an accurately controlled, stable and effective form of nitroprusside for clinical use.

SNP produces an extremely rapid, dose-dependent fall in systemic arterial blood pressure, dilating resistance and capacitance vessels equally. It is capable of inducing hypotension to any degree desired in normotensive individuals in addition to reducing pathological hypertension. Although originally believed to produce vasodilation by a nitrite-like action, comparative studies[12] have shown that the effect of SNP is approximately 10 times greater than other drugs of this group. Recent work suggests that nitroprusside acts by inhibiting intracellular metabolism, either by interference with sulphydryl systems[21] or by preventing the mobilisation of ionised calcium[14].

The evanescent action of SNP produces vasodilation and a profound, dose-dependent fall in blood pressure within one to two minutes. Return of blood pressure to normal is equally as rapid following discontinuation of therapy. The drug is therefore mainly suitable for use as an intravenous infusion to produce instantaneously controllable levels of blood pressure, against a background of moderate hypotension. This is usually best achieved with a combination of halothane, +-tubocurarine and controlled ventilation, with or without β-adrenergic blockade.

Although nitroprusside was originally believed to produce hypotension by inducing a minor degree of cyanide poisoning, this has now been disproved[12, 28]. Injection of a bolus dose of potassium cyanide into an anaesthetised dog initially produces a moderate elevation of systemic blood pressure, hypotension only occurring with a severe degree of cyanide poisoning. Nevertheless breakdown of the nitroprusside molecule within the bloodstream yields measurable quantities of free cyanide which must subsequently be metabolised. Following intravenous injection the intact nitro-prusside molecule appears to be responsible for producing vasodilation and hypo-tension.

Subsequent non-enzymatic breakdown of nitroprusside occurring in both red blood cells and plasma terminates the pharmacological effect of the drug (Fig. 14.1). Metabolism of the cyanide produced from SNP breakdown occurs mainly in the liver, the resulting thiocyanate being excreted in the urine. Two compartment breakdown of SNP has been confirmed by simultaneous measurement of plasma and red cell cyanide levels following bolus intravenous injection of the drug. Plasma cyanide levels peak before those in the red cells implying that at least some SNP breakdown is occurring extracellularly[32]. Nevertheless, as Smith and Krusyna[26] have shown, nitro-prusside breakdown within red cells is the more important, since free sulphydryl groups, present in far greater concentration intracellularly, are required in this reaction. They suggest that haemoglobin acts as a catalyst for SNP breakdown and that methaemoglobin is formed in the process. Of the five free cyanide ions formed from

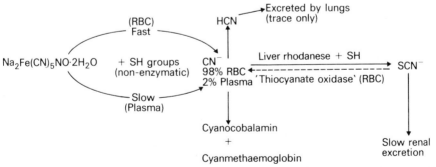

Fig. 14.1 Route of breakdown of sodium nitroprusside. CN^- = cyanide, SCN^- = thio-cyanate, SH = sulphydryl groups.

each molecule of nitroprusside, one combines with the simultaneously formed methaemoglobin to form cyanmethaemoglobin, leaving four potentially toxic cyanide ions.

Incubation of a fixed quantity of nitroprusside with whole blood for two hours at 37°C yields 98 % of the available cyanide[33]. Incubation with the red cell fraction alone yields only 80 % and with plasma alone 20 %. This 4:1 ratio demonstrates the relative importance of the two blood fractions in cyanide production from SNP. Under optimum conditions, after two hours, 98 % of the free cyanide is detectable within the red cells and only 2 % within the plasma, when SNP is incubated with whole blood. Since little or no effect upon oxygen transport is observed with intracellular cyanide levels measured following clinical concentrations of nitroprusside[4] the plasma levels, although relatively small, are important in determining the concentration gradient between plasma and other tissues and organs.

Following SNP infusion in dogs of a total dose of 1.5 mg kg^{-1} over one hour, plasma cyanide (HCN) levels peak at 40 min, reaching a mean value of 1.7 μmol l^{-1}[32]. The mean maximum red cell cyanide concentration of 120 μmol l^{-1} is not reached until the end of infusion. Both values decline rapidly, returning to pre-infusion concentrations 120 minutes after the cessation of infusion.

Nitroprusside and red cell metabolism

Two separate reactions are involved in the breakdown of nitroprusside within the blood, both of which are non-enzymatic and depend upon an adequate supply of sulphydryl groups. The first, a relatively fast reaction catalysed by haemoglobin occurs within the red cells, while the second slower reaction occurs in the plasma. Despite the preferentially high cyanide levels which occur within the red cells, both clinical and laboratory investigations in man[4] and dog[25] have failed to demonstrate significant effects on red cell oxygen transport at cyanide levels within the range normally measured during routine use of SNP. In one study[25] no significant alterations in either oxygen consumption, P$_{50}$ or oxygen content were recorded when the dose of SNP used was less than 1.5 mg kg^{-1} equivalent to a dose rate of 10 μg kg^{-1} min^{-1} over 2–3 hours. In another study[4] no measurable methaemoglobin or cyanmet-haemoglobin was detected nor were any alterations in either 2,3-DPG or carbonic anhydrase activity measured during routine use of the drug. Small increases in plasma lactate, mirrored by an increase in arterial base deficit (< 6 mmol l^{-1}) occur at doses of SNP approaching 1.5 mg kg^{-1}[25]. These effects are all spontaneously reversible without treatment. It would appear that the routine monitoring of base deficit in patients receiving prolonged SNP therapy provides a reliable indication of the development of even minor impairment of oxygen transport and delivery.

In an *in vitro* study, Vesey, Krapez and Cole[31] were able to demonstrate a dose-related reduction in P$_{50}$ but only at red cell cyanide concentrations three times the maximum recorded during clinical use. A parallel *in vivo* study[31] in patients undergoing hypotensive anaesthesia failed to demonstrate any change in P_{50}. They postulated that the effect on P_{50} might be produced either by cyanide interfering with 2,3-DPG binding to the β-chain of haemoglobin or possibly due to methaemoglobin formation leading to a fall in oxygen carrying capacity.

Metabolism and excretion

Plasma cyanide

There are several physiological pathways by which elimination of plasma cyanide occurs, the most important being hepatic metabolism. Free cyanide may also combine with methaemoglobin to form cyanmethaemoglobin, although this will only account for a maximum of 20% of the total cyanide produced from nitroprusside[28]. The formation of cyanocobalamin by the combination of cyanide with hydroxocobalamin is also responsible for detoxification of a proportion of cyanide while small amounts of free cyanide may be excreted unchanged in expired air and urine.

The hepatic enzyme rhodanese is capable of metabolising large quantities of cyanide, the rate-limiting factor in this reaction being the supply of free sulphydryl groups as substrate for the formation of thiocyanate (SCN). Michenfelder and Tinker[18] have clearly demonstrated that concomitant administration of sodium thiosulphate to dogs receiving prolonged infusion of SNP considerably reduces the rise in whole blood cyanide which would otherwise occur. Krapez *et al.*[13] have also shown that the rate of decrease of plasma cyanide by metabolism to thiocyanate in dogs following large bolus doses of nitroprusside can be considerably enhanced by sodium thiosulphate administration. These findings are of extreme importance in the treatment of cyanide toxicity or poisoning when rapid reduction of blood cyanide levels is vital.

Red cell cyanide

The subsequent metabolic pathway of cyanide contained in the red cells is as yet uncertain. Three possibilities exist:

1   Cyanide diffuses out of the red cell down a concentration gradient created by the metabolism of plasma cyanide to thiocyanate by rhodanese.

2   A separate metabolic pathway may exist within the red cell, e.g. the conversion of cyanide to an inactive form such as cyanate.

3   Cyanide is converted to thiocyanate within the red cell by another enzyme, β-mercaptopyruvate sulphur transferase. This enzyme however only appears to show low, if any, activity in man.

Although diffusion of cyanide from red cells to plasma appears to be a simple explanation for the reduction in intracellular cyanide concentrations, it may only in part be the answer. Following a bolus injection of potassium cyanide in dogs resulting in plasma and red cell cyanide levels of similar order to those obtained following 1.5 mg kg^{-1} of nitroprusside, while plasma cyanide concentrations returned to normal within 40 minutes, similar red cell concentrations were only reached after 2–3 hours. For simple diffusion of cyanide to explain the reduction in red cell cyanide, high plasma cyanide concentrations should be maintained until the red cell levels are normal.

Thiocyanate

Thiocyanate produced by hepatic metabolism of cyanide is subsequently excreted in the urine and impaired renal function may therefore result in thiocyanate accumulation. Thiocyanate itself is potentially toxic and was used originally in the treatment of hypertension. An hepatic enzyme system 'thiocyanate oxidase' was thought to convert thiocyanate to cyanide, a reversal of the rhodanese system, and that sub-clinical cyanide poisoning was then responsible for hypotension. A single report[22] of thiocyanate toxicity resulting in reversible hypothroidism occurred at a plasma thiocyanate level in excess of 1500 mmol l^{-1}. Maximum plasma thiocyanate levels reached in patients with normal renal function during routine nitroprusside therapy are < 150 mmol l^{-1} and are considerably less in non-smokers than in smokers[30].

Tachyphylaxis (acute tolerance)

The gradual increase in nitroprusside infusion rate necessary to produce the same degree of hypotension (tachphylaxis) only occurs in a small number of patients. Nevertheless, if persistent, this may lead to the use of unacceptably high levels of nitroprusside and the possible development of cyanide toxicity. Several possible mechanisms have been suggested to account for this tachyphylaxis[1a]. These have included pharmacological deterioration of the drug, unrecognised hypovolaemia, excessively light anaesthesia or the so-called central ischaemic reflex. The possible existence of an undetected phaeochromocytoma has also been suggested! The most likely reasons for tachyphylaxis, however, would appear to be either hyperactivity of the renin–angiotensin system producing vasoconstriction and tending to oppose the vasodilatory effects of nitroprusside, or an impairment of cyanide metabolism. Miller and his colleagues[19] demonstrated that the renin–angiotensin system was activated by moderate nitroprusside-induced hypotension and that hyperactivity of this system occurring in certain patients may account for a degree of resistance to nitroprusside.

The possibility of cyanide antagonism of nitroprusside vasodilation was suggested by Grayling[8], who demonstrated *in vitro* that while nitroprusside alone antagonised the increase in tension of the isolated rabbit aorta produced by noradrenaline, when nitroprusside was combined with cyanide in the presence of noradrenaline the tension increased. He postulated that cyanide antagonised nitroprusside either by a direct toxic effect or possibly by chemical antagonism of the nitroprusside molecule. The most likely effect would appear to be a pharmacological antagonism at the cellular level where nitroprusside is acting. Clinically this is substantiated by the fact that resistance may be due to an abnormally high cyanide level, since it is only seen when the cyanide concentration approaches that of the nitroprusside itself. As more SNP is given more cyanide is produced and the SNP becomes less effective. Although the use of high nitroprusside dose rates should be avoided, it is possible that resistance to the drug may be avoided by increasing the rate of metabolism of cyanide to thiocyanate[13].

Toxicity

The production of free cyanide as a result of nitroprusside metabolism is potentially toxic. Nevertheless this toxicity can be minimised by an awareness of the pharmaco-dynamics and pharmacokinetics of the drug, which have already been discussed. Several fatalities attributable to nitroprusside infusion have been reported, all of which were essentially due to cyanide poisoning[6, 11, 17]. All occurred however, soon after reintroduction of the drug into clinical anaesthetic practice in 1969, and were due to gross overdosage.

Table 14.1 illustrates the reported cases of toxicity[6, 11, 15, 17] and the doses of SNP used, all of which were greatly in excess of the maximum safe doses currently recommended. Most were probably due to the development of resistance to the drug. The continued administration of SNP in increasing doses despite any expected effect being reduced or absent is potentially toxic and should not be attempted. It is interesting that no recent reports of fatalities directly attributable to SNP have appeared, suggesting that it is being used with greater caution.

From these reported cases (Table 14.1) estimated plasma cyanide levels have been calculated, based upon the calculated ratio of red cell to plasma cyanide already

Table 14.1   Reported cases of cyanide toxicity.

Reference	SNP dose	Details	Estimated plasma HCN $(\mu mol\, l^{-1})$
Davies *et al.*[6]	400 mg ($10\,mg\,kg^{-1}$)	14-year-old male infused over 80 min: fatal	22
Jack[11]	750 mg ($11\,mg\,kg^{-1}$)	39-year-old male infused over 30 min: fatal	24
MacRae and Owen[15]	250 mg ($6.3\,mg\,kg^{-1}$)	42-year-old female infused over 90 min: severe reversible acidosis	9
Merrifield and Blundell[17]	750 mg ($10\,mg\,kg^{-1}$)	20-year-old male infused over 5 h: fatal	13 after 3 h (? 22 after 5 h)

discussed. This indicates a minimum fatal plasma cyanide level in the region of $20 \, \mu\mathrm{mol}\,l^{-1}$ which would be associated with a red cell level of $200\text{--}250 \, \mu\mathrm{mol}\,l^{-1}$ and would result in the development of an irreversible metabolic acidosis. By the application of similar calculations to the maximum safe doses recommended for SNP therapy[2, 16, 29] (Table 14.2) a total dose of $1.5 \, \mathrm{mg}\,\mathrm{kg}^{-1}$ would produce a plasma cyanide concentration in the region of $3 \, \mu\mathrm{mol}\,l^{-1}$. This is equivalent to the administration of $12 \, \mu\mathrm{g}\,\mathrm{kg}^{-1}\,\mathrm{min}^{-1}$ to a 70 kg man for 2 hours. In most cases, satisfactory hypotension can be achieved with doses considerably less than this.

Table 14.2 Maximum recommended doses of SNP.

Reference	SNP dose	Details	Estimated plasma HCN ($\mu\mathrm{mol}\,l^{-1}$)
B. M. J. Editorial[2]	$3 \, \mathrm{mg}\,\mathrm{kg}^{-1}\,\mathrm{hr}^{-1}$	Recommended rate	20 after 3 h
McDowall *et al.*[16]	$3.6 \, \mathrm{mg}\,\mathrm{kg}^{-1}$	Suggested lethal dose in man	8 after 1–3 h infusion
	$320 \, \mathrm{mg}\,\mathrm{hr}^{-1}$ ($4.6 \, \mathrm{mg}\,\mathrm{kg}^{-1}\,\mathrm{hr}^{-1}$)	Smallest toxic infused dose in man, calculated from baboon studies	10.2 after 1 h
Vesey, Cole and Simpson[29]	$1.5 \, \mathrm{mg}\,\mathrm{kg}^{-1}$	Recommended total dose	3.3 after 1–3 h infusion

In the few cases of apparent resistance to SNP, concomitant administration of another hypotensive agent, for example a sympathetic ganglion-blocking drug such as trimetaphan may enhance the effect. The use of preoperative or simultaneous administration of β adrenergic blockade may also help to reduce both the total dose of SNP required and the development of a compensatory tachycardia[1].

To exceed these recommended maximum safe doses, i.e. $1.5 \, \mathrm{mg}\,\mathrm{kg}^{-1}$ or $10 \, \mu\mathrm{g}\,\mathrm{kg}^{-1}\,\mathrm{min}^{-1}$ is likely to produce a severe metabolic acidosis which may become irreversible. In contrast, many anaesthetists now believe that the potential toxicity of SNP is no more serious than that due to many other drugs and that it initially occurred because of the free availability of the drug without the doses and dose rates having been firmly established.

Antidotes for cyanide poisoning

Although the classical use of sodium nitrite to produce methaemoglobin is still advocated for cyanide poisoning, other techniques have been suggested for intraoperative use. The use of large doses of vitamin B12 to facilitate detoxification of cyanide by the formation of cyanocobalamin has been advocated[24], since this does not appear to have any effect upon the hypotensive effects of nitroprusside. More recently, however, sodium thiosulphate in a dose of 150 mg kg^{-1} in water given intravenously over 20 minutes has been shown to enhance the metabolism of cyanide to thiocyanate[31]. This is thought to be due to free sulphydryl group availability being the rate limiting factor in the metabolism of cyanide by rhodanese within the liver and provides a practical way of decreasing cyanide levels rapidly in cases of suspected toxicity. The commercially available chelating agent, cobalt EDTA (Kelocyanor) is useful in cases of cyanide poisoning, but is both expensive and of limited usefulness within the clinical situation.

Prolonged infusion of sodium nitroprusside

The use of long-term nitroprusside infusions has been shown to be beneficial in a wide variety of conditions. By producing both arteriolar and venous dilation, SNP reduces both the afterload and preload of the heart, decreases myocardial oxygen consumption and improves left ventricular function and cardiac output[5]. Nitroprusside infusions have been advocated in cardiogenic shock following myocardial infarction[7], in myocardial ischaemia to decrease oxygen consumption[5] and in the emergency treatment of hypertension[3]. In all cases the rate of nitroprusside administration is usually considerably less than that required intra-operatively. The dose rate limits for prolonged SNP therapy have not been clearly established and depend upon adequate hepatic and renal function for metabolism and excretion of cyanide. Impaired hepatic function will produce high levels of free cyanide both within the red cells and as free cyanide in plasma, while renal failure may lead to high thiocyanate levels. In addition, the metabolism of cyanide is dependent upon an adequate supply of sulphydryl groups and simultaneous sodium thiosulphate administration may be necessary. In an attempt to determine the maximum safe dose rate for prolonged nitroprusside therapy, Michenfelder and Tinker[18] observed whole blood cyanide levels in five groups of dogs receiving 0.5–0.75 and 1.0 mg kg^{-1} hr^{-1}. The dogs in the fourth group received 1.0 mg kg^{-1} h^{-1} together with thiosulphate and in the fifth group the same nitroprusside dose with both thiosulphate and extra fluid therapy. They found that the cyanide concentrations remained below toxic levels in groups 1, 4 and 5 concluding that 0.5 mg kg^{-1} h^{-1} (equivalent to 8 μg kg^{-1} min^{-1}) was the safe upper limit for prolonged nitroprusside administration. They also concluded that simultaneous administration of thiosulphate may protect against the development of cyanide toxicity, and that the development of a metabolic acidosis and/or an increase in mixed venous oxygen concentration both reflect cyanide toxicity. In a more recent study in anuric dogs when thiocyanate and therefore also free sulphydryl group excretion was impaired[27], the same authors found that blood cyanide remained below toxic concentrations with higher infusion rates than those in dogs with normal renal function. They suggested that this was due to artificially elevated sulphydryl concentrations and enhanced hepatic metabolism as a result of impaired excretion.

We have found in several patients studied during prolonged nitroprusside infusion[10, P. J. Simpson & C. Vesey, unpubl. obs.] that cyanide metabolism is satisfactorily maintained at dose rates similar to those found by Michenfelder and Tinker[18]. Indeed, in one patient with normal hepatic function who received more than 2g of nitroprusside over 10 days for the treatment of cardigenic shock, red cell and plasma cyanide concentrations did not rise above 2 and $6\,\mu\text{mol}\,l^{-1}$ respectively [P. J. Simpson & C. Vesey, unpubl. obs.]. Plasma thiocyanate levels reached a plateau of $500\,\text{mmol}\,l^{-1}$, one third of the concentration reported to cause toxicity. Measurements of serum protein-bound iodine and cortisol at repeated intervals during treatment did not show any change. In contrast, another patient with pulmonary hypertension and hepatic failure received a total dose of 545mg of nitroprusside over 72 hours. Due to inability to metabolise cyanide, maximum plasma and red cell concentrations recorded in this patient were 2.75 and 260 respectively, both within the toxic range. Predictably his plasma thiocyanate level rose only slightly[P. J. Simpson & C. Vesey, unpubl. obs.]. Although no symptoms of acute toxicity were observed, care should be taken in those whose ability to metabolise or excrete cyanide following nitroprusside therapy may be impaired.

Although the documented evidence at present is small, it would seem that with normal hepatic and renal function the maximum safe dose rate for prolonged nitroprusside infusion should not exceed $8\,\mu\text{g}\,\text{kg}^{-1}\,\text{min}^{-1}$[18]. If a temporary increase above this level is necessary, the simultaneous use of sodium thiosulphate would appear prudent to minimise the development of toxic cyanide concentrations.

REFERENCES

1. ADAMS A. P., CLARKE T. N. S., EDMONDS-SEAL J., FOËX P., PRYS-ROBERTS C. & ROBERTS J. G. (1974) The effects of sodium nitroprusside on myocardial contractility and haemodynamics. *Br. J. Anaesth.* **46**, 807.

1a. AMARANATH L. & KELLERMEYER W. F. (1976) Tachyphylaxis to Sodium nitroprusside. *Anesthesiology* **44**, 345–8.

2. Editorial (1975) Nitroprusside in Anaesthesia. *Br. Med. J.* **2**, 524–5.

3. CACACE L. & THOMAS T. (1970) Treatment of hypertensive emergencies with sodium nitroprusside. *Drug Intell. Clin. Pharm.* **4**, 187–9.

4. CAILAR J. DU, MATHIEU-DAUDE J. C., DUSCHODE J., LAMARCHE Y. & CASTEL J. (1978) Nitroprusside, its metabolites and red cell function. *Can. Anaesth. Soc. J.* **25**, 92–105.

5. DA LUZ P. L., FORRESTER J. S., WYATT H. L., TYBERG J. V., CHAGRASULIS R., PARMLEY W. W. & SWAN H. J. C. (1975) Haemodynamic and metabolic effects of sodium nitroprusside on the performance and metabolism of the regionally ischaemic myocardium. *Circulation* **52**, 400–6.

6. DAVIES D. W., KADAR D., STEWARD D. J. & MUNROE I. R. (1975) A sudden death associated with the use of sodium nitroprusside for the induction of hypotension during anaesthesia. *Can. Anaesth. Soc. J.* **22**, 547–52.

7. FRANCIOSA J. A., GUILIA N. H., LUMAS C. J., RODRIGUERA E. & COHN J. A.

(1972) Improved left ventricular function during sodium nitroprusside infusion in acute myocardial infarction. *Lancet* **1**, 650–4.

8. GRAYLING G. W., MILLER E. D. & PEACH M. J. (1978) Sodium cyanide antagonism of the vasodilator action of sodium nitroprusside in the isolated rabbit aortic strip. *Anesthesiology* **49**, 21–5.

9. HERMANN L. (1886) Über die wirkung des nitroprussidnatriums. *Arch. Physiol.* **39**, 419.

10. HILLMAN K. & KRAPEZ J. (1978) Treatment of dissecting aortic aneurism and renin-induced hypertension with sodium nitroprusside. *Br. Med. J.* **2**, 799.

11. JACK R. (1974) The toxicity of sodium nitroprusside. *Br. J. Anaesth.* **46**, 952.

12. JOHNSON C. C. (1929) The actions and toxicity of sodium nitroprusside. *Arch. Int. Pharmacodynam.* **35**, 480–96.

13. KRAPEZ J. R., VESEY C. J., ADAMS L. & COLE P. V. (1981) Effects of cyanide antidotes used with sodium nitroprusside infusions: sodium thiosulphate and hydroxocobalamin given prophylactically to dogs. *Br. J. Anaesth.* **53**, 793–804.

14. KREYE V. A. W., BARON G. P. & LÜTH J. B. *et al.* (1975). Mode of action of sodium nitroprusside on vascular smooth muscle. *Naunyn-Schmiedebergs Arch. Pharmacol.* **288**, 381–402.

15. MACRAE W. & OWEN MARY (1974) Severe metabolic acidosis following hypotension induced with sodium nitroprusside. *Br. J. Anaesth.* **46**, 795–7.

16. MCDOWALL D. G., KEANEY J. P., TURNER J. M., LANE J. R. & OKUDA Y. (1974) The toxicity of sodium nitroprusside. *Br. J. Anaesth.* **46**, 327–32.

17. MERRIFIELD A. & BLUNDELL M. (1974) Toxicity of sodium nitroprusside. *Br. J. Anaesth.* **46**, 324.

18. MICHENFELDER J. D. & TINKER J. H. (1977). Cyanide toxicity and thiosulphate protection during chronic

administration of sodium nitroprusside in the dog. *Anesthesiology* **47**, 441–8.

19. MILLER E. D., ACKERLY J. A., VAUGHAN E. D., PEACH M J. & EPSTEIN R. C. (1977) The renin-angiotensin system during controlled hypotension with sodium nitroprusside. *Anesthesiology* **47**, 257–62.

20. MORACA P. P., BITTE E. M., HALE D. E., WASMUTH C. E. & POUTASSE E. F. (1962) Clinical evaluation of sodium nitroprusside as a hypotensive agent. *Anesthesiology* **23**, 193.

21. NEEDLEMAN P., JAKSCHILK B. & JOHNSON E. M. (1973) Sulphydryl requirements for relaxaticn of vascular smooth muscle. *J. Pharmacol. Exp. Ther.* **187**, 324–31.

22. NOUROK, D. S., GLASSOCK, R. J., SOLOMON, D. H. and MAXWELL, M. H. (1964). Hypothyroidism following prolonged S.N.P. therapy. *Am. J. Med. Sci.* **248**, 129–38.

23. PAGE I. H. (1951) The treatment of essential and malignant hypertension. *J. Am. Med. Assoc.* **147**, 1311–18.

24. POSNER M. A., RODKEY F. L. & TOBEY R. E. (1976) Nitroprusside induced cyanide poisoning: Antidotal effect of hydroxocobalamin. *Anesthesiology* **44**, 330–5.

25. SIMPSON P. J., ADAMS L., VESEY C. J. & COLE P. (1979) Some physiological and metabolic effects of sodium nitroprusside and cyanide in the dog. *Br. J. Anaesth.* **51**, 81–6.

26. SMITH R. P. & KRUSZYNA H. (1974) Nitroprusside produces cyanide poisoning via a reaction with haemoglobin. *J. Pharmacol. Exp. Ther.* **191**, 557–63.

27. TINKER J. H. & MICHENFELDER J. D. (1980) Increased resistance to nitroprusside-induced cyanide toxicity in anuric dogs. *Anesthesiology* **52**, 40–7.

28. VESEY C. J., COLE P. V., LINNELL J. C. & WILSON J. (1974) Some metabolic effects of sodium nitroprusside in man. *Br. Med.*

J. **2**, 140–2.

29. VESEY C. J., COLE P. V. & SIMPSON P. J. (1975) Sodium nitroprusside in anaesthesia. *Br. Med. J.* **3**, 229.

30. VESEY C. J., COLE P. V. & SIMPSON P. J. (1976) Cyanide and thiocyanate levels following sodium nitroprusside infusion in man. *Br. J. Anaesth.* **48**, 651–60.

31. VESEY C. J., KRAPEZ J. R. & COLE P. V. (1980) The effects of sodium nitro-

prusside and cyanide on haemoglobin function. *J. Pharm. Pharmacol.* **32**, 256–61.

32. VESEY C. J., SIMPSON P. J., ADAMS L. & COLE P. V. (1979) Metabolism of sodium nitroprusside and cyanide in the dog. *Br. J. Anaesth.* **51**, 89–97.

33. VESEY C. J. & WILSON J. (1978) Red cell cyanide. *J. Pharm. Pharmacol.* **30**, 20–6.

15 Drug Preservatives and Solvents

E. M. WALSH

Some parenteral drugs used in clinical anaesthesia and research are poorly soluble in water, whilst others may deteriorate during storage through chemical decomposition or microbial metabolism. To improve the water solubility and shelf-life of such drugs, manufacturers add organic and inorganic agents to their products. These additives or *pharmaceutic aids* are generally regarded as inert and non-toxic. In this chapter, a selection of pharmaceutic aids which have been or are used in parenteral drugs of interest to anaesthetists are described and attention is drawn to their possible unwanted or adverse effects, as well as ways in which they may influence the action of the drugs they preserve or solubilise.

PRESERVATIVES

Chemical preservatives

Parenteral drugs may deteriorate before use through oxidation or hydrolysis, especially if ultraviolet light, oxygen or heavy metal ions are present. Simple methods such as exclusion of ultraviolet light and oxygen from ampoules may help to prevent deterioration, but often chemicals with antioxidant properties have to be used to control the action of oxygen and heavy metal ions.

Antioxidants produce their effect by several types of mechanisms. 'True' antioxidants (butylated hydroxytoluene, alpha-tocopherol) prevent oxidation by combining with free radicals; reducing agents (ascorbic acid, sodium and potassium salts of

321

sulphurous acid) divert the process of oxidation by virtue of their relatively lower redox potential; and antioxidant synergists (citric acid, disodium edetate) act as chelating agents, combining with heavy metal ion catalysts. Not all types of antioxidants are found in parenteral drugs.

Chemical decomposition may also be increased by changes in hydrogen ion concentration. Such changes may affect the activity of the drug. Buffer systems, such as phosphate or citrate, are used to prevent these changes and to ensure the optimum hydrogen ion concentration for all drug constituents.

Antimicrobial preservatives

Injectable drugs can also deteriorate through the action of microbial metabolism. Bacteria and fungi may also pose an infection hazard to the patient. Simple physical precautions such as sterile preparation and storage and heat sterilisation can decrease microbial problems, but often chemical means must be used, especially in the cases of heat-labile drugs and of drugs dispensed from multidose containers.

Antimicrobial preservatives used in drugs are characterised by a wide range of chemical compounds and by a broad spectrum of antimicrobial activity. The selection of a particular preservative depends on the chemical and physical characteristics of the active drug and of the other constituents, and on the materials of the container. For example, interactions between preservative and other constituents, particularly macromolecules, or between preservative and container may reduce the potency of the preservative. Often there is an optimum concentration for a preservative in a given drug preparation, so that any dilution may alter the efficacy of the preservative.

Benzyl alcohol

Benzyl alcohol is used in parenteral drugs as an antimicrobial agent, usually in a concentration of 1 %. In man, benzyl alcohol is metabolised to benzoic acid and then mainly to hippuric acid and partly to benzoyl glucuronide.

Toxicity

Benzyl alcohol is a relatively non-toxic agent in several species when administered by the intravenous route[59]. However, at the extremes, 94 % benzyl alcohol is twenty-three times more toxic than 95 % ethyl alcohol in rats, but $1 \, ml \, kg^{-1}$ of 0.9 % benzyl alcohol has no effect on blood pressure, heart rate, respiration, electrocardiogram or haematological status of dogs or monkeys. The lethal intravenous dose of 0.9 % benzyl alcohol in anaesthetised dogs is $0.03–1.06 \, g \, kg^{-1}$.

In man, there is little published information on the effects, tolerance, safety and interactions of benzyl alcohol in parenteral drugs. Benzyl alcohol 0.9 % in one preparation of methylprednisolone sodium succinate (Solu-Medrol) was well tolerated intravenously in 24 subjects and no important side-effects were seen[81]. From this study and animal studies, 30 ml of 0.9 % benzyl alcohol can be injected intravenously without toxicity problems[59, 81], in fact there is a probable safety factor of 38 for rapid injection of this dose in a 50 kg adult human[59].

Cardiovascular effects

In isolated rabbit atrium, benzyl alcohol reduces or abolishes spontaneous dysrhythmias as well as strophanthin or adrenaline-induced dysrhythmias by lengthening the effective refractory period of atrial myocardium[31, 112]. Benzyl alcohol, like quinidine and procainamide, also has a negative inotropic effect on isolated rabbit atrium, but unlike these two drugs, its effect develops and wears off rapidly and there is no effect on the rate of spontaneous contraction[113]. In a different study on the same tissue, the diluent of a commercial preparation of + -tubocurarine (Tubocurarine chloride), containing 0.9 % benzyl alcohol and 0.1 % metabisulphite reduced contractility to 60 % of control value[14]. In whole isolated rabbit heart, benzyl alcohol has a similar depressive effect on ventricular contractile force, but to a lesser degree than procainamide or quinidine, and, whereas it does not affect heart rate, it does increase coronary flow[113].

The hypotensive effect of commercial preparations of + -tubocurarine may be caused by many factors including ganglion blockade and histamine release. The presence of a preservative which may have a negative inotropic effect on the heart may be another factor. Both commercial + -tubocurarine (Tubocurarine chloride) and its preservative, benzyl alcohol, reduce the contractility of rabbit atrial strips, and the effect is abolished by the addition of calcium chloride[14]. Pure crystalline + -tubocurarine does not have a negative inotropic effect except at high doses. Another commercial preparation (Tubocurarine chloride) and its diluent containing 0.9 % benzyl alcohol, had a similar effect on rabbit atrial strips[29].

However, in man, the same commercial preparations of benzyl alcohol-preserved + -tubocurarine produced significant reductions in mean arterial blood pressure, whereas the preservative on its own did not[99]. Again, in 38 pairs of patients, no difference was seen in the reduction of mean blood pressure after plain or benzyl alcohol-preserved preparations of + -tubocurarine[101].

Benzyl alcohol may also have effects on peripheral vascular resistance. Commercial atropine sulphate containing 1.5 % benzyl alcohol, when used in high dose on vagotomised dogs ventilated on 0.5 % halothane, reduced mean aortic blood pressure by 20 %, whereas unpreserved atropine reduced blood pressure by 9 %[87]. In both cases, myocardial indices remained unchanged, but calculated peripheral vascular resistance paralleled the fall in blood pressure.

Respiratory effects

In a study on volunteers, hyperventilation was demonstrated following the injection of a diazepam vehicle (propylene glycol, ethyl alcohol and benzyl alcohol) but not after saline[8]. When diazepam 0.35 mg kg^{-1} was given intravenously with and without benzyl alcohol in the solvent, only solutions containing benzyl alcohol gave a statistically significant increase in respiratory rate and minute volume. However, it is clinically more common for diazepam in this solvent to depress respiration[15, 19].

Central and peripheral nervous system effects

Benzyl alcohol may also produce a general anaesthetic effect. Surgical anaesthesia can be induced in rats with 5 mg benzyl alcohol g^{-1} body weight intraperitoneally and in dogs with 200 mg benzyl alcohol kg^{-1} body weight intravenously[31]. As well as a preservative effect, benzyl alcohol has a weak local anaesthetic action when used in dilute concentrations. In contrast, in excess of 4%, benzyl alcohol causes local irritation, oedema and pain[69]. Benzyl alcohol 0.9% may also cause inflammatory changes in central nervous tissues when introduced directly into the cerebrospinal fluid[25, 89].

Chlorbutol

Chlorbutol, or chlorbutanol, is used in parenteral anaesthetic drugs for its antibacterial and antifungal properties, usually in a concentration of 0.5%.

Cardiovascular effects

The cardiovascular effects of chlorbutol have been studied especially with preparations of atropine and +-tubocurarine which contain chlorbutol as a preservative. Atropine sulphate with 0.5% chlorbutol, reduced mean ascending aortic blood pressure and calculated systemic vascular resistance twice as much as pure crystalline atropine sulphate in vagotomised dogs ventilated on halothane[87]. Yet after both preparations of atropine, indices of myocardial contractility remained unchanged. In contrast, with a commercial preparation of +-tubocurarine (Amelizol), both the preparation itself and its preservative, chlorbutol 0.5%, reduced the contractile amplitude of stimulated right atrial strips of rabbit heart to a similar extent, whereas crystalline +-tubocurarine had a slight but significant positive inotropic effect[29].

In man, the significance of chlorbutol-induced effects is not clear. One study in only four subjects showed no change in mean blood pressure after injection of a chlorbutol-containing diluent, despite a reduction in pressure following administration of the complete preparation of +-tubocurarine (Tubocurarine chloride)[99].

Chlorocresol

Chlorocresol is a derivative of phenol and is used as a preservative for its potent antibacterial properties. At a concentration of 0.1 %, it is bacteristatic and at 0.2 % it is bactericidal. In humans, chlorocresol is conjugated with glucuronide or sulphate and is excreted in urine. Very little is excreted unchanged.

Chlorocresol has no toxic effects when used intravenously as a preservative in small volumes of drugs. However, relatively large doses of chlorocresol may be given when a drug containing chlorocresol is given in a higher dose than was originally intended by the manufacturer. For instance, a preparation of morphine sulphate preserved with 0.2 % chlorocresol, if given in a high dose technique, may lead to inadvertent administration of excess chlorocresol[70]. Also, relatively high concentrations of chlorocresol, or other preservatives, may be delivered more directly to the myocardium, when preservative-containing drugs are added to the oxygenator of the cardiopulmonary bypass pump, thus avoiding the usual dilution which occurs with the intravenous route.

Cardiovascular effects

Chlorocresol may produce cardiovascular effects in animals. The action on rabbit atrial strips of a commercial preparation of +-tubocurarine containing 0.1 % chlorocresol and 0.1 % potassium metabisulphite (Tubarine) was compared with crystalline +-tubocurarine[29]. The latter produced a slight but significant positive inotropic effect on stimulated atrial strips, whereas both the commercial preparation and its diluent, chlorocresol, reduced contractility. The antioxidant, potassium metabisulphite, also had a minor negative inotropic effect. Similar results were obtained in another study using the same drugs and tissues, but the addition of calcium to the experimental system reversed the depressive effects of commercial +-tubocurarine (Tubarine) and its preservative, chlorocresol[14].

Neural effects

The neural toxicity of chlorocresol is probably much less than of phenol, but chlorocresol is employed in chemical neurolysis for chronic pain. Drugs containing chlorocresol should not therefore be given unintentionally by the intrathecal, intracisternal or extradural routes[69]. The recent widespread increase in spinal and epidural opiate analgesia has raised the question of whether preserved opiates or other drugs should be given by these routes[20, 71]. This question has not been answered conclusively, but it would seem a sound principle to avoid preservatives with known neurotoxic effects. Very few histological studies have been published on this question and only with other drugs and preservatives[26].

Allergic responses

Chlorocresol is used as a preservative in heparin because it is effective in an acid medium. There have been reports of patients developing Arthus-type reactions to subcutaneous heparin and, in one case, subsequent intravenous heparin precipitated a systemic reaction[52, 82]. In both reports, sensitivity to bovine heparin may have been a factor. The possible significance of the preservative in heparin was considered in a later investigation of nine patients who had reacted to mucous heparin preserved with 0.15 % chlorocresol[43]. Of the nine patients receiving chlorocresol-preserved mucous heparin, two reacted systematically after intravenous injection, with either cardio-vascular collapse or an urticarial reaction, and seven patients on subcutaneous heparin developed localised reactions. Subsequent intradermal tests showed that the patient who had collapsed gave positive reactions to both chlorocresol-preserved and plain heparin, whereas in the patient who had had the urticarial reaction, unpreserved heparin did not provoke a response and treatment was successfully continued with this preparation. Tests on the patients who had reacted locally showed that four of the seven did not have a positive reaction to preservative-free heparin.

Chlorocresol-preserved heparin may also give pain at the injection site and a systemic reaction[1]. When unpreserved heparin was subsequently given intra-venously, there was no reaction, and later intradermal tests were positive for chlorocresol-heparin but negative for the preservative-free preparation.

Phenol

Phenol is used as a preservative for injectable drugs because of its antibacterial properties. It is bacteriostatic at concentrations below 0.2 % and bactericidal above 0.2 %. In man, phenol is mainly excreted unchanged or in conjugated form in the urine. About 20 % may be metabolised to hydroquinone and pyrocatechol.

Neural and cardiovascular effects

Used in low concentrations in small volumes of drugs, phenol does not produce toxic effects. However, at higher concentrations, phenol is neurotoxic and is used in the treatment of chronic pain. Large doses of phenol given parenterally may lead to central nervous stimulation and subsequent depression and cardiovascular collapse. These changes may be, in part, the result of increased acetylcholine release from nerve-endings caused by phenol[83]. The administration of large doses in humans has occurred through inadvertent intravascular injection of 6 % phenol during pain relief procedures and by the use of drugs containing phenol in techniques not originally specified by the manufacturer. For instance, glucagon used for hypoglycaemic therapy was dissolved in a solution containing 0.2 % phenol. If this preparation is used in high doses for the treatment of shock, a 100 mg dose of glucagon includes 200 mg phenol. Consequently, it was recommended that glucagon be dissolved in physiological saline when used in this way[22]. In much smaller doses 50 μg kg^{-1} glucagon (10 μg kg^{-1} phenol), gave no adverse effects when the diluent alone was injected, and a positive inotropic effect was obtained when glucagon dissolved in the phenol-based diluent was injected[98].

Parahydroxybenzoic acid esters

Parahydroxybenzoic acid has only slight antiseptic activity, but when esterified with alcohols, such as methanol, ethanol, propanol or butanol, the resulting compounds are much more active. These esters are known as 'parabens' and are used in parenteral drugs to prevent growth of moulds, fungi and yeasts. They have little antibacterial activity. Parabens preservatives have a low order of toxicity in many animals and man. In the latter, parabens are metabolised to parahydroxybenzoic acid which is relatively non-toxic.

Allergic effects

Allergic reactions have occurred infrequently to paraben-preserved drugs. For instance, a preparation of hydrocortisone containing methyl- and propylparabens produced bronchospasm and pruritus in an asthmatic patient[78]. Other hydrocortisone preparations did not cause a reaction and subsequent direct and passive transfer tests for immediate hypersensitivity to several parabens were positive. Local anaesthetic agents containing parabens may also produce reactions: a patient who had had a pruritic reaction to paraben-preserved lignocaine subsequently gave positive intra-dermal reactions to methylparaben[66].

The chemical similarity of parabens to parahydroxybenzoic acid, a known allergen and a metabolite of parabens, may explain the allergic potential of these preservatives. Reactions to amide-type local anaesthetics, although rare, may be due to the amide itself or to their commonly used preservative, methylparaben[75].

Neural effects

Like other phenolic derivatives used as preservatives, parabens may be painful on injection even at low concentrations but they have a subsequent local anesthetic effect. Direct application of 0.1 or 0.2 % methylparaben reversibly blocked nerve conduction in the spinal roots and the vagus nerve of the cat[79].

Salts of sulphurous acid

Sodium and potassium salts of sulphurous acid such as metabisulphite, bisulphite and sulphite, are used as antimicrobial agents and antioxidants. As antimicrobials, these salts act by liberating sulphur dioxide and sulphurous acid, and, as antioxidants, they prevent oxidation by being strong reducing agents with a low redox potential relative to the active drug. Salts of sulphurous acid are metabolised by oxidation to sulphates which are excreted in the urine. In mammals, clearance of sulphites depends on the activity of sulphite oxidase which is inhibited by excess sulphite[40].

Large doses of sulphites are rarely, if ever, given intravenously in man, but some peritoneal dialysis fluids may contain 0.012–0.05% sodium metabisulphite. Until equilibration is reached between blood and peritoneal dialysis fluid, 120–500 mg sodium metabisulphite may be absorbed from each litre of dialysis fluid. When such peritoneal dialysis fluid was injected into rabbits, absorption of bisulphite was rapid and three out of five rabbits died[41]. But other animal studies, using 0.05% sodium bisulphite have not supported this finding[108].

SOLVENTS

Most drugs used in anaesthesia or of interest to anaesthetists are soluble in water, but some are poorly soluble. The addition of certain pharmaceutic aids, such as glycols, macrogols and non-ionic surfactants may increase the solubility of such drugs. Solubilising agents, often considered as inert, may have pharmacological actions of their own and may exert synergistic or antagonistic effects on the drug they carry.

Glycols

Glycols are dihydric alcohols with hydroxyl groups on separate carbon atoms. Low molecular weight glycols are soluble in water and can be used as solubilisers or solvents for poorly water-soluble drugs. Only propylene glycol is used since other glycols, such as ethylene glycol and di- and tri-ethylene glycol, are too toxic for pharmaceutical use[36].

Propylene glycol

Toxicity

Propylene glycol is generally considered a non-toxic glycol, since it is converted mainly to naturally-occurring carbohydrate metabolites[89]. In man, 25% of an oral dose of 1 ml kg^{-1} propylene glycol is excreted unchanged in the urine within 10 hours[44]. In animals, oral propylene glycol has a low order of toxicity[35, 95, 107]. Long-term intravenous studies of up to 4 ml kg^{-1} propylene glycol for 4 weeks produced no changes in organ weights, function tests or biochemical analyses, but some haematuria did develop (Roche Products, pers. comm.). Acute intravenous studies in dogs of single doses up to 8 ml kg^{-1} propylene glycol were tolerated without harmful effects.

Table 15.1 Some drugs used in anaesthsia containing pharamceutic acids.

Name of drug	Trade name	Manufacturer	Pharmaceutic aid
Alphaxolone/alphadolone	Althesin	Glaxo	Cremophor EL
Diamorphine HCl		Macarthy	Phenol
Di-isopropyl phenol	Diprivan	ICI	Cremophor EL
Etomidate	Hypnomidate	Janssen	Propylene glycol
Fazadinium bromide	Fazadon	Duncan, Flockhart	Alpha-thioglycerol
Heparin sodium	Heparin (mucous) Injection multidose	Weddel	Chlorocresol
Ketamine	Ketalar (50 mg ml^{-1})	Parke-Davis	Benzethonium chloride
Lorazepam	Ativan Injection	Wyeth	Polyethylene glycol
			Propylene glycol
Metaraminol tartrate	Aramine	MSD	Methyl and propyl parabens
Morphine sulphate		Macarthy	Chlorocresol
Naloxone HCl	Narcan	Winthrop	Methyl and propyl parabens
Nitroglycerin	Tridil	American Hospital Supply (UK)	Propylene glycol
Pancuronium bromide	Pavulon	Organon-Teknika	Benzyl alcohol
Papaveretum	Omnopon	Roche	Methyl and propyl parabens
Papaveretum		Macarthy	Phenylmercuric nitrate
Pentobarbitone sodium	Nembutal Soluble	Abbott	Propylene glycol
Procaine HCl		Macarthy	Bisulphite and Chlorocresol

There is little published information on parenteral toxicity of propylene glycol in man, especially in longer-term studies. Increasing doses of propylene glycol up to 65 ml over 16 days in four patients did not affect electrolyte balance or crude liver function tests[74].

Central nervous system effects

Early acute studies in dogs showed propylene glycol to have some anaesthetic activity, but that the anaesthetic dose was 85 % of the lethal dose[44]. More recent studies in mice have demonstrated propylene glycol to have anticonvulsant activity[55], weak but significant CNS depressive effects, such as increased hexobarbital sleeping times and decreased motor activity[116], and also disturbance of righting reflexes[21]. No narcotic effect was detected, however, when 4 ml kg^{-1} propylene glycol was injected intraperitoneally in rats, rabbits or dogs[31]. There is no published evidence to suggest that propylene glycol accompanying intravenous drugs in humans, may have CNS depressive effects, however CNS depression has been reported following excessive oral doses of vitamins dissolved in propylene glycol[68].

Cardiovascular effects

The effects of propylene glycol have been studied in isolated and intact animal tissues. In isolated frog heart, perfusion concentrations of propylene glycol between 1 μg and 10 mg ml^{-1} gave a reduced stroke volume, bradycardia and, ultimately, diastolic arrest[86]. Perfusion of isolated rabbit atrium with 0.76–7.6 mg ml^{-1} propylene glycol reduced contractile force by 20 % without a change in rate of contraction[112], whereas in isolated rabbit heart, rate was unaltered but contractile force and coronary flow increased by 60 % and these effects were not altered by propanolol[113].

Sodium phenytoin, which has been used as an antiarrhythmic agent, in a preparation consisting of 40 % propylene glycol and 10 % ethanol (Dilantin) was found to reduce blood pressure, increase pulse rate and QRS intervals and alter cardiac rhythm in cats[65]. Both propylene glycol and dilute Dilantin solvent produced similar changes which could be prevented by prior treatment with phenytoin. In contrast, propylene glycol showed pronounced antidysrhythmic and antifibrillatory effects in spontaneous and drug-induced dysrhythmias, when injected into rats and dogs, and also caused initial mild hypotension[31].

Haematological effects

An aqueous solution of 2 % propylene glycol is iso-osmotic with plasma, but *in vitro* it produces 100 % haemolysis in 45 minutes[42]. Haemolysis may be prevented by the addition of 0.9 % sodium chloride in aqueous solutions of up to 30 % propylene glycol[88]. *In vivo* studies in rabbits, showed that 2 g kg^{-1} propylene glycol in 0.9 %

saline intravenously had no effect on erythrocyte count or fragility, packed cell volume, haemoglobin concentration or total white cell count, but polymorphs and platelets increased and lymphocyte count and clotting time decreased[10]. However, another study in rabbits and dogs using 400 mg kg^{-1} of intravenous propylene glycol did show haemolysis[31].

Muscular effects

Propylene glycol may affect the function of smooth muscle in the gut and uterus[86]. In human isolated uterine muscle, isotonic contractility was reduced by propylene glycol[11]. A brief general muscular rigidity with marked muscle tremor in the hind limbs has been observed in rabbits following intravenous injection of 4 ml kg^{-1} of 50% propylene glycol[10, 95].

Venous effects

Many parenteral drugs containing propylene glycol cause pain and thrombophlebitis, but it is often difficult to determine whether drug or solvent is responsible. High concentrations of propylene glycol, such as 78%, do cause tissue necrosis by an osmotic effect[67], but modern drugs usually contain less than 45% propylene glycol. For individual drugs, the presence of propylene glycol and other solvents may affect the incidence of pain and thrombophlebitis following injection. For instance, etomidate (Hypnomidate) in 30% propylene glycol may cause pain less frequently than aqueous etomidate but the difference may not be significant[114, 115] and may arise from the different pH and osmolality of the preparations[48]. In comparison, etomidate in 20% Cremophor EL did not give pain on injection in twenty children[57].

Likewise, whereas diazepam in 40% propylene glycol gave pain in 44% of patients on injection[94] and in 66–78% after two weeks[72, 94], diazepam in Cremophor EL produced pain in 14% of patients on injection and in 38% after two weeks[94]. Cremophor EL added to preparations of diazepam in glycol, may reduce the incidence of pain on injection[12]. One study, however, showed the Cremophor preparation to cause a 64% incidence of pain[97]. In contrast, diazepam in Intralipid (Diazemals) caused pain in less than 10% of patients[54, 94].

Thrombophlebitis may also be caused by drugs containing propylene glycol[16, 47, 61, 72, 94, 97]. Diazepam in 40% propylene glycol caused thrombophlebitis in 3.5–48% of patients in the first few days[47, 61, 94], but the incidence rose after 2–4 weeks[47, 72, 94, 97]. In contrast, the same drug in either Cremophor EL or Intralipid caused thrombophlebitis in less than 10% of patients[54, 72, 94]. The ear veins of adult rats have been used to examine the venous effects of propylene glycol[38]. It was found that diazepam with propylene glycol solvent produced histological changes in the veins similar to those caused by 1% propylene glycol alone.

Metabolic effects

There is some evidence that long-term oral propylene glycol may increase liver cholesterol[2, 50] and affect liver enzymes and proteins[24, 111]. Propylene glycol seems to affect drug metabolism selectively. For instance, it does not affect hexobarbital metabolism[24, 116] or the microsomal enzyme-inducing effects of phenobarbital, but it may accelerate diphenylhydantoin metabolism[116]. Thus, this solvent cannot be regarded as inert in pharmacological studies. Some caution must be exercised when interpreting effects of drugs containing propylene glycol on triglyceride metabolism[46]. Although pentobarbitone in 20% propylene glycol and 10% ethanol was found to produce elevated plasma triglycerides in experimental animals, the increase was shown to be spurious and arose from interaction of propylene glycol with the laboratory reagents. Propylene glycol does not interfere with some methods of triglyceride estimation such as the neutral fat enzymatic hydrolysis method (Boehringer Mannheim assay kit).

Effects of drug potency

Solvents may affect the potency of various drugs. For instance, ED_{50} values for loss of righting reflex in mice vary not only with the benzodiazepine used but also the solvent used[21]. This effect may arise from changes in drug solubilisation following injection or from a synergistic or antagonistic effect of the solvent itself. Lower ED_{50} values were found for benzodiazepines in propylene glycol compared with aqueous carboxymethyl cellulose suspension.

Macrogols

The term macrogol describes a wide range of polyethylene or polyoxyethylene glycols which are formed by the condensation of ethylene oxide and water. Molecular weights of macrogols range from 200 to 6000, and, for ease of reference, macrogols are described according to their average molecular weight. For instance, macrogol 200 or polyethylene glycol 200 has an average molecular weight of between 190 and 210. Physical properties are related to molecular weight: lower macrogols are liquid and hydrophilic, higher ones are solid and lipophilic.

Polyethylene glycols

Polyethylene glycols have several pharmaceutic uses which include solubilisation of poorly water-soluble drugs, stabilisation of emulsions and the complexing of blood-clotting factors. Liquid macrogols are excreted in the urine mainly unchanged. Some is metabolised, but ethylene glycol is not a metabolite[96]. In the rat, one intravenous dose of ^{14}C-labelled polyethylene glycol 4000 was excreted in the urine within 24 hours[13].

Effects in animals

Polyethylene glycol 200 and 400 have been shown to produce effects in various isolated and intact animal organs[86]. Repeated injections of polyethylene glycol 4000, a macrogol used as a complexing agent, had no toxic effect in beagles even at the highest dose of 90 mg kg^{-1} day^{-1} for one year[13].

Human toxicity

Macrogols are believed to have a low toxicity in humans. Published instances of suspected toxicity have arisen from one particular antibiotic used before 1959. Of thirty-two patients with renal disease treated with nitrofurantoin in polyethylene glycol 300 (Furadantoin i.v. Solution), seven patients developed severe metabolic acidosis and nephropathy and two of these patients died[73]. The clinical appearances and renal histologies were similar to those seen following ethylene glycol ingestion. In experimental animals given polyethylene glycol, urinary organic acid excretion increased but ethylene glycol or its possible metabolite, oxalic acid, were not identified in the urine[73]. In another report, two patients with renal disease, but normal renal function, developed similar clinical problems whilst on the same preparation and one patient died[100]. Decomposition of the polyethylene glycol solvent prior to injection may have been a factor in these cases.

Polyethylene glycol in anaesthetic drugs

Studies of polyethylene glycol in anaesthetic agents in humans have largely involved the clinical comparison of polyethylene glycol with other solvents for particular drugs. For instance, compared with other studies of aqueous etomidate, etomidate in polyethylene glycol produced similar recovery times and changes in blood pressure but reduced the incidence of pain on injection[48]. A significantly lower incidence of pain with etomidate in polyethylene glycol compared with aqueous etomidate has also been reported by others[114, 115]. This difference may arise from the dissimilar pH and osmolality of the two preparations[48]. The partial substitution of propylene glycol with polyethylene glycol 300 as the solvent for diazepam reduced the incidence of pain on intramuscular injection[60].

Non-ionic surfactants

Surfactants, or surface-active agents, comprise a large and diverse group of chemicals which is characterised by the presence of both hydrophilic moieties such as oxyethylene and hydroxyl groups, and lipophilic moieties such as fatty acids or hydrocarbon polymers. By adjusting the ratio of these groups in a molecule, the desired hydrophilic–lipophilic balance can be obtained and one of a number of properties will predominate.

All surfactants in aqueous dispersion concentrate at boundaries of immiscible liquids with hydrophilic and lipophilic moieties orientated to their preferred medium. At a critical concentration, they also form micelles which consist of 50–150 molecules of surfactant orientated according to the lipophilic property of the surrounding liquid. Non-ionic surfactants are characterised by the absence of ionised groups. In other respects they have a similar range of uses compared with ionised surfactants and are relatively less affected by pH or electrolytes. There are several chemically distinct non-ionic surfactants consisting of fatty acid esters and ethers of glycols, glycerol, macrogols and sorbitol. Only some of these are used in parenteral drugs.

Cremophor EL and related surfactants

Cremophor EL production involves the reaction of ethylene oxide with castor oil at high temperatures in the presence of an alkali. Approximately 35–40 moles of ethylene oxide react with each mole of castor oil to form 1 mole of Cremophor EL[5]. Castor oil itself is a mixture of triglycerides expressed without heat from the seeds of the castor oil plant (*Ricinus communis*, Euphorbiaceae). The residual seed cake or *pomace*, which is not used, contains the highly toxic albuminoid protein, ricin[69]. Ricinoleic acid forms 90 % of the component fatty acids of the castor oil triglycerides; oleic acid is also present but in small amounts[49]. Cremophor EL consists of lipophilic (83 %) and hydrophilic (17 %) elements of a complex nature, which may vary between production batches. These constituents have been analysed[77].

If the hydrophilic elements of Cremophor EL are removed by butanol extraction, the remaining lipophilic part is known as Tensid, Micellophor or ORPE (oleum ricini polyethoxylate) and is the solvent for propanidid (Epontol). Originally Epontol contained Cremophor EL, but in 1966 Micellophor was introduced because it was less viscous. A study of Epontol with the old and new solvent in one thousand patients showed no differences in blood pressure and heart rate changes or in the incidence of allergic effects with either preparation[27].

Animal toxicity

Compared with rabbit, mouse and pig, the dog and cat are the more sensitive to intravenous Cremophor EL, owing to non-specific release of histamine from mast cells[63, 109].

In dogs, histamine release as manifested by itching, diarrhoea and hypotension, may be prevented or attenuated by antihistamines[109]. Several types and fractions of

Cremophor EL have been injected into dogs to determine the cause of histamine release[64]. Samples from four different batches of Cremophor EL, as well as Cremophor RH40 and technical grade oxyethylated castor oil (Mulgofen EL 620), all gave a high incidence of reactions with significant decreases in blood pressure and liberation of histamine. Similar effects were produced by the lipophilic fraction of Cremophor RH40 and by oxyethylated oleic acid. However, the hydrophilic fraction of Cremophor RH40 and oxyethylated glycerol caused neither hypotension nor histamine release, whereas oxyethylated ricinoleic acid decreased blood pressure but did not release histamine. Several non-ionic surfactants were also investigated in dogs to determine whether all or some of these agents produce reactions. Tween 80 (polyoxyethylene sorbitan mono-oleate) and oxyethylated glycerol mono-oleate ester produced a higher incidence of reactions, decreases in blood pressure and release of histamine than did Cremophor EL, but Lutensol AP 10 (oxyethylated nonylphenol), a chemically unrealted surfactant, produced similar degrees of hypotension without release of histamine and, alone of all agents, caused death in all eight dogs studied.

Chronic intravenous Cremophor EL in rats for 4 weeks resulted in accumulation of Cremophor EL or its derivatives in spleen, kideny, thymus and lymph nodes after $80 \, \mathrm{mg \, kg^{-1} \, day^{-1}}$ Cremophor EL and also in the liver after $540 \, \mathrm{mg \, kg^{-1} \, day^{-1}}$. These changes resolved after 6 weeks and there were no changes in body weights, haematological or biochemical measurements, urinalyses, vision, hearing or macroscopic pathology[6].

Human toxicity

Cremophor EL normally releases clinically insignificant amounts of histamine[28]. Cremophor EL $0.15 \, \mathrm{ml \, kg^{-1}}$ intravenously in eight patients failed to release histamine despite previous exposures to induction agents containing Cremophor EL during which four of the patients had released insignificant amounts of histamine. Changes associated with histamine release such as cardiovascular collapse, decreased basophils and increase in gastric acidity were not seen after Cremophor EL or Micellophor alone in man[28, 62].

Metabolism

When a drug containing Cremophor or Micellophor is injected intravenously, some of the drug circulates in the free state and the rest associates with micelles and plasma proteins. In the case of propanidid in Epontol, approximately 60 % remains in the free state, and the degree of association between propanidid and Micellophor depends on the drug's plasma concentration, protein binding capacity, metabolism and excretion[92]. Because Cremophor EL is a complex substance, it is difficult to study the metabolism of all its constituents by isotope tracer studies. Studies on rats have shown that Cremophor EL is metabolised by lipases by attack on ester bonds to produce ricinoleic acid, triglyceride and a polyoxyethylene fraction (Glaxo Laboratories, pers. comm.). Some de-esterification is also effected by liver enzymes. The polyoxyethylene metabolite is resistant to further change and is rapidly eliminated in the urine; it has a plasma half-life of 13 minutes. The half-life of Cremophor EL in rat plasma is about 22 hours, indicating that de-esterification is the rate-limiting step. Work in man indicates a similar half-life and route of elimination.

Cardiovascular effects

The effects of Cremophor EL on isolated and intact animal tissues have been studied[86, 109]. In man, twelve fit, unpremedicated patients prior to anaesthesia did not show significant cardiovascular changes following incremental doses of Cremophor EL over 20 minutes[90]. Only non-clinical doses of 20 ml of Cremophor EL produced significant changes. Other studies with Micellophor 0.15 ml kg^{-1} in twelve subjects and Cremophor EL in eight, showed no alteration in blood pressure or heart rate[28, 62].

Respiratory effects

No significant respiratory effects of Cremophor EL have been demonstrated in man either after a bolus dose of 0.15 ml kg^{-1}[28], or after 50 ml given over 16 minutes[90]. In the dog, 16 mg kg^{-1} Cremophor EL by intra-carotid injection, increased the rate but not the depth of respiration by 23% immediately and by 78% after 10 minutes, but hypotension was also produced[45].

Plasma viscosity

Drugs containing Cremophor EL or Micellophor, such as Althesin, Epontol and Stesolid MR (diazepam), as well as Cremophor EL itself, reduce plasma viscosity[39]. Reductions of 45% were found at the low shear rate of 11.5 sec^{-1} *in vitro*, using concentrations of Cremophor EL equivalent to those found in plasma during anaesthesia. Under clinical conditions a reduction of 42% was seen in eleven patients 5 minutes after injection and the effect lasted 50 minutes. Triton X-100, a non-ionic polyoxyethylated surfactant, produced a similar effect *in vitro*. Plasma viscosity results from the aggregation of protein molecules and formation of surface films. Surfactants produce an envelope of structured water around protein molecules, thus disrupting molecular aggregates and reducing viscosity.

Surface tension

The surfactant property of Cremophor EL may affect the drop size of infusions of drugs containing Cremophor EL, since the volume of a drop is directly proportional to the surface tension of the liquid. Cremophor EL and other surface-active agents reduce surface tension, consequently reducing drop volume. When an infusion of 20% Althesin was controlled by a drop counter, only 50% of the fluid volume, as predicted from the manufacturer's information on the intravenous set, was actually delivered[110].

Plasma lipids

Patients receiving long-term infusions of drugs containing Cremophor EL may develop hyperlipidaemia and an abnormal lipoprotein electrophoretic pattern[4, 34]. Regular intravenous injections of the surfactant Triton over 4 months in dogs produced a similar pattern with subsequent atherosclerosis, diffuse lipoidosis, depletion of fat stores and death[91].

Adverse reactions to Cremophor-containing drugs

Although anaesthetic drugs containing Cremophor release clinically undetectable amounts of histamine, some patients have serious reactions in which classical signs of hypersensitivity may develop. The incidence of such reactions to Althesin and Epontol have been estimated[18, 27]. Such reactions also occur after other induction agents such as thiopentone and methohexitone[7, 17]. However, in the case of Cremophor-containing drugs, several reactions have been observed both on first exposure[3, 7, 27, 58, 62] as well as on repeated exposure[27, 51, 56, 85]. Reactions on first exposure may be due, in part, to direct pharmacological release of histamine from mast cells. However, in some cases, complement C3 activation is an important factor[53, 106]. In those patients who react on subsequent exposures, some develop reactions of the delayed histaminoid type, others reactions of classical hypersensitivity involving IgE, and in others, the occurrence of a reaction within 4 weeks of first exposure suggests an unconventional mechanism such as a short-term memory phenomenon involving lymphocyte receptors and IgD[103].

Some anaphylactoid reactions to Althesin have occurred after previous exposure to Epontol[30, 80, 102]. This has led to the possibility that the related solvents may have been a common factor in precipitating these reactions. Alternatively, an underlying primary or secondary immunopathological condition may lower the threshold of an immune response to an intravenous drug[7, 105]. Whether surfactants lower this threshold further is unknown.

Other drugs which contain Cremophor EL or related polyoxyethylated fatty acid derivatives, have produced anaphylactoid reactions of variable severity. For example, there are a few reported instances of immune or hypersensitivity reactions to diazepam in propylene glycol[32, 82], despite its widespread use, yet diazepam in Cremophor El (Stesolid MR) has been associated with cardio-respiratory collapse with reported incidences of between 1 in 1700 and 1 in 10 000[16, 53, 93]. Aqueous colloid solution of phytomenadione, (Aqua Mephyton Injection and Konakion) which contains a polyoxyethylated fatty acid derivative have also produced hypersensitivity reactions. Severe reactions, resembling hypersensitivity and anaphylaxis and including cardiac and respiratory arrest, have occurred during and immediately after intravenous Aqua Mephyton, in some cases on first exposure[23]. Rapid intravenous injection of Konakion, which contains Cremophor EL, may cause facial flushing, sweating, feelings of chest constriction, cyanosis and peripheral vascular collapse[23]. It seems unlikely that phytomenadione, a synthetic analogue of a naturally occurring vitamin with a molecular weight of 450, is solely responsible for these reactions. The similarity of the reactions to those seen with Althesin and Epontol, in particular reactions occurring on first exposure, may imply that the non-ionic surfactant used in these preparations is an important factor. It may be possible that Cremophor EL and related solvents act as haptens or increase the immunogenicity of the active drug[104].

The value of intradermal sensitivity tests for Althesin reactions has been questioned[33]. Most reported tests in patients who have had reactions to intravenous agents have shown no clear response to Cremophor EL or Micellophor, or to the induction agents[9, 56, 62, 102]. However, some patients have shown skin reactions to both induction agent and solvent[76].

Since investigation of anaphylactoid reactions to induction agents and solvents may involve risk to subjects and patients, the use of the mini-pig (Göttingen-derived strain) has been proposed as a model for human responses[37]. As in man, Cremophor EL in this pig does not release histamine; Althesin may lead to insignificant rises in plasma histamine; yet repeated injections of Althesin may produce severe responses. Alphaxalone/alphadolone and propanidid, both with Cremophor or with ethyl alcohol/propylene glycol solvents were injected, but only alphaxalone/alphadolone in alcohol/glycol solvent on one occasion produced a reaction on first exposure. A second injection of Cremophor EL, Althesin or Epontol given 7 days after the first, produced a high frequency of responses. Alphaxalone/alphadolone, but not propanidid, in the alcohol/glycol solvent also produced adverse responses, but neither repeated thiopentone nor the alcohol/glycol solvent produced abnormal reactions. Adverse reactions to Cremophor EL occurred less frequently if injection interval was extended from 1 to 2 weeks, whereas an interval of more than 4 days and less than 3 weeks appeared to be important with Althesin. It would seem from these studies that Cremophor EL as well as Cremophor/Micellophor-containing drugs and alphaxalone/alphadolone in alcohol/glycol solvent can produce reactions on second exposure in this model. The implications and relevance in man of these studies have yet to be ascertained.

CONCLUSIONS

Despite the widely-held view that pharmaceutic aids are inert, there are many, albeit sporadic, reports of effects of a toxic or pharmacologic nature which have been attributed to these agents. Some of these reports have been described in this chapter. Many deal with effects seen *in vitro* or in animals, the relevance of which to humans is not certain. There are fewer reports of undesirable effects in humans, but of these, allergic reactions pose a serious threat to patients. Most other effects of a pharmacological type are not, on the whole, of importance in clinical situations, since the small doses of pharmaceutic aids usually given are insufficient to produce significant effects. However, the effects may assume a greater importance in certain circumstances and even toxic effects may develop. For instance, larger doses of pharmaceutic aids may be given in techniques involving large volumes of drugs either given acutely or given over long periods, such as induction and maintenance of anaesthesia and perioperative infusions of drugs. In these situations or if the patient is ill or if metabolic pathways used by the aids are impaired, harmful effects could develop. Also, if a drug which was introduced for use in a specific technique is given in a different dosage or by another route not positively recommended by the manufacturer, problems could arise from the presence of preservatives or solvents. Manufacturers and users of drugs should therefore carefully consider any possible effects of drug vehicles, but what safeguards should there be in the production and use of pharmaceutically-aided drugs?

Since man is the ultimate recipient of drugs containing these aids and the relevance of animal models to humans is not certain, all existing as well as new aids should be tested in man in the doses and by the routes proposed by manufactuers in the same way that active drug constituents are. The establishment of the absence of toxic effects in animals is probably insufficient. The resulting information should be made known to users through the usual channels and details of substances added to drugs by the manufacturer should be given in product information. At present (1981), US manufacturers are obliged to publish the formulation of their products, but in the UK this is not the case. Indeed very few of the drugs listed in Tables 15.1 or 15.2 had positive details of their preservatives or solvents in their Data Sheets or package inserts.

Ideally, manufacturers could avoid possible and real problems by not using chemical pharmaceutic aids (Table 15.2), but if it is essential to use them, they should avoid substances with biological effects even if these effects are only seen in unusual clinical situations. They should also caution users to give the drug only by the route and dose schedule they recommend.

Researchers for their part, when using drugs containing pharmaceutic aids, should exclude the possibility that these substances have effects of their own or that they have any influence on the uptake, distribution, metabolism or excretion of the active drug under study. Full details of all drug constituents should be given in publications when comparing different preparations of the same drug or different drugs with different

Table 15.2 Some drugs used in anaesthesia, not containing preservatives or solvents.

Name of drug	Trade name	Manufacturer
Droperidol	Droleptan	Janssen
Heparin sodium	Heaprin (mucous) Injection ampoules	Weddel
Ketamine	Ketalar (10 mg ml^{-1})	Parke-Davis
Bupivacaine HCl	Marcain Plain	Duncan, Flockhart
Phenoperidine HCl	Operidine	Janssen
Protamine sulphate	Protamine Sulphate Injection	Weddel
Heparin sodium	Pularin ampoules	Duncan, Flockhart
Fentanyl	Sublimaze	Janssen
Tubocurarine chloride	Tubarine Injection	Calmic
Tubocurarine chloride	Tubocurarine Injection	Duncan, Flockhart

solvents and preservatives. Also if new dose schedules or routes are proposed, researchers should consider drug vehicle effects.

Total intravenous anaesthesia avoids the atmospheric pollution which is difficult to prevent with inhalational techniques, thereby reducing harmful effects on operating theatre staff. But the incidence and reality of these effects have been much debated. In comparison, at least some of the effects of pharmaceutic aids are much more real and dangerous to patients. For instance, some drugs of diverse chemical composition but with similar solvents are known to have an incidence of reactions as high as 1 per 1000, with some reactions of life-threatening seriousness. Less serious effects may occur in some circumstances. If these undesirable effects are the result of solvents or preservatives even to a minor extent, we may be exposing patients to a more serious type of pollution whilst attempting to avoid the uncertain effects on staff of atmospheric pollution from inhalational anaesthetics.

REFERENCES

1. AINLEY E. J., MACKIE I. G. & MACARTHUR D. (1977) Adverse reaction to chlorocresol-preserved heparin. *Lancet* 1, 705.
2. AMMA M. K. P., DANI H. M. & AHLUWALIA P. (1978) 1,2-Propanediol-induced changes in plasma and tissue lipids of rats. *Lipids* 13, 455–7.
3. AVERY A. F. & EVANS A. (1973) Reactions to Althesin. *Br. J. Anaesth.* 45, 301–2.
4. BAGNARELLO A. G., LEWIS L. A., MCHENRY M. C., WEINSTEIN A. J., NAITO H. K., MCCULLOUGH A. J., LEDERMAN R. J. & GAVAN T. L. (1977) Unusual serum lipoprotein abnormality induced by the vehicle of miconazole. *New Engl. J. Med.* 296, 497–9.
5. B.A.S.F. Technical Leaflet (1980). Cremophor EL. Ludwigshafen: B.A.S.F.
6. B.A.S.F. Toxicity Report (1977). Summary of a 4-week toxicity report of Cremophor EL on rats after intravenous application. Ludwigshafen: B.A.S.F.

7. BEAMISH D. & BROWN D. T. (1980) Delayed adverse responses to both methohexitone and Althesin. *Anaesthesia* **35**, 279–81.

8. BENKE A., BALOGH A. & REICH-HILSCHER B. (1979) Über die atmungs-spezifische Wirkung des Lösungs-vermittlers von Diazepam (Valium). *Anaesthesist* **28**, 24–8.

9. BRADBURN C. C. (1970) Severe hypotension following induction with propanidid. *Br. J. Anaesth.* **42**, 362–3.

10. BRITTAIN R. T. & D'ARCY P. F. (1962) Hematologic effects following the intravenous injection of propylene glycol in the rabbit. *Toxicol. Appl. Pharmacol.* **4**, 738–44.

11. BUENO-MONTANO M., McGAUGHEY H. S., HARBERT G. M. & THORNTON W. N. (1966) Drug preservatives and uterine contractility. *Am. J. Obstet. Gynecol.* **94**, 1–5.

12. BURTON G. W., LENZ R. J., THOMAS T. A. & MIDDA M. (1974) Cremophor EL as a diluent for diazepam. *Br. Med. J.* **3**, 258.

13. CARPENTER C. P., WOODSIDE M. D., KINKEAD E. R., KING J. M. & SULLIVAN L. J. (1971) Response of dogs to repeated intravenous injection of polyethylene glycol 4000 with notes on excretion and sensitization. *Toxicol. Appl. Pharmacol.* **18**, 35–40.

14. CARRIER O. & MURPHY J. C. (1970). The effects of d-tubocurarine and its commercial vehicles on cardiac function. *Anesthesiology* **33**, 627–34.

15. CATCHLOVE R. F. H. & KAFER E. R. (1971) The effects of diazepam on the ventilatory response to carbon dioxide and on steady-state gas exchange. *Anesthesiology* **34**, 9–13.

16. CHRISTENSEN B. G. & HANSEN T. (1977) Diazepam injeksjoner og thromboflebitt. *Tidsskr. Nor. Laegeforen.* **97**, 1767–8.

17. CHUNG D. C. W. (1976) Anaphylaxis to thiopentone: a case report. *Can. Anaesth. Soc. J.* **23**, 319–22.

18. CLARKE R. S. J., FEE J. H. & DUNDEE J. W. (1978) Hypersensitivity reactions to intravenous anaesthetics. In Watkins J. & Milford Ward A. (eds.), *Adverse Response to Intravenous Drugs*, pp. 41–7. Academic Press, New York.

19. CLERGUE F., DESMONTS J. M., DUVALDESTIN P., DELAVAULT E. & SAUMON G. (1981) Depression of respiratory drive by diazepam as premedication. *Br. J. Anaesth.* **53**, 1059–63.

20. CRAIG D. B. & HABIB G. G. (1977) Flaccid paraparesis following obstetrical epidural anesthesia. Possible role of benzyl alcohol. *Anesth. Analg. (Cleve)* **56**, 219–21.

21. CRANKSHAW D. P. & RAPER C. (1971) The effect of solvents on the potency of chlordiazepoxide, diazepam, medazepam and nitrazepam. *J. Pharm. Pharmacol.* **23**, 313–21.

22. CRONK J. D. (1971) Phenol with glucagon in cardiotherapy. *New Engl. J. Med.* **284**, 219–20.

23. *Data Sheet Compendium 1979–80.* Association of the British Pharmaceutical Industry. Pharmind Publications Ltd, London.

24. DEAN M. E. & STOCK B. H. (1974) Propylene glycol as a drug solvent in the study of hepatic microsomal enzyme metabolism in the rat. *Toxicol. Appl. Pharmacol.* **28**, 44–52.

25. DE LAND F. H. (1973) Intrathecal toxicity studies with benzyl alcohol. *Toxicol. Appl. Pharmacol.* **25**. 153–6.

26. DELANEY T. J., ROWLINGSON J. C., CARRON H. & BUTLER A. (1980) Epidural steroid effects on nerves and meninges. *Anesth. Analg. (Cleve)* **59**, 610–14.

27. DOENICKE A. (1974) Propanidid. In Arias A., Llourada R., Nalda A. & Lunn J. N. (eds.), *Recent Progress in Anaesthesiology and Resuscitation: Proceedings of IV European Congress of Anaesthesiology, Madrid, 1974*, pp. 107–13. Excerpta Medica, Amsterdam.

28. DOENICKE A., LORENZ W., BEIGL R.,

BEZECNY H., UHLIG G., KALMAR L., PRAETORIUS B. & MANN G. (1973) Histamine release after intravenous application of short-acting hypnotics: a comparison of etomidate, Althesin (C.T. 1341) and propanidid. *Br. J. Anaesth.* **45**, 1097–104.

29. DOWDY E. G., HOLLAND W. C., YAMANAKA I. & KAYA K. (1971) Cardioactive properties of d-tubocurarine with and without preservatives. *Anesthesiology* **34**, 256–61.

30. DYE D. & WATKINS J. (1980) Suspected anaphylactic reaction to Cremophor EL. *Br. Med. J.* **280**, 1353.

31. EICHBAUM F. W. & YASAKA W. J. (1976) Antiarrhythmic effect of solvents: propylene glycol, benzyl alcohol. *Basic Res. Cardiol.* **71**, 355–70.

32. FALK R. H. (1977) Allergy to diazepam. *Br. Med. J.* **1**, 287.

33. FISHER M. (1979) Sensitivity testing for Althesin. *Anaesthesia* **34**, 906–7.

34. FORREST A. R. W., WATRASIEWICZ K. & MOORE C. J. (1977) Long-term Althesin infusion and hyperlipidaemia. *Br. Med. J.* **2**, 1357–8.

35. GAUNT I. F., CARPANINI F. M. B., GRASSO P. & LANSDOWN A. B. G. (1972) Long-term toxicity of propylene glycol in rats. *Food Cosmet. Toxicol.* **10**, 151–62.

36. GEILING E. M. G. & CANNON P. R. (1938) Pathologic effects of Elixir of Sulfanilamide (diethylene glycol) poisoning. *J. Am. Med. Assoc.* **111**, 919–26.

37. GLEN J. B., DAVIES G. E., THOMSON D. S., SCARTH S. C. & THOMPSON A. V. (1979) An animal model for the investigation of adverse responses to i.v. anaesthetic agents and their solvents. *Br. J. Anaesth.* **51**, 819–26.

38. GRAHAM C. W., PAGANO R. R. & KATZ R. L. (1977) Thrombophlebitis after intravenous diazepam—can it be prevented? *Anesth. Analg. (Cleve)* **56**, 409–13.

39. GRAMSTAD L. & STOVNER J. (1979) Plasma viscosity and Cremophor-containing anaesthetics. *Br. J. Anaesth.* **51**, 1175–8.

40. GUNNISON A. F. & PALMES E. D. (1976) A model for the metabolism of sulfite in mammals. *Toxicol. Appl. Pharmacol.* **38**, 111–26.

41. HALABY S. F. & MATTOCKS A. M. (1965) Absorption of sodium bisulfite from peritoneal dialysis solutions. *J. Pharm. Sci.* **54**, 52–5.

42. HAMMARLUND E. R. & PEDERSEN-BJERGAARD K. (1961) Hemolysis of erythrocytes in various iso-osmotic solutions. *J. Pharm. Sci.* **50**, 24–30.

43. HANCOCK B. W. & NAYSMITH A. (1975) Hypersensitivity to chlorocresol-preserved heparin. *Br. Med. J.* **3**, 746–7.

44. HANZLIK P. J., NEWMAN H. W., VAN WINKLE W., LEHMAN A. J. & KENNEDY N. K. (1939) Toxicity, fate and excretion of propylene glycol and some other glycols. *J. Pharmacol. Exp. Ther.* **67**, 101–13.

45. HARNIK E. (1969) Hyperventilation following the injection of propanidid in dogs. *Proc. R. Soc. Med.* **62**, 1018.

46. HATA Y., SHIGEMATSU H., TONOMO Y., EHATA Y., GOTO Y. & MIYAJIMA E. (1978) Interference of an anesthetic preparation with plasma triglyceride determinations. *Jap. Circ. J.* **42**, 689–94.

47. HEGARTY J. E. & DUNDEE J. W. (1978) Local sequelae following the i.v. injection of three benzodiazepines. *Br. J. Anaesth.* **50**, 78–9.

48. HENDRY J. G. B., MILLER B. M. & LEES N. W. (1977) Etomidate in a new solvent: a clinical evaluation. *Anaesthesia* **32**, 996–9.

49. HILDITCH T. P. & WILLIAMS P. N. (1964) *The Chemical Constitution of Natural Fats*, 4th edition, pp. 248–9. Chapman & Hall, London.

50. HOENIG V. & WERNER F. (1980) Is propylene glycol an inert substance? *Toxicol. Lett.* **5**, 389–92.

51. HORTON J. N. (1973) Adverse reaction to Althesin. *Anaesthesia* **28**, 182–3.

52. HUME M., SMITH-PETERSEN M. & FREMONT-SMITH P. (1974) Sensitivity to intrafat heparin. *Lancet* 1, 261.

53. HÜTTEL M. S., SCHOU OLESEN A. & STOFFERSEN E. (1980) Complement-mediated reactions to diazepam with Cremophor as solvent (Stesolid MR). *Br. J. Anaesth.* 52, 77–9.

54. JENSEN S., HÜTTEL M. S. & SCHOU OLESON A. (1981) Venous complications after i.v. administration of Diazemuls (diazepam) and Dormicum (midazolam). *Br. J. Anaesth.* 53, 1083–5.

55. JEPPSSON R. & LJUNGBERG S. (1975) Anticonvulsant activity in mice of diazepam in an emulsion formulation for intravenous administration. *Acta Pharmacol. Toxicol. (Copenh.)* 36, 312–20.

56. JOHNS G. (1970) Cardiac arrest following induction with propanidid. A case report. *Br. J. Anaesth.* 42, 74–7.

57. KAY B. (1976) A clinical assessment of the use of etomidate in children. *Br. J. Anaesth.* 48, 207–11.

58. KESSEL J. & ASSEM E. S. K. (1974) An adverse reaction to Althesin. *Br. J. Anaesth.* 46, 209.

59. KIMURA E. T., DARBY T. D., KRAUSE R. A. & BRONDYK H. D. (1971) Parenteral toxicity studies with benzyl alcohol. *Toxicol. Appl. Pharmacol.* 18, 60–8.

60. KORTTILA K., SOTHMAN A. & ANDERSSON P. (1976) Polyethylene glycol as a solvent for diazepam. *Acta Pharmacol. Toxicol. (Copenh.)* 39, 104–17.

61. LANGDON D. E., HARLAN J. R. & BAILEY R. L. (1973) Thrombophlebitis with diazepam used intravenously. *J. Am. Med. Assoc.* 223, 184–5.

62. LORENZ W., DOENICKE A., MEYER R., REIMANN H-J., KUSCHE J., BARTH H., GEESING H., HUTZEL M. & WEISSENBACHER B. (1972) Histamine release in man by propanidid and thiopentone: pharmacological effects and clinical consequences. *Br. J. Anaesth.* 44, 355–69.

63. LORENZ W., MEYER R., DOENICKE A., SCHMAL A., REIMANN H-J., HUTZEL M., & WERLE E. (1971) On the species specificity of the histamine release from mast cell stores by Cremophor EL. *Naunyn Schmiedebergs Arch. Pharmacol.* 269, 417–18.

64. LORENZ W., REIMANN H-J., SCHMAL A., DORMANN P., SCHWARTZ B., NEUGEBAUER E. & DOENICKE A. (1977). Histamine release in dogs by Cremophor EL and its derivatives. *Agents Actions* 7, 63–7.

65. LOUIS S., KUTT H. & McDOWELL F. (1967) The cordiocirculatory changes caused by intravenous Dilantin and its solvent. *Am. Heart J.* 74, 523–9.

66. LUEBKE N. H. & WALKER J. A. (1978) Discussion of sensitivity to preservatives in anesthetics. *J. Am. Dent. Assoc.* 97, 656–7.

67. MARGOLIS G., HALL H. E. & NOWILL W. K. (1953) An investigation of Efocaine, a long-acting local anesthetic agent: I: Animal studies. *Arch. Surg.* 67, 715–30.

68. MARTIN G. & FINBERG L. (1970) Propylene glycol: a potentially toxic vehicle in liquid dosage form. *J. Pediatr.* 77, 877–8.

69. *Martindale, The Extra Pharmacopoeia* (1982) Edited by J. E. F. Reynolds. 28th edition The Pharmaceutical Press. London.

70. MATHEWS E. (1977) Preservatives in drugs. *Lancet* I, 1004.

71. MATHEWS E. (1979) Epidural morphine. *Lancet* I, 673.

72. MATTILA M. A. K., RUOPPI M. KORHONEN M., LARNI H. M., VALTONEN L. & HEIKKINEN H. (1979) Prevention of diazepam-induced thrombophlebitis with Cremophor as a solvent. *Br. J. Anaesth.* 51, 891–4.

73. McCABE W. R., JACKSON G. G. & GRIEBLE H. G. (1959) Treatment of chronic pyelonephritis. *Arch. Intern. Med.* 104, 710–19.

74. McGAVACK T. H. & VOGEL M. (1944)

Propylene glycol as a menstruum for the administration of steroid hormones. *J. Lab. Clin. Med.* **29**, 1256–65.

75. MCLESKEY C. H. (1981) Allergic reaction to an amide local anaesthetic. *Br. J. Anaesth.* **53**, 1105.

76. MEHTA S. (1973) Anaphylactic reaction to Althesin. *Anaesthesia* **28**, 669–72.

77. MÜLLER K. (1966) The analysis of Cremophor EL. *Tenside* **3**, 37–45.

78. NAGEL J. E., FUSCALDO J. T. & FIREMAN P. (1977) Paraben allergy. *J. Am. Med. Assoc.* **237**, 1594–5.

79. NATHAN P. W. & SEARS T. A. (1961) Action of methyl hydroxybenzoate on nervous conduction. *Nature* **192**, 668.

80. NOTCUTT W. G. (1973) Adverse reaction to Althesin. *Anaesthesia* **28**, 673–4.

81. NOVAK E., STUBBS S. S., SANBORN E. C. & EUSTICE R. M. (1972) The tolerance and safety of intravenously administered benzyl alcohol in methylprednisolone sodium succinate formulations in normal human subjects. *Toxicol. Appl. Pharmacol.* **23**, 54–61.

82. O'TOOLE R. D. (1973) Heparin: adverse reaction. *Ann. Intern. Med.* **79**, 759.

83. OTSUKA M. & NONOMURA Y. (1963) The action of phenolic substances on motor nerve endings. *J. Pharmacol. Exp. Ther.* **140**, 41–5.

84. PADFIELD A. & WATKINS J. (1977) Allergy to diazepam. *Br. Med. J.* **1**, 575–6.

85. RADFORD S. G., LOCKYER J. A., SEAR J. W. & SIMPSON P. J. (1980) Repeat exposure to Althesin. *Br. Med. J.* **281**, 60.

86. REHDER K. & SCHMIDT L. (1957) Pharmakologische Wirkungen einiger organischer Lösungsmittel. *Arzneimittelforsch.* **7**, 703–5.

87. REITAN J. A., JAMES O. F. & MARTUCCI R. W. (1977) Cardiovascular effects of atropine sulfate preparations in vagotomized dogs under halothane anesthesia. *Anesth. Analg. (Cleve.)* **56**, 338–43.

88. RUDDICK J. A. (1972) Toxicology, metabolism and biochemistry of 1,2-propanediol. *Toxicol. Appl. Pharmacol.* **21**, 102–11.

89. SAIKI J. H., THOMPSON S., SMITH F. & ATKINSON R. (1972) Paraplegia following intrathecal chemotherapy. *Cancer* **29**, 370–4.

90. SAVAGE T. M., FOLEY E. I. & SIMPSON B. R. (1973) Some cardiorespiratory effects of Cremophor EL in man. *Br. J. Anaesth.* **45**, 515–17.

91. SCANU A., ORIENTE P., SZAJEWSKI J. M., MCCORMACK L. J. & PAGE I. H. (1961) Triton hyperlipemia in dogs. *J. Exp. Med.* **114**, 279–93.

92. SCHOLTAN W. & LIE S. Y. (1966) Kolloidchemische Eigenschaften eines neuen Kurznarkoticums. *Arzneimittelforsch.* **16**, 679–91.

93. SCHOU OLESEN A. & HÜTTEL M. (1978). Kredsløbskollaps ved intravenøs brug af Stesolid MR. *Ugeskr. Laeger.* **140**, 2644–5.

94. SCHOU OLESEN A. & HÜTTEL M. S. (1980) Local reactions to i.v. diazepam in three different formulations. *Br. J. Anaesth.* **52**, 609–11.

95. SEIDENFELD M. A. & HANZLIK P. J. (1932) The general properties, actions and toxicity of propylene glycol. *J. Pharmacol. Exp. Ther.* **44**, 109–21.

96. SHAFFER C. B., CRITCHFIELD F. H. & NAIR J. H. (1950) The absorption and excretion of liquid polyethylene glycol. *J. Am. Pharmaceut. Assoc. Sci. Ed.* **39**, 340–4.

97. SIEBKE H., ELLERTSEN B. B. & LIND B. (1976) Reactions to intravenous injections of diazepam. *Br. J. Anaesth.* **48**, 1187–9.

98. SPODICK D. H., BYRNE M. J. & PIGOTT V. M. (1971) Phenol in glucagon diluent. *New Engl. J. Med.* **284**, 500–501.

99. STOELTING R. K. (1971) Blood-pressure responses to d-tubocurarine and its preservatives in anesthetized patients. *Anesthesiology* **35**, 315–17.

100. SWEET A. Y. (1958) Fatality from intra-

venous nitrofurantoin. *Pediatrics* **22**, 1204.

101. TORDA T. A., BARRY B. J., McCULLOCH C. H. & GIBB D. B. (1973) Blood pressure, d-tubocurarine and the effect of preservatives. *Anaesth. Intensive Care* 1, 293–6.

102. TWEEDIE D. G. & ORDISH P. M. (1974) Reactions to intravenous agents (Althesin and pancuronium). *Br. J. Anaesth.* **46**, 244.

103. WATKINS J., ALLEN R. & MILFORD WARD A. (1978) Adverse response to alphadolone/alphaxalone: possible role of IgD. *Lancet* **2**, 736.

104. WATKINS J., CLARK A., APPLEYARD T. N. & PADFIELD A. (1976) Immune-mediated reactions to Althesin (alpha-xalone). *Br. J. Anaesth.* **48**, 881–6.

105. WATKINS J., PADFIELD A. & ALDERSON J. D. (1978) Underlying immuno-pathology as a cause of adverse responses to two intravenous anaesthetic agents. *Br. Med. J.* **2**, 1180–81.

106. WATKINS J., UDNOON S., APPLEYARD T. N. & THORNTON J. A. (1976) Identification and quantition of hyper-sensitivity reactions to intravenous anaesthetic agents. *Br. J. Anaesth.* **48**, 457–61.

107. WEIL C. S., WOODSIDE M.D., SMYTH H. F. & CARPENTER C. P. (1971) Results of feeding propylene glycol in the diet to dogs for two years. *Food Cosmet. Toxicol.* **9**, 479–90.

108. WILKINS J. W., GREENE J. A. & WELLER J. M. (1968) Toxicity of intraperitoneal bisulfite. *Clin. Pharmacol. Ther.* **9**, 328–

32.

109. WIRTH W. & HOFFMEISTER F. (1965) Pharmacological studies on Epontol. *Anaesthesiology and Resuscitation* **4**, 17–47.

110. WRAIGHT W. J. & COX D. J. (1980) Fluid deprivation due to Althesin solution affecting drop size. *Br. Med. J.* **280**, 904.

111. YAMAMOTO T. & ADACHI Y. (1978) Effect of oral administration of propylene glycol on the induction of enzymes and proteins in microsomes and cytosol of the rat liver. *Gastroenterol. Jap.* **13**, 359–65.

112. YASAKA W. J., EICHBAUM F. W. & OGA S. (1979) Antiarrhythmic effects of solvents: II: Effects of propylene glycol and benzyl alcohol on the effective refractory period of isolated rabbit atria. *Cardiovasc. Res.* **13**, 711–16.

113. YASAKA W. J., EICHBAUM F. W. & OGA S. (1979) Antiarrhythmic effects of solvents: III: Effects of propylene glycol and benzyl alcohol on contractile force of isolated rabbit heart. *Cardiovasc. Res.* **13**, 717–22.

114. ZACHARIAS M., CLARKE R. S. J., DUNDEE J. W. & JOHNSTON S. B. (1978) Evaluation of three preparations of etomidate. *Br. J. Anaesth.* **50**, 925–9.

115. ZACHARIAS M., DUNDEE J. W., CLARKE R. S. J. & HEGARTY J. E. (1979) Effect of preanaesthetic medication on etomidate. *Br. J. Anaesth.* **51**, 127–32.

116. ZAROSLINSKI J. F., BROWNE R. K. & POSSLEY L. H. (1971) Propylene glycol as a drug solvent in pharmacologic studies. *Toxicol. Appl. Pharmacol.* **19**, 573–8.

Index